SAUNDER
VETERIN...

SMALL ANIMAL
DENTISTRY

Commissioning Editor: Joyce Rodenhuis, Rita Demetriou-Swanwick
Development Editor: Sarah Keer-Keer, Louisa Welch
Project Manager: Jess Thompson
Designer/Text Design: Charles Gray/Keith Kail
Illustrations Manager: Merlyn Harvey
Illustrator: Deborah Maizels

SAUNDERS SOLUTIONS IN
VETERINARY PRACTICE

SMALL ANIMAL
DENTISTRY

Series Editor: **Fred Nind** BVM&S, MRCVS

Cecilia Gorrel

BSc MA VetMB DDS MRCVS HonFAVD DipEVDC
European and RCVS Recognized Specialist in Veterinary Dentistry

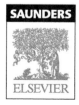

SAUNDERS

ELSEVIER

Edinburgh   London   New York   Oxford   Philadelphia   St Louis   Sydney   Toronto   2008

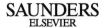

SAUNDERS
ELSEVIER

First published 2008

ISBN: 978-0-7020-2871-7

British Library Cataloguing in Publication Data
A catalogue record for this book is available from the British Library

Library of Congress Cataloging in Publication Data
A catalog record for this book is available from the Library of Congress

Notice
Knowledge and best practice in this field are constantly changing. As new research and experience broaden our knowledge, changes in practice, treatment and drug therapy may become necessary or appropriate. Readers are advised to check the most current information provided (i) on procedures featured or (ii) by the manufacturer of each product to be administered, to verify the recommended dose or formula, the method and duration of administration, and contraindications. It is the responsibility of the practitioner, relying on their own experience and knowledge of the patient, to make diagnoses, to determine dosages and the best treatment for each individual patient, and to take all appropriate safety precautions. To the fullest extent of the law, neither the Publisher nor the Author assumes any liability for any injury and/or damage to persons or property arising out or related to any use of the material contained in this book.
Neither the Publisher nor the Author assumes any responsibility for any loss or injury and/or damage to persons or property arising out of or related to any use of the material contained in this book. It is the responsibility of the treating practitioner, relying on independent expertise and knowledge of the patient, to determine the best treatment and method of application for the patient.

The Publisher

Printed in the United States of America
Transferred to Digital Printing, 2018

your source for books, journals and multimedia in the health sciences
www.elsevierhealth.com

Working together to grow
libraries in developing countries

www.elsevier.com | www.bookaid.org | www.sabre.org

ELSEVIER   BOOK AID International   Sabre Foundation

The publisher's policy is to use paper manufactured from sustainable forests

Contents

APPENDICES

Acknowledgements

I would like to thank:

- Graeme Blackwood (my better half) for continuous encouragement, proofreading and help with illustrations
- Sue Vranch (born Derbyshire) for her meticulous proofreading and constructive criticism
- My friends, notably Jacqueline Hosford and Carole Hulbert, for their support and encouragement
- My business partner Peter Southerden and the rest of the dentistry and oral surgery team (Sue Vranch, Lisa Milella and Alex Smithson) for their involvement in the treatment of most of the reported cases
- All the veterinarians who refer cases to me.

This book could not have happened without you!

Introduction

Saunders Solutions in Veterinary Practice series is a new range of veterinary textbooks which will grow into a mini library over the next few years, covering all the main disciplines of companion animal practice.

Readers should realize that it is not the authors' intention to cover all that is known about each topic. As such the books in the *Solutions Series* are not standard reference works. Instead, they are intended to provide practical information on the more frequently encountered conditions in an easily accessible form based on real-life case studies. They cover that range of cases that fall between the boringly routine and the referral. The books will help practitioners with a particular interest in a topic or those preparing for a specialist qualification. The cases are arranged by presenting sign rather than by the underlying pathology, as this is how veterinary surgeons will see them in practice.

Each case also includes descriptions of underlying pathology and details of the nursing required, both in the veterinary clinic and at home. It is hoped that the books will also, therefore, be of interest to veterinary students in the later parts of their course and to veterinary nurses.

Continuing professional development (CPD) is mandatory for many veterinarians and a recommended practice for others. The *Saunders Series* will provide a CPD resource which can be accessed economically, shared with colleagues and used anywhere. They will also provide busy veterinary practitioners with quick access to authoritative information on the diagnosis and treatment of interesting and challenging cases. The robust cover has been made resistant to some of the more gruesome contaminants found in a veterinary clinic because this is where we hope these books will be used.

Joyce Rodenhuis and Mary Seager were the inspiration for the Series, and both the Series editor and the individual authors are grateful for their foresight in commissioning the series and their unfailing support and guidance during their production.

DENTISTRY

When I graduated as a veterinary surgeon, dentistry was an unpopular backwater subject. Dental surgery was basic, brutal and unpopular.

Now the discipline has blossomed. The high levels of pain associated with some forms of dental disease have been recognized. Realizing the profound improvement in a patient's behaviour and well-being after effective dental treatment for a chronically painful condition can bring a wonderful warm glow to the heart of the practitioner which is not quickly forgotten.

Instrumentation has been developed which makes dental procedures easier and the range of procedures that can be undertaken has steadily expanded.

Veterinary surgeons have risen to this challenge, recognizing that dental cases form a significant part of any general practitioner's case load. It is hoped that this book will help practitioners to handle these cases in an effective way, minimizing the frustrations and stress that can be associated with unsatisfactory technique. The book will also help to identify what is possible and practical for the general practitioner and what is best left to a referral specialist.

Fred Nind
Series Editor

Author's note

Oral health is important for the general health and well-being of dogs and cats. Owners are often unaware that their pet is uncomfortable or even in pain. It is only when disease has been treated that they note a difference in their animal. At recheck it is common that owners report a dramatic change in behaviour. Although I had always known that oral disease impacted negatively on general health and well-being, it was only while amalgamating the cases for this book that I grasped the full impact of the detrimental effects that oral and dental diseases can have on the patient. The dramatic improvement after treating oral and dental conditions is what makes dentistry and oral surgery so worthwhile.

The aim of this book is to increase the understanding and thereby improve treatment of oral and dental conditions commonly encountered in canine and feline general practice. It is not a standard referenced textbook and does not cover all aspects of dentistry and oral surgery.

The format is a short summary of the aetiology and pathogenesis of common conditions and diseases, followed by case descriptions. The case descriptions aim to highlight diagnostic procedures, treatment options, anticipated problems and the importance of monitoring. There are often different treatment options available for the same condition; the choice depends on a number of factors, e.g. the systemic health of the patient, compliance with home care regimens, lifestyle (i.e. working or pet dog). The goal of veterinary dentistry is a comfortable animal with a functional bite; aesthetics is only a minor consideration.

Dentistry encompasses conditions of all structures of the oral cavity, namely teeth (hard tissues and periodontium), oral mucosa, salivary glands, etc. Some conditions can be managed successfully in general practice and some need referral to a specialist for treatment. The general practitioner needs to recognize the conditions, be able to perform a full diagnostic work-up, realize the clinical significance of the findings and institute treatment (in-house or referral) as required.

Oral conditions and diseases are a diagnostic challenge. Several disease conditions are generally present simultaneously. Presenting signs are rarely specific, i.e. malodour, changes in eating patterns and dysphagia are indications that there is a problem in the oral cavity, but they are not specific for a particular disease. Manifestations of disease are often not detected on conscious clinical examination. Full oral and dental examination, including dental radiography, under general anaesthesia is required for diagnosis, to evaluate the extent of disease and plan treatment. In my experience, it is common that an animal is referred to me with a diagnosis that is not the cause of the problem. The importance of a full oral exam under general anaesthesia cannot be underestimated. It should be performed for all animals with suspected oral disease.

In summary, oral/dental diagnosis and treatment planning should not be based on presenting signs. If this is attempted, the risk of misdiagnosis and incorrect treatment is high. Animals presented with suspected oral/dental disease require a full oral examination under general anaesthesia as a minimum prior to diagnosis and treatment.

As a quick reference, Table 1 links common clinical findings detected at examination under general anaesthesia to the cases reported in this book.

Sections 1 and 2 of this book summarize relevant oral and dental anatomy, and detail oral examination and recording, and radiography. The work-up is identical for all cases and is designed to detect underlying, not immediately apparent, pathological conditions which lie at the root of the patient's problem. All findings should be recorded on a dental record. A problem list can then be drawn up and further investigations performed as indicated. Radiography is essential in most cases.

Table 1 Clinical findings under general anaesthesia

Cavities
Chapter 20 – Clinical lesions and signs of discomfort
Chapter 21 – Idiopathic canine root resorption
Chapter 39 – Caries

Discoloured teeth
Chapter 21 – Idiopathic canine root resorption
Chapter 34 – Multiple tooth and jaw fracture

Drainage tracts
Chapter 32 – Uncomplicated crown fracture with periapical complications
Chapter 35 – Iatrogenic tooth damage

Enamel dysplasia
Chapter 38 – Enamel dysplasia

Excessive dental wear (attrition and/or abrasion)
Chapter 34 – Multiple tooth and jaw fracture
Chapter 37 – Excessive wear

Gingivitis
Chapter 6 – Natural progression of disease
Chapter 7 – Periodontitis in a cat
Chapter 8 – Importance of periodontal probing depth (PPD)
Chapter 9 – Systemic effects of periodontitis
Chapter 10 – Iatrogenic injuries
Chapter 12 – Chronic gingivostomatitis as a consequence of periodontitis and iatrogenic injuries
Chapter 15 – Idiopathic chronic gingivostomatitis with extraction leading to partial cure
Chapter 18 – No clinical signs of root resorption
Chapter 20 – Clinical lesions and signs of discomfort
Chapter 21 – Idiopathic canine root resorption
Chapter 23 – Persistent primary teeth
Chapter 24 – Interceptive extractions
Chapter 27 – Tooth shortening and endodontic therapy
Chapter 28 – Tooth shortening and endodontics, then extraction
Chapter 29 – Extraction of permanent teeth
Chapter 30 – Iatrogenic malocclusion
Chapter 32 – Uncomplicated crown fracture with periapical complications
Chapter 33 – Complicated crown fracture with periapical disease
Chapter 34 – Multiple tooth and jaw fracture
Chapter 35 – Iatrogenic tooth damage
Chapter 36 – Complicated crown fracture of an immature tooth
Chapter 37 – Excessive wear
Chapter 38 – Enamel dysplasia
Chapter 39 – Caries

Gingivostomatitis
Chapter 12 – Chronic gingivostomatitis as a consequence of periodontitis and iatrogenic injuries
Chapter 13 – Chronic gingivostomatitis associated with FeLV and FIV
Chapter 14 – Idiopathic chronic gingivomatitis with extraction leading to cure
Chapter 15 – Idiopathic chronic gingivostomatitis with extraction leading to partial cure
Chapter 16 – Canine chronic gingivostomatitis

Hard (bony) swelling
Chapter 33 – Complicated crown fracture with periapical disease
Chapter 35 – Iatrogenic tooth damage

Jaw fracture
Chapter 9 – Systemic effects of periodontitis
Chapter 10 – Iatrogenic injuries

Malocclusion
Chapter 23 – Persistent primary teeth
Chapter 24 – Interceptive extractions
Chapter 27 – Tooth shortening and endodontic therapy
Chapter 28 – Tooth shortening and endodontics, then extraction
Chapter 29 – Extraction of permanent teeth
Chapter 30 – Iatrogenic malocclusion

Missing teeth
Chapter 6 – Natural progression of disease
Chapter 18 – No clinical signs of root resorption
Chapter 19 – Virtually edentulous, no clinical signs of root resorption
Chapter 20 – Clinical lesions and signs of discomfort
Chapter 21 – Idiopathic canine root resorption
Chapter 34 – Multiple tooth and jaw fracture
Chapter 35 – Iatrogenic tooth damage

Non-healing extraction sites
Chapter 7 – Periodontitis in a cat
Chapter 13 – Chronic gingivostomatitis associated with FeLV and FIV

Oronasal communication
Chapter 9 – Systemic effects of periodontitis

Periodontitis
Chapter 7 – Periodontitis in a cat
Chapter 8 – Importance of periodontal probing depth (PPD)
Chapter 9 – Systemic effects of periodontitis
Chapter 10 – Iatrogenic injuries

It is suggested that readers of this book familiarize themselves with Sections 1 and 2 before moving on to Sections 3–7.

Sections 3–7 deal with the following common conditions:

- Periodontal disease
- Chronic gingivostomatitis
- Root resorption
- Malocclusion
- Pulp and periapical disease.

For each condition or disease entity, there is a short summary of aetiopathogenesis and then case descriptions. The case descriptions include straightforward cases as well as more complex ones. Each case also contains a theory refresher, which allows each one to be read as a self-contained clinical report. Inevitably, this incurs some repetition of the theory within different cases.

In order to get the full benefit from the book, it is necessary to read Sections 1 and 2 as a whole. The cases in Sections 3–7 can then be used as a reference guide to help in determining both an accurate diagnosis and a treatment plan. The cases are presented in such a way that the reader can draw up their own problem list and treatment plan based on my detailed oral examination findings, and then compare that with what was actually done.

Cecilia Gorrel

SECTION 1

ANATOMY AND PHYSIOLOGY

1 The tooth and its periodontium

THE TOOTH

Some fundamental points on the teeth of small animals are outlined as follows:
- The basic anatomy resembles that of man
- There are differences in the number of teeth
- There are differences in the shape of teeth:
  - The crowns are more tapered
  - There are sharp cutting surfaces
  - There are fewer chewing surfaces
- There are differences in spacing:
  - Teeth are further apart
  - Any contact points are small and not as tight.

Tooth consists of:
- Crown – generally above the gum line
- Root(s) – generally below the gum line
- Enamel
- Dentine
- Cementum
- Pulp (endodontic system).

Figure 1.1 depicts the basic structure of a tooth and its periodontium.

Enamel:
- Thin layer as compared to man
- Hardest and most mineralized tissue in the body
- Inorganic content amounts to 96–97% of weight
- Has no nerve or blood supply
- Has no reparative or regenerative capacity.

Dentine:
- Comprises the bulk of the mature tooth
- Inorganic content amounts to 70% of wet weight
- Tubular structure
- Slow continuous deposition of dentine throughout life (secondary dentine)
- Rapid deposition in response to trauma (reparative/tertiary dentine).

Cementum:
- Avascular bone-like tissue
- Less calcified than enamel or dentine
- Slow continuous deposition throughout life
- Capable of resorptive and reparative processes.

Pulp:
- Composed of connective tissue
- Lined by odontoblasts
- Pulp chamber = pulp tissue contained in the crown
- Root canal(s) = section of root containing pulp tissue
- Root apex = where the root canal opens into the periapical tissues:
  - Single, wide opening in the immature tooth
  - Numerous foramina in the mature tooth.

THE PERIODONTIUM

The periodontium is an anatomical unit, which functions to attach the tooth to the jaw and provide a suspensory apparatus resilient to normal functional forces.
Periodontium consists of:
- Gingiva
- Periodontal ligament
- Cementum
- Alveolar bone.

Gingiva:
- Forms a cuff around each tooth:
  - Free gingiva
  - Attached gingiva
- Margin of free gingiva forms invagination between tooth and gingiva = sulcus
- Normal sulcus depth is 1–3 mm in dogs and 0.5–1 mm in cats.

3

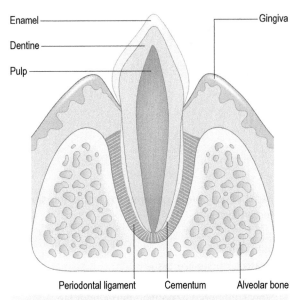

Figure 1.1 Basic anatomy of the tooth and periodontium. From Gorrel C (2004): Veterinary Dentistry for the General Practitioner, with permission of Elsevier.

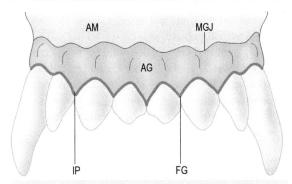

Figure 1.2 The visible landmarks of clinically normal gingiva. MGJ = mucogingival junction or line; AM = alveolar mucosa; AG = attached gingiva; FG = free gingiva; IP = interdental papilla. From Gorrel C (2004): Veterinary Dentistry for the General Practitioner, with permission of Elsevier.

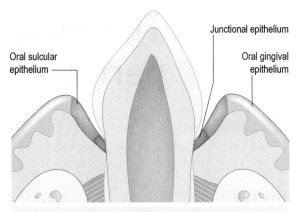

Figure 1.3 The gingival cuff. The oral surface is lined by a parakeratinized squamous cell epithelium, the oral gingival epithelium. The gingival sulcus is lined by the oral sulcular epithelium, which is closely apposed, but not adherent to the tooth. The junctional epithelium or epithelial attachment is adherent to the tooth surface. Both the sulcular epithelium and the junctional epithelium are non-keratinized squamous cell epithelia. From Gorrel C (2004): Veterinary Dentistry for the General Practitioner, with permission of Elsevier.

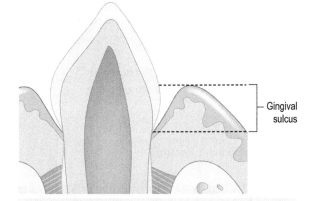

Figure 1.4 The gingival sulcus. It is measured from the free gingival margin to the base of the sulcus using a periodontal probe. From Gorrel C (2004): Veterinary Dentistry for the General Practitioner, with permission of Elsevier.

Figures 1.2, 1.3 and 1.4 depict the basic structures of the gingiva and gingival sulcus.

Periodontal ligament:
- Connective tissue that anchors the tooth to the bone
- Acts as a suspensory ligament for the tooth
- Is in a continual state of physiological activity.

Cementum:
- Avascular bone-like tissue
- Less calcified than enamel or dentine

- Slow, continuous deposition throughout life
- Capable of resorptive and reparative processes.

Alveolar bone:
- Ridges of the jaw that support the teeth
- Teeth are contained in deep depressions (alveolar sockets) in the bone
- Consists of four layers:
  - Periosteum
  - Compact bone

- Cancellous bone
- Cribriform plate (lines the alveolar sockets)
- Vessels and nerves perforate the cribriform plate to supply the periodontal ligament
- Develops during tooth eruption
- Undergoes atrophy with tooth loss
- Responds (usually resorption) readily to external and systemic influences
- The margin of the crest of the alveolar bone is normally located 1 mm below the cemento-enamel junction.

DENTAL FORMULAE

Dog:
- Primary teeth: 2 × {I 3/3 : C 1/1 : P 3/3} = 28
- Permanent teeth: 2 × {I 3/3 : C 1/1 : P 4/4 : M 2/3} = 42.

Cat:
- Primary teeth: 2 × {I 3/3 : C 1/1 : P 3/2}=26
- Permanent teeth: 2 × {I 3/3 : C 1/1 : P 3/2 : M 1/1} = 30.

TOOTH DEVELOPMENT AND MATURATION

- Crown formation (primary and permanent teeth) occurs within the alveolar bone.
- Enamel formation is completed before the tooth erupts.
- Dentine formation is just beginning when the tooth erupts.
- Root development occurs mainly after tooth eruption.

The primary teeth start forming in utero and erupt between 3 and 12 weeks of age. The permanent crowns start forming at or shortly after birth and mineralization of the crowns is complete by around 11 weeks of age. Resorption and exfoliation of the primary teeth and replacement by the permanent dentition occurs between 3 and 7 months of age in the dog, and between 3 and 5 months of age in the cat. Once the crowns of the permanent teeth have erupted, root development continues for several months. The approximate ages when teeth erupt in dogs and cats are shown in Table 1.1.

Once the enamel has formed, the ameloblasts (the cells which produce the enamel matrix) are lost and further development of enamel does not occur. The

Table 1.1 Approximate ages (in weeks) when teeth erupt in dogs and cats

	Primary teeth		Permanent teeth	
	Puppy	Kitten	Dog	Cat
Incisors	4–6	3–4	12–16	11–16
Canines	3–5	3–4	12–16	12–20
Premolars	5–6	5–6	16–20	16–20
Molars	–	–	16–24	20–24

only natural form of repair that can occur to enamel after eruption is surface mineralization, through deposition of minerals, mainly from saliva, into the superficial enamel layer. Although enamel formation is completed by the time the tooth erupts, dentine production is just beginning. Moreover, root development (i.e. growth in length and formation of a root apex) is by no means complete at the time of eruption. Figure 1.5 depicts maturation of a permanent tooth following eruption.

NORMAL RADIOGRAPHIC ANATOMY

- All normal anatomical landmarks are not demonstrable on any given radiograph.
- It is important to be familiar with them so they can be identified and correctly interpreted when they are visualized.
- There are also wide structural variations within normal limits.
- Contralateral radiographs should always be taken for comparison.

The teeth and their supporting tissues
Enamel:
- Thin radiodense band that covers the crown
- It tapers to a fine edge at the cervical margin of the tooth
- Often incompletely visualized on radiographs.

Dentine:
- Accounts for the bulk of the hard tissues of the mature tooth
- It is less radiodense than enamel.

Cementum:
- Thin layer covering root surfaces
- It is even less radiodense than dentine

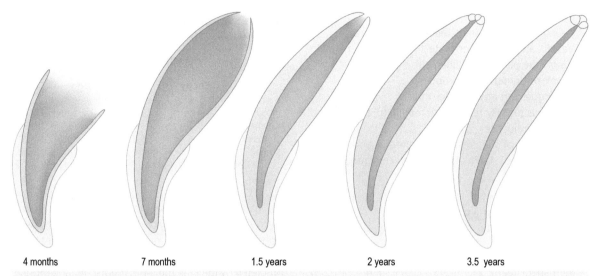

| 4 months | 7 months | 1.5 years | 2 years | 3.5 years |

Figure 1.5 Maturation of a permanent canine tooth after eruption. Enamel formation is complete at the time of eruption, while dentine production and root development (root elongation and formation of an apex) are just beginning. The apical foramen of an immature tooth is a single, wide opening. As the individual ages, closure of the apex (apexogenesis) occurs by continuous deposition of dentine and cementum until, in mature teeth, the root apex consists of numerous small openings or foramina, allowing the passage of blood vessels, lymphatics and nerves. From Gorrel C (2004): Veterinary Dentistry for the General Practitioner, with permission of Elsevier.

- It is only visible radiographically when it has undergone hyperplasia, i.e. not normally seen on radiographs.

Pulp cavity:
- Consists of the pulp chamber (in crown) and the root canal(s)
- It is visualized as a continuous radiolucent space in the centre of the tooth
- The size and width of the pulp chamber and root canal(s) will vary:
  - With the age of the animal
  - If pulpal disease (inflammation, necrosis) occurs.

Periodontium:
- The lamina dura represents the wall of the alveolar tooth socket
- It is seen as a radiodense line, which runs parallel to the root of the tooth
- It is not always visible on radiographs, but a break in the path of a visible lamina dura usually implies periodontal pathology

- The periodontal ligament space is depicted by a fine radiolucent line that is situated between the lamina dura and the root of the tooth
- The cortical bone on the crest of the alveolar ridge is continuous with the lamina dura.

Nutrient canals
- Seen as radiolucent lines of uniform width ± radio-dense borders
- Contain the blood vessels and nerves that supply the teeth, interdental spaces and gingiva:
  - Incisive
  - Infraorbital
  - Mandibular
  - Smaller canals extending into the interdental spaces
  - Smaller canals communicating with the periapical foramina.

Foramina
Important foramina to remember are:
- The anterior palatine (incisive) foramen
- The infraorbital foramina
- The mental foramina.

2 Occlusion

Occlusion is the term used to describe how the teeth contact each other (occlude with each other). Malocclusion is an abnormality in the position of the teeth. Malocclusion can result from jaw length/width discrepancies (skeletal malocclusion), from tooth malpositioning (dental malocclusion), or a combination. Malocclusion is common in the dog, but also occurs in cats. The clinical significance of malocclusion is that it may cause discomfort and sometimes pain to the affected animal. In some cases, it may be the direct cause of severe oral pathology. It is consequently important to diagnose malocclusion early in the life of the animal so that preventative measures can be taken.

The development of the occlusion is determined by both genetic and environmental factors. While the specific genetic mechanisms regulating malocclusion are unknown, a polygenic mechanism is likely and explains why not all siblings in successive generations are affected by malocclusion to the same degree, if they are affected at all. With a polygenic mechanism, the severity of clinical signs is linked to the number of defective genes.

It is known that the following are inherited:
- Jaw length
- Tooth bud position
- Tooth size.

It is also known that the development of the upper jaw, mandible and teeth is independently regulated genetically. Disharmony in the regulation of these structures results in malocclusion. Alteration of jaw growth by hormonal disorder, trauma or functional modification may also result in skeletal malocclusion. Although tooth bud position is inherited, various events during development and growth may alter the definitive tooth position.

NORMAL OCCLUSION

The shape of the head (mesocephalic, dolicocephalic, brachycephalic) affects the positioning of the teeth.

MESOCEPHALIC DOG

The mandible is shorter and less wide than the upper jaw. This means that:
- There is a scissor bite of the incisor teeth (Fig. 2.1).
- There is interdigitation of the canine teeth (Fig. 2.2).
- The incisor scissor bite and canine interdigitation form the dental interlock, which coordinates rostral growth of the upper jaw and mandible.
- There is interdigitation of the premolars (Fig. 2.3).
- There are premolar and molar relationships (Fig. 2.4).

MESOCEPHALIC CAT

The incisor and canine occlusion of the adult mesocephalic cat is the same as in the dog. The premolar and molar occlusion differs (Fig. 2.5) from the dog as follows:
- The most rostral premolar is the maxillary second premolar (the cat lacks the first maxillary premolar and the first two mandibular premolars).
- The buccal surface of the first mandibular molar occludes with the palatal surface of the maxillary fourth premolar.
- The maxillary first molar is located distopalatal to the maxillary fourth premolar and does not occlude with any other tooth.
- The cat does not have any teeth with occlusal (chewing) surfaces.

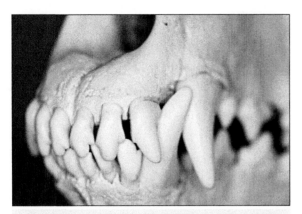

Figure 2.1 Mesocephalic dog – scissor bite of the incisor teeth. The upper incisors are rostral to the lower, with the incisal tips of the mandibular incisors contacting the cingulae of the upper incisors.

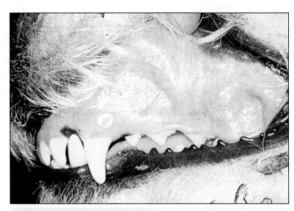

Figure 2.2 Mesocephalic dog – interdigitation of the canine teeth. The mandibular canine fits into the diastema (space) between the upper third incisor and the upper canine, touching neither, i.e. there should be equal space on either side of the mandibular canine crown.

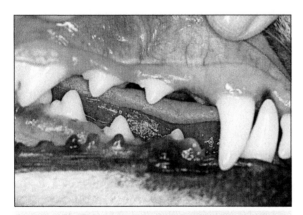

Figure 2.3 Mesocephalic dog – interdigitation of the premolars. The mandibular first premolar should be the most rostral of the premolars. Cusps (tips) of the premolars oppose the interdental spaces of the opposite arcade, with the mandibular first premolar being the most rostral. This interdigitation is called the 'pinking shear' effect.

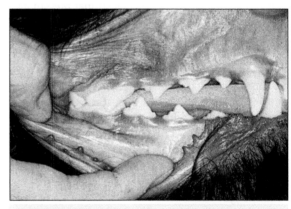

Figure 2.4 Premolar and molar relationships in the mesocephalic dog. The mesiobuccal surface of the first mandibular molar occludes with the palatal surface of the maxillary fourth premolar and the distal occlusal surface of the mandibular first molar occludes with the palatal occlusal surface of the maxillary first molar.

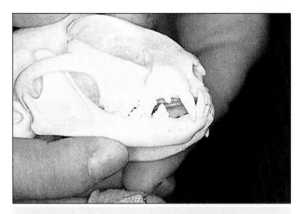

Figure 2.5 Premolar and molar relationships in the cat. The most rostral premolar is the maxillary second premolar. The buccal surface of the first mandibular molar occludes with the palatal surface of the maxillary fourth premolar. The maxillary first molar is located distopalatal to the maxillary fourth premolar and does not occlude with any other tooth.

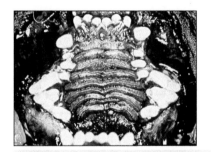

Figure 2.6 Brachycephalic animals have a shorter than normal upper jaw. A short jaw results in reduced interdental spaces with rotation and/or overlap of teeth. From Gorrel C (2004): Veterinary Dentistry for the General Practitioner, with permission of Elsevier.

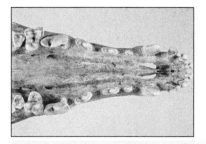

Figure 2.7 Dolicocephalic breeds have a longer than normal upper jaw. The increased jaw length results in interdental spaces that are wider than normal. From Gorrel C (2004): Veterinary Dentistry for the General Practitioner, with permission of Elsevier.

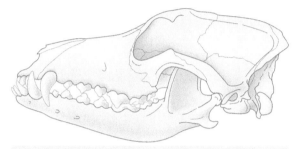

Figure 2.8 Mandibular prognathic bite. The lower jaw is too long with respect to the short upper jaw. From Gorrel C (2004): Veterinary Dentistry for the General Practitioner, with permission of Elsevier.

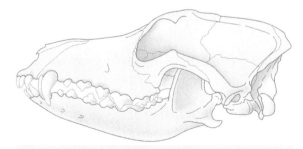

Figure 2.9 Mandibular brachygnathic bite. The mandible is too short in relation to the long upper jaw. From Gorrel C (2004): Veterinary Dentistry for the General Practitioner, with permission of Elsevier.

BRACHYCEPHALIC AND DOLICOCEPHALIC DOG AND CAT

Brachycephalic animals have a shorter than normal upper jaw (Fig. 2.6). Dolicocephalic animals have a longer than normal upper jaw (Fig. 2.7). In both cases, the mandible is not responsible for any rostrocaudal discrepancy. All will have some degree of malocclusion as compared to a mesocephalic animal (Figs 2.8 and 2.9).

DIAGNOSTIC TECHNIQUES

3 Oral examination and recording

Conscious examination yields limited information:
- Gross abnormalities may be detected
- Occlusal evaluation.

Definitive oral examination requires general anaesthesia:
- All detected abnormalities should be recorded
- Clinical record and dental chart are essential.

CONSCIOUS EXAMINATION

- Gentle technique
- Limited to visual inspection and some digital palpation
- Occlusion must be evaluated in the conscious animal.

Examination involves assessing not only the oral cavity proper, but also palpation of:
- The face (facial bones and zygomatic arch)
- Temporomandibular joint
- Salivary glands (mandibular/sublingual; the parotids are usually only palpable if enlarged)
- Lymph nodes (mandibular, cervical chain).

The mouth is first examined by gently holding the jaws closed and retracting the lips (do not pull on the fur to retract lips) to look at the soft tissues and buccal aspects of the teeth. *This is the optimal time to evaluate occlusion.*

Below is a checklist for evaluation of occlusion:
- Head symmetry
- Incisor relationship
- Canine occlusion
- Premolar alignment
- Distal premolar/molar occlusion
- Individual teeth positioning.

Finally, open the animal's mouth. Most animals allow at least a cursory inspection of the oral cavity once the jaws have been opened. The mucous membranes of the oral cavity should be examined as well as the teeth.

Mucous membranes:
- Colour and texture
- Evidence of bleeding problems (petechiation, purpura, ecchymoses)
- Signs of trauma
- Evidence of vesicles and/or ulceration.

Teeth and periodontium:
- Number of teeth
- Tooth fracture
- Gingival recession
- Furcation exposure.

Assess the oropharynx (soft palate, palatoglossal arch, tonsillary crypts, tonsils and fauces) if possible.

EXAMINATION UNDER GENERAL ANAESTHESIA

The oropharynx should be examined prior to endotracheal intubation. Normal anatomical features of the oral cavity need to be identified and inspected. A series of useful checklists are given below.

Oropharynx:
- Soft palate
- Palatoglossal arch
- Tonsillary crypts
- Tonsils
- Hamular process of the pterygoid
- Fauces.

Lips and cheeks:
- Mucocutaneous junction
- Vestibules

- Philtrum
- Frenula (maxillary and mandibular)
- Salivary papilla (parotid and zygomatic).

Oral mucous membranes:
- Alveolar mucosa
- Mucogingival line
- Attached gingiva
- Free gingiva.

Hard palate:
- Incisive papilla
- Incisive duct openings
- Palatine raphe and rugae.

Floor of mouth and tongue:
- Sublingual caruncle
- Lingual frenulum
- Lingual salivary gland (cat)
- Tongue papillae (types and distribution).

Teeth:
- Primary, permanent or mixed dentition
- Missing and/or supernumerary teeth
- Abnormalities in size and/or shape
- Abnormalities in angulation and/or position
- Wear patterns (abrasion, attrition)
- Pathology, e.g. caries, enamel hypoplasia, tooth fracture.

Periodontium

The periodontium of each tooth needs to be assessed to:
- Identify the presence of periodontal disease (gingivitis and periodontitis)
- Differentiate between gingivitis (inflammation of the gingiva) and periodontitis (inflammation of the periodontal tissues resulting in loss of attachment and eventually tooth loss)
- Identify the precise location of disease processes
- Assess the extent of tissue destruction where there is periodontitis.

Instruments required include:
1. Periodontal probe
2. Dental explorer
3. Dental mirror.

The following indices and criteria should be evaluated for each tooth:

1. Gingivitis and gingival index
2. Periodontal probing depth (PPD)
3. Gingival recession
4. Furcation involvement
5. Mobility
6. Periodontal (clinical) attachment level (PAL/CAL).

In animals with large accumulations of dental deposits (plaque and calculus) on the teeth, it may be necessary to remove these to assess periodontal status accurately.

Gingivitis and gingival index

The presence and degree of gingivitis is assessed based on:
- Redness
- Swelling
- Presence or absence of bleeding on probing of the gingival sulcus.

Various indices can be used to give a numerical value to the degree of gingival inflammation present. In the clinical situation, a simple bleeding index is the most useful (Fig. 3.1):
- A periodontal probe is gently inserted into the gingival sulcus at several locations around the whole circumference of each tooth, and given a score of 0 if there is no bleeding and a score of 1 if the probing elicits bleeding.

An index which relies on both visual inspection and bleeding, namely the *modified* Löe and Silness gingival

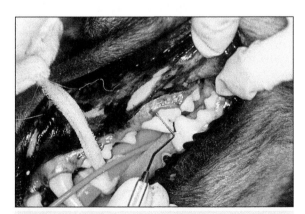

Figure 3.1 Gingivitis scoring using the 'bleeding index'. A periodontal probe is gently inserted into the gingival sulcus at several locations around the whole circumference of each tooth, and given a score of 0 if there is no bleeding and a score of 1 if the probing elicits bleeding.

Table 3.1 The modified Löe and Silness gingival index

Gingival index 0	Clinically healthy gingiva.
Gingival index 1	Mild gingivitis: slight reddening and swelling of the gingival margin; no bleeding on gentle probing of the gingival sulcus.
Gingival index 2	Moderate gingivitis: the gingival margin is red and swollen; gentle probing of the gingival sulcus results in bleeding.
Gingival index 3	Severe gingivitis: the gingival margin is very swollen with a red or bluish red; there is spontaneous haemorrhage and/or ulceration of the gingival margin.

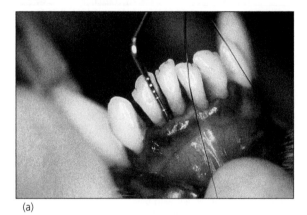

(a)

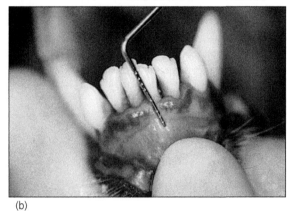

(b)

Figure 3.2 Periodontal probing depth (PPD). From Gorrel C (2004): Veterinary Dentistry for the General Practitioner, with permission of Elsevier.

(a) PPD is measured by inserting a periodontal probe into the gingival sulcus until firm resistance is felt. The distance from the free gingival margin to the depth of the sulcus or pocket is the periodontal probing depth. It should be measured and recorded at several sites around the circumference of each tooth.

(b) The probe has been placed on the surface of the gingiva to depict the depth to which it had been inserted.

index, can also be used (Table 3.1). It is more accurate than the bleeding index, but more time-consuming. It is the most common index used in research.

Periodontal probing depth (PPD)

PPD measures the depth of the sulcus (Fig. 3.2):

- A graduated periodontal probe is gently inserted into the base of the gingival sulcus, i.e. until resistance is felt.
- The depth from the free gingival margin to the base of the sulcus is measured in millimetres at several locations around the whole circumference of the tooth. The probe is moved gently horizontally, walking along the floor of the sulcus.

The gingival sulcus is 1–3 mm deep in the dog and 0.5–1 mm in the cat. Measurements in excess of these values usually indicate the presence of periodontitis, when the periodontal ligament has been destroyed and alveolar bone resorbed, thus allowing the probe to be inserted to a greater depth. The term used to describe this situation is periodontal pocketing. All sites with periodontal pocketing should be accurately recorded. Gingival inflammation resulting in swelling or hyperplasia of the free gingiva will, of course, also result in measuring sulcus depths in excess of normal values. In these situations, the term pseudo-pocketing is used, as the periodontal ligament and bone are intact (i.e. there is no evidence of periodontitis) and the increase in PPD is due to swelling or hyperplasia of the gingiva.

Gingival recession

Gingival recession is the distance (in mm) from the cemento-enamel junction to the free gingival margin. It

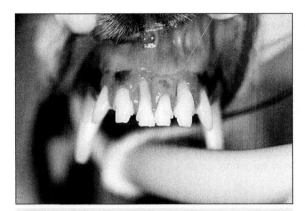

Figure 3.3 Gingival recession is measured from the cemento-enamel junction to the gingival margin using a graded periodontal probe. The right upper first incisor has an extensive (most of the root surface is exposed) gingival recession affecting its buccal aspect. From Gorrel C (2004): Veterinary Dentistry for the General Practitioner, with permission of Elsevier.

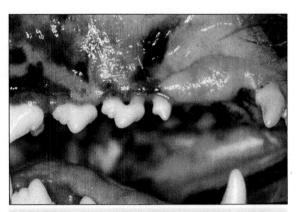

Figure 3.4 Furcation involvement. The furcation sites of multirooted teeth should be examined with either a periodontal probe or a dental explorer so that the degree of furcation involvement can be graded. The right maxillary second premolar has a grade 3 furcation, i.e. the explorer or probe can be passed through from buccal to palatal. From Gorrel C (2004): Veterinary Dentistry for the General Practitioner, with permission of Elsevier.

Table 3.2 Grading of furcation involvement

Grade 0	No furcation involvement.
Grade 1	Initial furcation involvement: the furcation can be felt with the probe/explorer, but horizontal tissue destruction is less than one-third of the horizontal width of the furcation.
Grade 2	Partial furcation involvement: it is possible to explore the furcation but the probe/explorer cannot be passed through it from buccal to palatal/lingual. Horizontal tissue destruction is more than one-third of the horizontal width of the furcation.
Grade 3	Total furcation involvement: the probe/explorer can be passed through the furcation from buccal to palatal/lingual.

is also measured (Fig. 3.3) using a graduated periodontal probe. At sites with gingival recession, PPD may be within normal values despite loss of alveolar bone due to periodontitis.

Furcation involvement

Furcation involvement refers to the situation where the bone between the roots of multirooted teeth is destroyed due to periodontitis (Fig. 3.4). The furcation sites of multirooted teeth should be examined with either a periodontal probe or a curved dental explorer. The grading of furcation involvement is listed in Table 3.2.

Tooth mobility

The grading of mobility is listed in Table 3.3.

Table 3.3 Grading of tooth mobility

Grade 0	No mobility
Grade 1	Horizontal movement of 1 mm or less
Grade 2	Horizontal movement of more than 1 mm*
Grade 3	Vertical as well as horizontal movement is possible

*Note that multirooted teeth are scored more severely and a horizontal mobility in excess of 1 mm is usually considered a Grade 3, even in the absence of vertical movement.

- It is assessed using a suitable instrument, e.g. the blunt end of the handle of a dental mirror or probe.
- It should not be assessed using fingers directly, since the yield of the soft tissues of the fingers will mask the extent of tooth mobility.

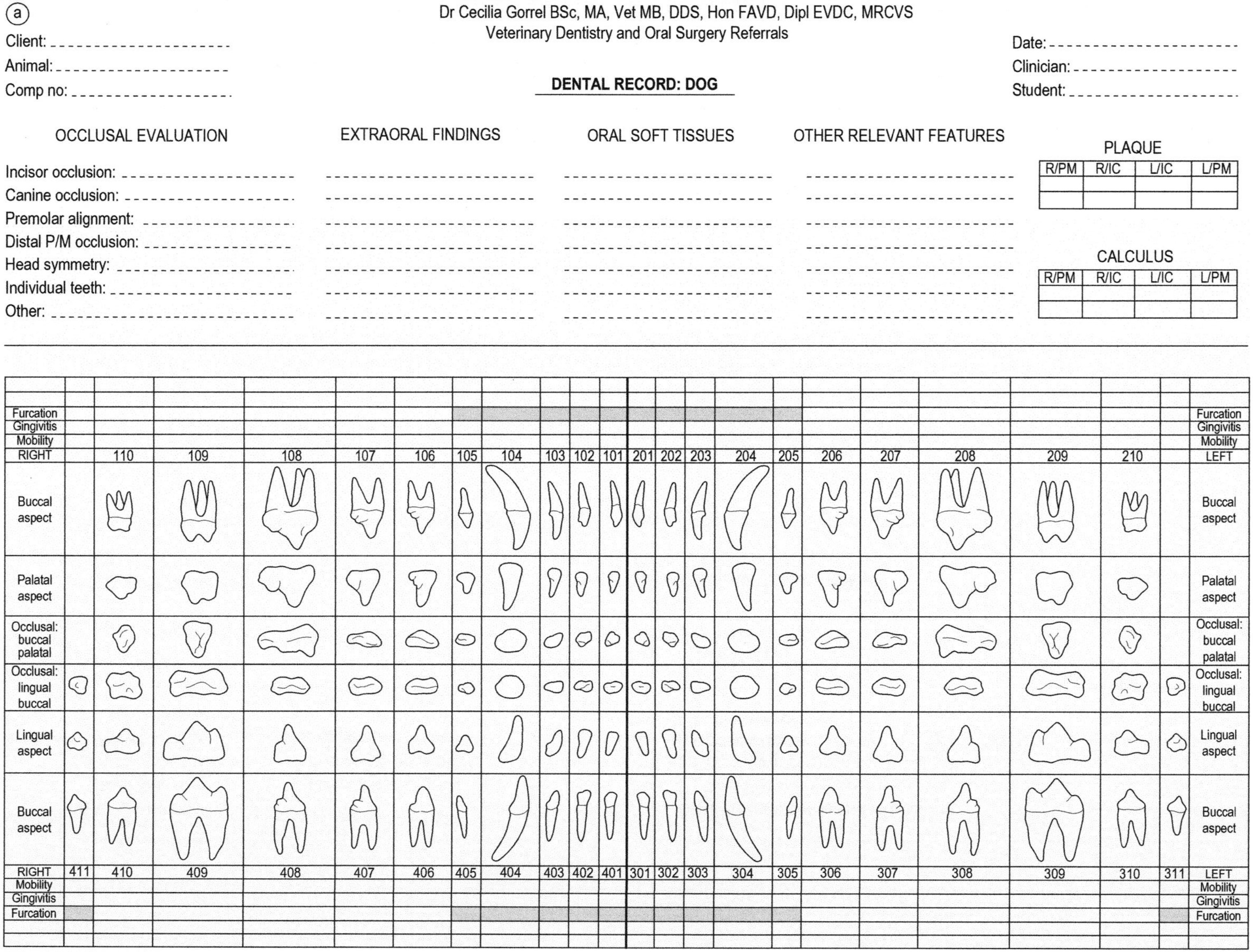

Figure 3.5 Dental record sheets.

(a) Blank record sheet. From Gorrel C, Derbyshire S (2005): Veterinary Dentistry for the Nurse and Technician, with permission of Elsevier.

ORAL PROBLEM LIST

THERAPEUTIC PLAN

PERIODONTICS

- [ ] Sonic scaling
- [ ] Subgingival curettage
- [ ] Pumice polishing
- [ ] Periodontal surgery
- [ ] Ultrasonic scaling
- [ ] Periodontal debridement
- [ ] Air polishing

ORAL SURGERY (Note sites on graph - X)

- [ ] Closed extraction(s):
- [ ] Open extraction(s):
- [ ] Incisional biopsy
- [ ] Other/comments
- [ ] Excisional biopsy

OTHER DENTAL PROCEDURES

COMPLICATIONS/COMMENTS

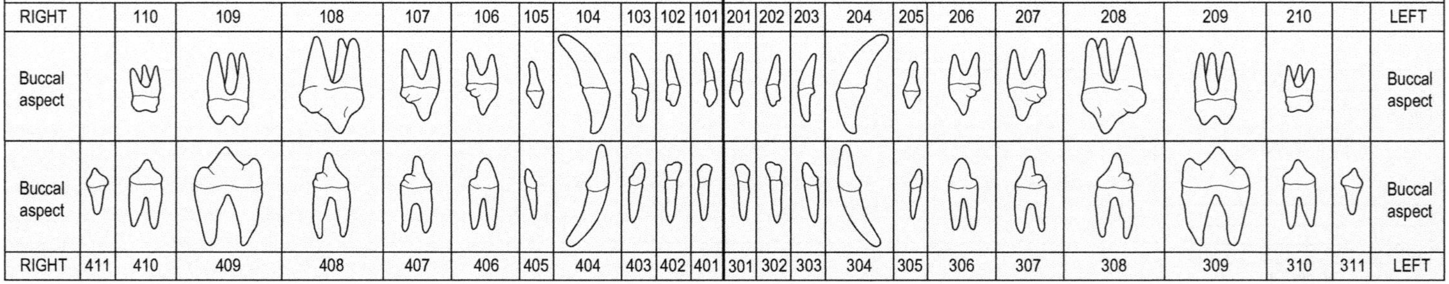

RIGHT	411	410	409	408	407	406	405	404	403	402	401	301	302	303	304	305	306	307	308	309	310	311	LEFT
Buccal aspect																							Buccal aspect
Buccal aspect																							Buccal aspect
RIGHT	110	109	108	107	106	105	104	103	102	101	201	202	203	204	205	206	207	208	209	210			LEFT

Figure 3.5 Dental record sheets. (*continued*)

(b)

Dr Cecilia Gorrel BSc, MA, Vet MB, DDS, Hon FAVD, Dipl EVDC, MRCVS
Veterinary Dentistry and Oral Surgery Referrals

Client:
Animal:
Comp no:

DENTAL RECORD: CAT

Date:
Clinician:
Student:

OCCLUSAL EVALUATION		EXTRAORAL FINDINGS	ORAL SOFT TISSUES	OTHER RELEVANT FEATURES
Incisor occlusion:	Normal occlusion			
Canine occlusion:		NAD	NAD	None
Premolar alignment:				
Distal P/M occlusion:				
Head symmetry:				
Individual teeth:				
Other:				

PLAQUE

R/PM	R/IC	L/IC	L/PM

CALCULUS

R/PM	R/IC	L/IC	L/PM

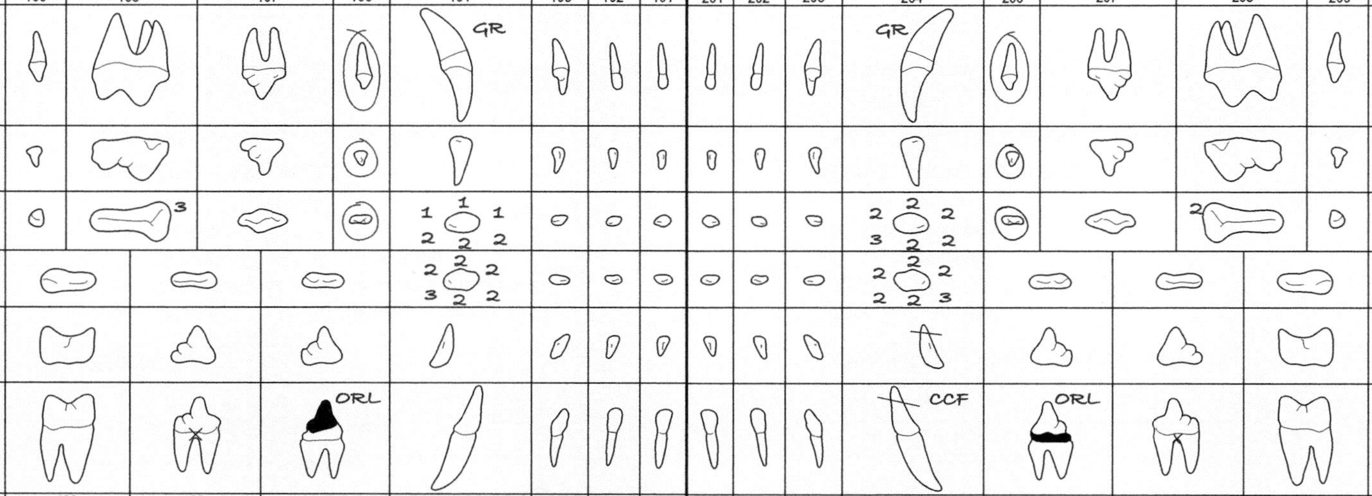

GR					3mm							2mm					GR
Furcation																	Furcation
Gingivitis	I	II	I		II	I	I	I	I	I	I	II		I	II	I	Gingivitis
Mobility																	Mobility
RIGHT	109	108	107	106	104	103	102	101	201	202	203	204	206	207	208	209	LEFT
Buccal aspect																	Buccal aspect
Palatal aspect																	Palatal aspect
Occlusal: buccal palatal		3			1 1 1 / 2 2 2							2 2 2 / 3 2 2			2		Occlusal: buccal palatal

Occlusal: lingual buccal				2 2 2 / 3 2 2							2 2 2 / 2 2 3				Occlusal: lingual buccal
Lingual aspect															Lingual aspect
Buccal aspect															Buccal aspect
RIGHT	409	408	407	404	403	402	401	301	302	303	304	307	308	309	LEFT
Mobility					1	1	2	2	1	1					Mobility
Gingivitis	I	I	I	I	I	I	I	I	I	I	I	I	I	I	Gingivitis
Furcation		2													Furcation
GR															GR

Figure 3.5 Dental record sheets. *(continued)*
(b) Completed form. After Gorrel C, Derbyshire S (2005): Veterinary Dentistry for the Nurse and Technician, with permission of Elsevier.

ORAL PROBLEM LIST

1. ORL 307, 407
2. CCF 304
3. Periodontitis 104, 204
4. 106 and 206 are missing
5. Mild generalized gingivitis

PERIODONTICS

☐ Sonic scaling ☑ Ultrasonic scaling
☑ Subgingival curettage ☐ Periodontal debridement
☑ Pumice polishing ☐ Air polishing
☐ Periodontal surgery

OTHER DENTAL PROCEDURES

Full-mouth radiographic series taken.

THERAPEUTIC PLAN (after reviewing radiographs)

1. Periodontal therapy
2. Extract 304, 307, 407

ORAL SURGERY (Note sites on graph - X)

☐ Closed extraction(s):
☑ Open extraction(s): 304, 307 and 407
☐ Incisional biopsy ☐ Excisional biopsy
☐ Other comments

COMPLICATIONS/COMMENTS

Needs recall for EUA and full-mouth radiographs in one year's time.

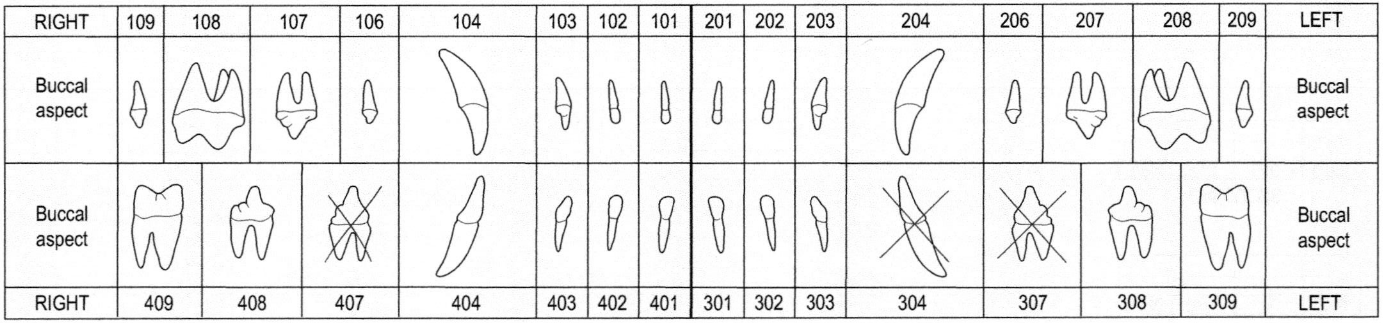

Figure 3.5 Dental record sheets. (continued)

Table 3.4 Modified Triadan System, a three-digit numbering system

Permanent dentition

Right upper = 1	Left upper = 2
Right lower = 4	Left lower = 3

Primary dentition

Right upper = 5	Left upper = 6
Right lower = 7	Left lower = 8

Table 3.5 Common abbreviations

NAD	No abnormality detected
ORL	Odontoclastic resorptive lesion
GR	Gingival recession
GH	Gingival hyperplasia
UCF	Uncomplicated crown fracture
CCF	Complicated crown fracture
UCRF	Uncomplicated crown and root fracture
CCRF	Complicated crown and root fracture
W	Wear (abrasion or attrition) facet

Periodontal/clinical attachment level (PAL/CAL)

Periodontal attachment level records the distance from the cemento-enamel junction (or from a fixed point on the tooth) to the base or apical extension of the pathological pocket.

- PAL can be measured with a periodontal probe.
- It can also be calculated, i.e. PPD + gingival recession/PPD – gingival hyperplasia.
- It is a more accurate assessment of tissue loss in periodontitis than PPD.

Recording

The information resulting from the examination and any treatment performed needs to be recorded. A basic dental record consists of written notes and a completed dental chart. Additional diagnostic tests and radiographs are included as indicated.

A dental chart is a diagrammatic representation of the dentition, where information (findings and treatment) can be entered in a pictorial and/or notational form. It provides a simple way of recording most of your findings and treatments. However, it is only a chart and needs to be supplemented by clinical notes, radiographs, etc. to make a complete dental record.

Copies of the dog and cat dental record sheets used in our clinic are depicted in Fig. 3.5a and b. The front is used to record clinical findings, and the back is used to enter diagnosis, draw up a treatment plan and record the treatment performed. The nurse or technician who performs the clinical examination completes the front page. The veterinarian checks the clinical findings and interprets any radiographs taken, and then fills in the back page of the chart. Figure 3.5a depicts a blank record sheet and Fig. 3.5b shows a completed form.

We number the teeth using the modified Triadan System, which is a three-digit numbering system. The first digit denotes the quadrant of the mouth and whether the tooth is part of the permanent or primary dentition (Table 3.4).

The second and third digits together denote the tooth. In dogs, the teeth are numbered consecutively from the rostral midline to the caudal end of each quadrant. In cats, where the complement of teeth is reduced (the first maxillary premolar and the first and second mandibular premolars are absent), some numbers are skipped in the premolar region.

On the completed cat dental record sheet (Fig. 3.5b), plaque and calculus accumulation can be noted as mild, moderate or severe. We do not routinely score the degree of accumulation of plaque or calculus, as they will be removed during the periodontal therapy.

Note that only abnormalities are recorded on the chart. Gingivitis has been recorded using the modified Löe and Silness gingival index. Sites with increased periodontal probing depths are marked on the occlusal view.

Abbreviations are used when filling in the record sheet. It is important that a list of what the abbreviations mean is available. A list of commonly used abbreviations is given in Table 3.5.

4 Radiography

Radiography is a vital diagnostic tool in veterinary dentistry. Radiographs are required to:
- Reach a diagnosis
- Plan optimal treatment
- Perform certain procedures
- Assess the outcome of treatment performed.

General anaesthesia is required for radiography. Ideally, clinical examination and recording should precede the radiographic evaluation. It is also useful to clean the teeth before any radiographs are taken. Dental calculus, because it is radiodense, can obscure pathological lesions on a radiograph.

DENTAL RADIOGRAPHY

For a dental radiograph to be diagnostic, it should be an accurate representation of the size and shape of the tooth without superimposition of adjacent structures (Fig. 4.1). Intra-oral (film placed inside mouth and X-ray beam directed from outside the mouth through the tooth and adjacent structures onto the film) radiographic techniques are therefore required. The two basic techniques are:
1. Parallel technique for the mandibular premolars and molars
2. Bisecting angle technique for all other teeth.

Contralateral (same teeth, opposite side) views should routinely be taken for comparison.

FULL-MOUTH RADIOGRAPHS

Full-mouth radiographs describe a series of films where each tooth of the dentition is accurately depicted in at least one view. A full-mouth radiographic series of all animals undergoing dental examination provides valuable information, but is not always practically or financially viable. However, it is strongly recommended that all adult cats have full-mouth radiographs taken as part of the oral and dental examination. Odontoclastic resorptive lesions are common in cats and clinical examination without radiography will only detect end-stage lesions.

In cats, it is necessary to take a minimum of eight views, but 10 views are recommended, to ensure that all teeth are properly visualized. These are as follows:

Essential radiographic views
- Incisor view in the upper jaw
- Lateral view for each of the canines of the upper jaw
- Left and right maxillary premolar and molar views
- Mandibular incisor and canine view
- Left and right mandibular premolar and molar views.

Recommended radiographic views
- Lateral view for each of the canines of the mandible (in addition to the eight essential views).

The choice of film size for each view is subjective. The smallest film that will depict the area of interest should be used to facilitate film positioning. Adult periapical size film can be used for all cat views.

In the case of dogs, full-mouth radiographs are encouraged, especially at first examination. If this is not possible then radiographs should be taken where indicated based on the findings during the clinical examination. In the event of full-mouth radiographs, the size of film and the number of films used will depend upon the breed of dog and the shape of its face.

EQUIPMENT AND MATERIALS FOR CONVENTIONAL INTRA-ORAL RADIOGRAPHY

- X-ray machine
- X-ray film

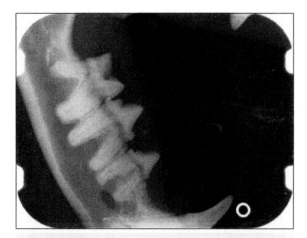

Figure 4.1 A diagnostic view. For a dental radiograph to be diagnostic, it should be an accurate representation of the size and shape of the tooth without superimposition of adjacent structures. Intra-oral placement of dental film and parallel technique gives an accurate representation of the mandibular third and fourth premolars and the first molar, as well as detail of the mandibular bone in a cat. In this view, the component structures of the tooth and its supporting tissues are well defined. The enamel is seen as an incompletely visualized radiodense band that covers the crown and tapers to a fine edge at the cervical margin of the tooth. The dentine is less radiodense than enamel and accounts for the bulk of the hard tissues of the tooth. The cementum is not visible. The pulp cavity is the continuous radiolucent space in the centre of the tooth which extends from the coronal portion to the apex of the roots. The wall of the alveolar tooth socket (the lamina dura) is the radiodense line which runs parallel to the root of the tooth. The periodontal ligament space is the fine radiolucent line between the lamina dura and the root of the tooth. The cortical bone on the crest of the alveolar ridge is continuous with the lamina dura. The mandibular canal is clearly visible.

- Processing facilities
- Mounts or envelopes for film storage.

The X-ray unit

A dental X-ray machine (Fig. 4.2) is preferable to a veterinary X-ray machine. However, most veterinary X-ray machines can be used for dental radiography, but the film-focus distance will need to be adjusted to between 30 and 50 cm.

X-ray film

To allow intra-oral film placement and achieve high definition, dental film (Fig. 4.3) should be used. Dental film is single emulsion, non-screen, and is available in three sizes (occlusal, adult periapical and child periapical) and

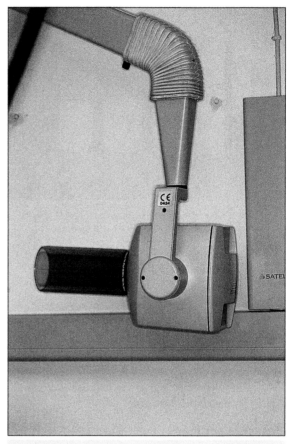

Figure 4.2 A dental X-ray unit installed in the designated dental theatre is the ideal situation. These units are available as free standing or wall mounted. Wall mounting is usually preferable to save space.

different speeds. The dental film is packed in either a paper or a plastic envelope, and the film is flanked by black paper and backed by a thin lead sheet (foil) that reduces scattered radiation.

Orientation

Ensure the correct side of the film envelope is facing the incident beam; the envelope is marked or labelled. If exposed through the back of the envelope, the lead sheet will absorb much of the X-ray beam, resulting in an underexposed radiograph with the pattern of the lead sheet imposed on it.

Each film has a raised dot in one corner. The dot helps with orientation when viewing and mounting dental radiographs if the following procedure is adhered to. Firstly, the dot should face the incident beam. Secondly, the film should be placed in the mouth so that the dot

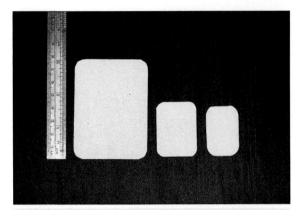

Figure 4.3 Sizes of dental film. Dental film is available in three sizes, namely occlusal (5 cm × 7 cm), periapical (3 cm × 4 cm) and paediatric (2 cm × 3 cm). The smallest film that depicts the area of interest should be used to facilitate film positioning in the mouth.

is always facing a specific direction. We position the dot so that it is always facing forward in the mouth. Another way of doing it is to ensure that the film is placed so that the dot is always in the same position, i.e. facing forward in the mouth on one side and backward in the mouth on the contralateral side.

Exposure settings

Dental film requires higher exposure settings than screen film, but gives better definition. The actual settings required vary with different X-ray machines and with different film-focal distances, as well as with the speed of dental film used.

Dental X-ray units provide guideline exposures for different size patients and different teeth. The X-ray unit is brought as close to the tooth that is being radiographed as possible, so setting film-focus distance is not required.

If you are using a veterinary X-ray unit and D speed dental film, set the film-focal distance between 30 and 50 cm and try the following exposures:

Cat/small dog	60–70 kV	20–25 mA
Medium/large dog	70–80 kV	20–25 mA
Rabbit/guinea-pig	50–60 kV	10–20 mA
Chinchilla	50–60 kV	5–15 mA.

Irrespective of the type of X-ray unit available, it is advisable to take series of trial exposures on animals of different size to make up exposure charts prior to undertaking dental radiography on patients.

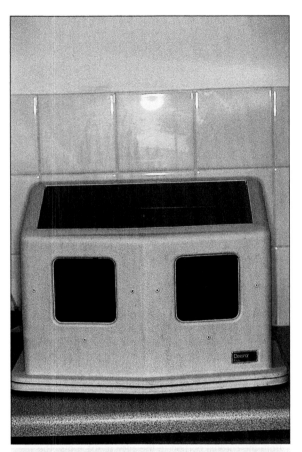

Figure 4.4 The Rinn box. A chair-side 'darkroom' for processing dental film is a simple and inexpensive way of processing dental film. Thorough rinsing under running water (rubbing the film gently with your fingers until it no longer feels 'soapy') after developing and fixing is essential to avoid fixation stains.

Dental film processing

Automated processors are available for dental film processing, but excellent results can be obtained with the use of a chair-side processor (Fig. 4.4).

Handling and mounting of dental radiographs

It is important to handle and mount processed dental films with care. Fingerprints can damage the emulsion on the film surface and the film is easily scratched. After rinsing thoroughly, adequate time should be allowed for the film to dry before being mounted or else it will adhere to the mount. It is also important to archive the film in such a way that it can be easily retrieved and

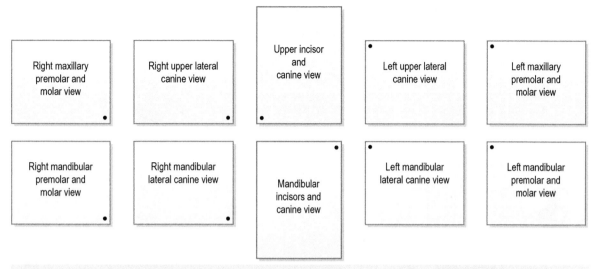

Figure 4.5 Mounting if films are exposed with the dot facing forward in the mouth. Dental radiographs are viewed and mounted as if you were facing the animal and looking into its mouth. The raised dot should face you when viewing the film. Based on the anatomy of the jaws and teeth, it is then possible to identify upper and lower jaw views. If the films are always exposed with the dot facing forward in the mouth, then all views on the right side will have the dot in a different position from the left-side views. This diagram depicts how we would mount a full-mouth series of cat radiographs when all the films have been exposed with the dot facing forward. This is our preferred method. From Gorrel C, Derbyshire S (2005): Veterinary Dentistry for the Nurse and Technician, with permission of Elsevier.

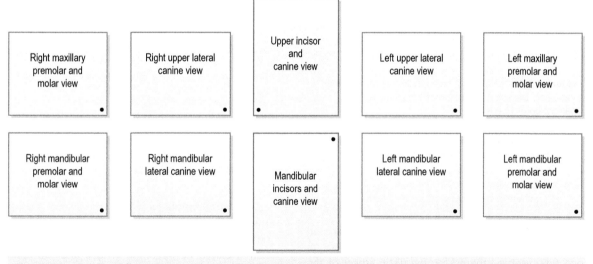

Figure 4.6 Mounting if films are exposed with the dot in the same position. If the films are always exposed with the dot in the same position, then all the views on one side will have the dot on the distal aspect of the teeth and the views on the other side will have it in the mesial aspect of the teeth. This diagram depicts how we would mount a full-mouth series of cat radiographs if the films had been exposed with the dot always in the same position. From Gorrel C, Derbyshire S (2005): Veterinary Dentistry for the Nurse and Technician, with permission of Elsevier.

identified. Remember that these films make up part of the patient's clinical records.

Dental radiographs are viewed and mounted as if you were facing the animal and looking into its mouth (Figs 4.5 and 4.6). The raised dot should face you when viewing the film. Based on the anatomy of the jaws and teeth, it is then possible to identify upper and lower jaw views. If the films were always exposed with the dot facing forward in the mouth, then all views on the right side will have the dot in a different position from the

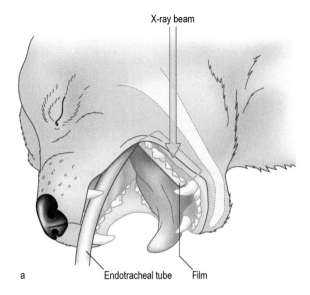

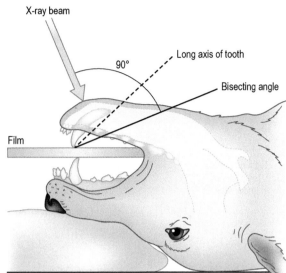

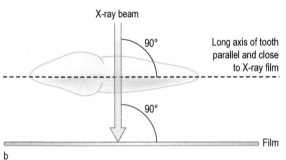

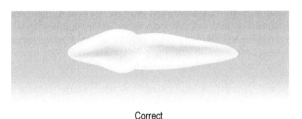

Figure 4.7 The parallel technique. From Gorrel C (2004): Veterinary Dentistry for the General Practitioner, with permission of Elsevier.

(a) With the patient in lateral recumbency (with the side to be radiographed uppermost), the film is placed between the tongue and the teeth and pushed as far down into the sublingual fossa as possible.

(b) The X-ray beam is then directed from lateral to medial at right angles to the long axis of the tooth.

Figure 4.8 The bisecting angle technique. To avoid foreshortening or elongation of the image, an imaginary plane is drawn halfway between the plane of the film and a plane through the long axis of the tooth, i.e. at the bisecting angle, and the X-ray beam is directed perpendicular to this plane. In this way, both sides of the triangles formed are the same length and the resulting image of the tooth is similar to the real tooth. From Gorrel C (2004): Veterinary Dentistry for the General Practitioner, with permission of Elsevier.

left-side views (Fig. 4.5). If the films were always exposed with the dot in the same position, then all the views on one side will have the dot on the distal aspect of the teeth and the other side will have it on the mesial aspect of the teeth (Fig. 4.6).

INTRA-ORAL RADIOGRAPHIC TECHNIQUES

The film is placed intra-orally and the incident beam directed through the tooth onto the film.

- The parallel technique is used to radiograph the mandibular premolars and molars (Fig. 4.7).
- All other teeth are radiographed using the bisecting angle technique (Fig. 4.8).

The parallel technique:

- The patient is placed in lateral recumbency (with the side to be radiographed uppermost).
- Film is placed between the tongue and the teeth and pushed as far down into the sublingual fossa as possible.
- The X-ray beam is then directed from lateral to medial at right angles to the long axis of the tooth.

The bisecting angle technique:

- Film is positioned at an angle behind the tooth.
- An imaginary plane is drawn halfway between the plane of the film and a plane through the long axis of the tooth, i.e. at the bisecting angle, and the X-ray beam is perpendicular to this plane; this is

important to avoid foreshortening or elongation of the teeth in the resulting image.

To achieve correct positioning requires a mental image of the normal orientation, length and morphology of the tooth roots. Two tongue spatulas, fingers or instrument handles can be used to visualize these planes outside the mouth and so aid the positioning of the beam. A common problem is to 'miss the apex' of a tooth (especially on canine teeth) due to poor estimation of root length or position.

It may be helpful to position the patient as follows:
- Sternal recumbency for the incisors in the upper jaw
- Lateral or sternal recumbency for the canines, premolars and molars in the upper jaw
- Dorsal recumbency for the mandibular incisors
- Dorsal or lateral recumbency for mandibular canines.

The premolar and molar views of the upper jaw of the cat are difficult. Often, the zygomatic arch is superimposed over the roots and apices of the teeth. Placing a foam wedge or small sandbag under the nose, thus tilting the head up so that the dental arch is parallel with the table, will help avoid this.

Another common problem is superimposition of the mesiobuccal and mesiopalatal roots of the upper fourth premolar in both dogs and cats. It is often necessary to take more than one view, changing the angle of the incident beam slightly (either rostrally or caudally), to be able to visualize both roots separately.

EXTRA-ORAL FILM PLACEMENT

Extra-oral views are not ideal for dental examination, mainly due to superimposition of the contralateral side, which obscures the image and causes distortion of the image. However, it may be possible to obtain diagnostic radiographs of the maxillary and mandibular premolars and molars using extra-oral film placement, especially in dogs with wide skulls. Some examiners routinely use extra-oral film placement to radiograph the maxillary premolars and molars in the cat. The technique is depicted in Fig. 4.9.

THE PARALLAX EFFECT

As a radiograph is two-dimensional, it is not possible to tell which of two objects in the image is nearer to the viewer. It is often necessary to know at what depth an object is – for example, in locating an ectopic unerupted tooth. When a second image is taken, after rotating the

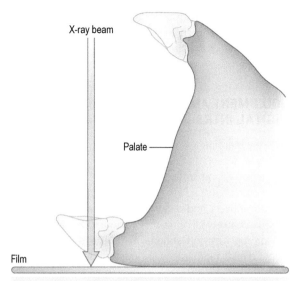

Figure 4.9 Extra-oral film placement. The film is placed on the table and the animal is placed in dorsolateral recumbency with the side to be radiographed closest to the film, i.e. the lower side of the animal's head. The mouth is held wide open using a radiolucent device, e.g. a plastic needle cap. Tilting the head rotates the contralateral side away and an open mouth should mean the beam passes only through the soft tissue of the contralateral side. The tilting will place maxillary teeth almost parallel to the film, but the beam still requires adjustment according to the bisecting angle technique to reduce image distortion. From Gorrel C (2004): Veterinary Dentistry for the General Practitioner, with permission of Elsevier.

beam position around the object's axis, the image of the object will move relative to other structures. When the object appears to move in the same direction as the shift in the X-ray head, it is placed lingually (nearer to the film); if it moves in the opposite direction, it is more buccally positioned (further from the film). This technique is also useful to separate and identify two overlying roots, e.g. the mesiobuccal and palatal roots of an upper carnassial tooth in carnivores.

The SLOB rule (same direction lingual, opposite direction buccal) may help you remember the parallax effect. To use the SLOB rule you need to know the original and second beam position. An object that has moved in the same direction as you have moved the incident beam is lingually located. Conversely, an object that has moved in the opposite direction to that which the incident beam has been moved is buccally located.

An easy way to visualize this is to place two similarly sized objects one in front of the other, both in front of a white wall. Use a semi-darkened room. Stand in front of both objects, take a torch and shine the beam at both objects, noting the position of the shadows on the wall. Then move the torch to the left or right and observe how the shadows of the two objects move relative to each other.

EQUIPMENT AND MATERIALS FOR DIGITAL INTRA-ORAL RADIOGRAPHY

- X-ray machine
- Digital sensors
- Computer and software.

Both indirect and direct digital systems are available on the market for intra-oral radiography. The digital sensor replaces conventional film. The advantages of using digital radiography include speed, reduction in exposure requirements and easier storage of patient data. I would strongly recommend investing in a digital system.

RADIOGRAPHIC INTERPRETATION

The radiographs should be viewed on a viewing box with minimal peripheral light and preferably using magnification. The radiographs of the contralateral structures, to those being evaluated, are used for comparative purposes. A good knowledge of the radiographic appearance of normal structures of the upper jaw and mandible is imperative to avoid misdiagnosis. Normal radiographic features (teeth and bone) are outlined in Chapter 1 and pathological radiographic features are covered in Sections 3–7.

SECTION 3

PERIODONTAL DISEASE

5 Periodontal disease – an introduction

Periodontal disease is the result of the inflammatory response to dental plaque, i.e. oral bacteria, and is limited to the periodontium. It is probably the most common disease seen in small animal practice, with the great majority of dogs and cats over the age of 3 years having a degree of disease that warrants intervention.

Periodontal disease is a collective term for a number of plaque-induced inflammatory lesions that affect the periodontium. It is a unique infection in that it is not associated with a massive bacterial invasion of the tissues. Gingivitis is inflammation of the gingiva and is the earliest sign of disease. Individuals with untreated gingivitis *may* develop periodontitis. The inflammatory reactions in periodontitis result in destruction of the periodontal ligament and alveolar bone. The result of untreated periodontitis is ultimately exfoliation of the affected tooth. Thus, gingivitis is inflammation that is not associated with destruction (loss) of supporting tissue – it is reversible. In contrast, periodontitis is inflammation where the tooth has lost a variable degree of its support (attachment) – it is irreversible.

Infection of the periodontium may cause discomfort to the affected animal. There is also strong evidence that a focus of infection in the oral cavity can cause disease of distant organs. Consequently, prevention and treatment of periodontal diseases is, contrary to common belief, not a cosmetic issue, but a general health and welfare issue!

AETIOLOGY

The primary cause of gingivitis and periodontitis is accumulation of dental plaque on the tooth surfaces. Calculus (tartar) is only a secondary aetiological factor.

Classic experiments have demonstrated that accumulation of plaque on the tooth surfaces reproducibly induces an inflammatory response in associated gingival tissues, and that removal of the plaque leads to disappearance of the clinical signs of this inflammation.

Dental plaque

Dental plaque is a biofilm composed of aggregates of bacteria and their by-products, salivary components, oral debris, and occasional epithelial and inflammatory cells. Plaque accumulation starts within minutes on a clean tooth surface. The initial accumulation of plaque occurs supragingivally but will extend into the sulcus and populate the subgingival region if left undisturbed.

The formation of plaque involves two processes, namely the initial adherence of bacteria and then the continued accumulation of bacteria due to a combination of bacterial multiplication and further aggregation of bacteria to those cells that are already attached. As soon as a tooth becomes exposed to the oral cavity, its surfaces are covered by the pellicle (an amorphous coating of salivary proteins and glycoproteins). The pellicle alters the charge and free energy of the tooth surfaces, which increases the efficiency of bacterial adhesion. Certain specific bacteria such as *Streptococcus sanguis* and *Actinomyces viscosus* can adhere directly to the pellicle. These bacteria produce extracellular polysaccharides, which then aggregate other bacteria that are not otherwise able to adhere.

The plaque associated with healthy gingiva is mainly comprised of aerobic and facultative anaerobic bacteria. As gingivitis develops, plaque extends subgingivally. Aerobes consume oxygen and a low redox potential is created, which makes the environment more suitable for the growth of anaerobic species. The aerobic population does not decrease, but with increasing numbers of anaerobes, the aerobic/anaerobic ratio decreases. The subgingival florae associated with periodontitis are predominantly anaerobic and consists of *Porphyromonas* spp., *Prevotella* spp., *Peptostreptococcus* spp., *Fusobacterium* spp. and spirochetes. High levels of *Porphyromonas* spp. and spirochetes are consistently associated with progressive periodontitis in the dog. The bacterial florae of cats with and without gingivitis and periodontitis are similar to those found in humans and dogs under similar conditions.

To summarize, the first bacteria to adhere to the pellicle are aerobic Gram-positive organisms. In dogs and cats, the main bacteria in supragingival plaque are *Actinomyces* and *Streptococcus* spp. As the plaque thickens, matures and extends further down the gingival sulcus, the environment becomes suitable for growth of anaerobic organisms, motile rods and spirochetes.

Dental calculus

Dental calculus is mineralized plaque. However, a layer of plaque always covers calculus. Both supragingival and subgingival plaque becomes mineralized. Supragingival calculus per se does not exert an irritant effect on the gingival tissues. The main importance of calculus in periodontal disease seems to be its role as a plaque-retentive surface. This is supported by well-controlled animal and clinical studies that have shown that the removal of subgingival plaque on top of subgingival calculus will result in healing of periodontal lesions and the maintenance of healthy periodontal tissues.

PATHOGENESIS

The pathogenic mechanisms involved in periodontal disease include:
- Direct injury by plaque microorganisms
- Indirect injury by plaque microorganisms via inflammation.

The microbiota in periodontal pockets is in a continual state of flux; periodontitis is a dynamic infection caused by a combination of bacterial vectors that change over time. As a result, the molecular events that trigger and sustain the inflammatory reactions constantly change. Many microbial products have little or no direct toxic effect on the host. However, they possess the potential to activate non-immune and immune inflammatory reactions that cause the tissue damage. It is now well accepted that *it is the host's response to the plaque bacteria, rather than microbial virulence per se*, that directly causes the tissue damage.

In gingivitis, the plaque-induced inflammation is limited to the soft tissue of the gingiva. Sulcus depths are normal (i.e. periodontal probing depths are 1–3 mm in the dog and 0.5–1 mm in the cat). As periodontitis occurs, the inflammatory destruction of the coronal part

of the periodontal ligament allows apical migration of the epithelial attachment and the formation of a pathological periodontal pocket (i.e. periodontal probing depths increase). If the inflammatory disease is permitted to progress, the crestal portion of the alveolar process begins to resorb. Alveolar bone destruction type and extent are diagnosed radiographically. The resorption may proceed apically on a horizontal level. Horizontal bone destruction is often accompanied by gingival recession, so periodontal pockets may not form. If there is no gingival recession the periodontal pocket is supra-alveolar, i.e. above the level of the alveolar margin. The pattern of bone destruction may also proceed in a vertical direction along the root to form angular bony defects. The periodontal pocket is now intra- or subalveolar, i.e. below the level of the crestal bone.

Disease progression is generally an episodic occurrence rather than a continuous process. Tissue destruction occurs as acute bursts of disease activity followed by relatively quiescent periods. The acute burst is clinically characterized by rapid deepening of the periodontal pocket as periodontal ligament fibres and alveolar bone are destroyed by the inflammatory reactions. The quiescent phase is not associated with clinical or radiographic evidence of disease progression. However, complete healing does not occur during this quiescent phase, because subgingival plaque remains on the root surfaces and inflammation persists in the connective tissue. The inactive phase can last for extended periods.

Other conditions, such as physical or psychological stress and malnutrition, may impair protective responses, such as the production of antioxidants and acute phase proteins, and can aggravate periodontitis, but do not actually cause destructive tissue inflammation. A genetic predisposition to destructive inflammation of the periodontium may be important in some individuals.

Significance

Undisturbed plaque accumulation results in gingivitis. While some individuals with untreated gingivitis will develop periodontitis, not all animals with untreated gingivitis do so. It cannot be predicted which individuals with gingivitis will develop periodontitis. However, animals in which clinically healthy gingivae are maintained will not develop periodontitis. Consequently, *the aim in periodontal disease prevention and treatment is to establish and maintain clinically healthy gingivae to prevent periodontitis.*

TREATMENT

General considerations

The treatment of periodontal disease is aimed at controlling the cause of the inflammation, i.e. dental plaque. Conservative or cause-related periodontal therapy consists of removal of plaque and calculus, and any other remedial procedures required, under general anaesthesia, in combination with daily maintenance of oral hygiene. In other words, the treatment of periodontal disease has two components:

1. Maintenance of oral hygiene
2. Professional periodontal therapy.

Maintenance of oral hygiene is performed by the owner and is often called home care. Its effectiveness depends on the motivation and technical ability of the owner and the cooperation of the animal.

Professional periodontal therapy is performed under general anaesthesia and includes supra- and subgingival scaling, rootplaning and tooth crown polishing.

The term 'dental prophylaxis' or 'prophy' has been used to encompass clinical examination and professional periodontal therapy. This is misleading, since the real prophylaxis, i.e. steps taken to prevent disease development and progression, is not the professional periodontal therapy carried out under general anaesthesia but the daily home care regime to remove plaque. If no home care is instituted, then plaque will rapidly reform after a professional periodontal therapy procedure and the disease will progress. The owner must be made aware that home care is the most essential component in both preventing and treating periodontal disease.

The aim of treatment differs whether the patient has gingivitis only or if there is also periodontitis.

Gingivitis

Gingivitis is by definition *reversible*. Removal or adequate reduction of plaque will restore inflamed gingivae to health. Once clinically healthy gingivae have been achieved, these can be maintained by daily removal or reduction in the accumulation of plaque. In short, the treatment of gingivitis is to restore the inflamed tissues to clinical health and then to maintain clinically healthy gingivae, thus preventing periodontitis. The purpose of the professional periodontal therapy in the gingivitis patient is removal of dental deposits, mainly calculus (which is not removed by toothbrushing). Once the teeth

have been cleaned it remains up to the owner to remove the plaque that re-accumulates on a daily basis.

Summary for treatment of gingivitis:
- Educating the owner to understand the disease process
- Training and motivating the owner to perform daily home care
- Instituting a daily home care regimen by the owner – ideally, toothbrushing with a pet toothpaste in conjunction with a dental hygiene product
- Professional periodontal therapy (supra- and subgingival scaling and polishing) under general anaesthesia to remove dental deposits (plaque and calculus)
- Regular check-ups to ensure that the owner is following recommendations and to boost the owner's motivation.

Periodontitis

Untreated gingivitis may progress to periodontitis. In most instances in a practice situation, periodontitis is *irreversible*. It is important to remember that periodontitis is a site-specific disease, i.e. it may affect one or more sites of one or several teeth. The aim of treatment is thus to prevent development of new lesions at other sites and to prevent further tissue destruction at sites which are already affected.

Professional periodontal therapy removes dental deposits above and below the gingival margin. It then rests with the owner to ensure that plaque does not re-accumulate. Meticulous supragingival plaque control, by means of daily toothbrushing and adjunctive antiseptics when indicated, will prevent migration of the plaque below the gingival margin. If the subgingival tooth surfaces are kept clean, the sulcular epithelium will reattach.

In patients with suspected periodontitis, I recommend instituting daily toothbrushing 3–4 weeks prior to the planned professional periodontal therapy if the animal will allow it. This will result in less inflamed tissue at the time of professional therapy and will allow assessment of the ability of the owner to perform home care. If home care is not possible, the professional treatment will need to be more radical, e.g. extraction of teeth that could potentially have been retained with good home care.

Periodontal surgery is the term used for certain specific surgical techniques aimed at preserving the periodontium. Periodontal surgery techniques include closed curettage, gingivoplasty, various flap techniques, osseous surgery, guided tissue regeneration and, of course, implants. The techniques create accessibility for professional scaling and polishing, and establish a gingival morphology that facilitates plaque control by home care regimes. Some techniques are aimed at regeneration of periodontal attachment lost, e.g. guided tissue regeneration.

Periodontal surgery is never first-line treatment for periodontal disease. Conservative management of periodontal disease (i.e. thorough supra- and subgingival scaling, rootplaning and polishing), in combination with daily meticulous home care, is always the first step. Periodontal surgery should only be performed where the owner has shown the ability to keep the mouth clean. If a client cannot maintain good oral hygiene measures in his pet, then in the interest of the well-being of the animal there is no indication for surgery.

Summary for treatment of periodontitis:
- Educating the owner to understand the disease process
- Training and motivating the owner to perform daily home care
- Instituting a daily toothbrushing regimen by the owner
- Professional periodontal therapy – this includes supra- and subgingival scaling and polishing, rootplaning and extraction of unsalvageable teeth under general anaesthesia
- Regular check-ups to ensure that the owner is following recommendations and to boost the owner's motivation
- Periodontal surgery may be indicated (if the owner has shown the ability to maintain adequate plaque control).

Natural progression of disease

INITIAL PRESENTATION

Halitosis.

PATIENT DETAILS

A 14-month-old, neutered male whippet.

CASE HISTORY

The dog was seen in primary practice for a non-oral problem (suturing of a skin laceration after running through a barbed wire fence while chasing rabbits). The owners were concerned about a possible oral infection as the dog had halitosis. They were worried about the risk of infecting their children as the dog was licking them in the face.

ORAL EXAMINATION – CONSCIOUS

The dog was amenable to conscious oral examination, which confirmed the halitosis and revealed a generalized gingivitis.

ORAL EXAMINATION – UNDER GENERAL ANAESTHETIC

See the front page of the dental record for details of findings (Fig. 6.1a) and the back page of the dental record for details of the treatment performed (Fig. 6.1b).

In summary, examination under general anaesthesia confirmed the moderate generalized gingivitis (Fig. 6.2a, b). There was no evidence of periodontitis, i.e. no gingival recession and no increased periodontal probing depth at any site (Fig. 6.3). There was moderate accumulation of calculus, especially on the buccal aspect of the upper fourth premolar and first molar bilaterally (Fig. 6.2a).

FURTHER INVESTIGATIONS

Radiographs were taken at sites of the missing premolars (105, 305 and 405) to confirm that they were congenitally absent.

ORAL PROBLEM LIST

1. Generalized gingivitis, uncomplicated by periodontitis
2. Congenital absence of 105, 305 and 405.

THEORY REFRESHER

Periodontal disease is a collective term for a number of plaque-induced inflammatory lesions that affect the periodontium.

In gingivitis, the plaque-induced inflammation is limited to the soft tissue of the gingiva. Sulcus depths are normal (i.e. periodontal probing depths are 1–3 mm in the dog and 0.5–1 mm in the cat). As periodontitis occurs, the inflammatory destruction of the coronal part of the periodontal ligament allows apical migration of the epithelial attachment and the formation of a pathological periodontal pocket (i.e. periodontal probing depths increase). If the inflammatory disease is permitted to progress, the crestal portion of the alveolar process begins to resorb. Alveolar bone destruction type and extent are diagnosed radiographically. The resorption may proceed apically on a horizontal level. Horizontal bone destruction is often accompanied by gingival recession, so periodontal pockets may not form. If there is no gingival recession, the periodontal pocket is supra-alveolar, i.e. above the level of the alveolar margin. The

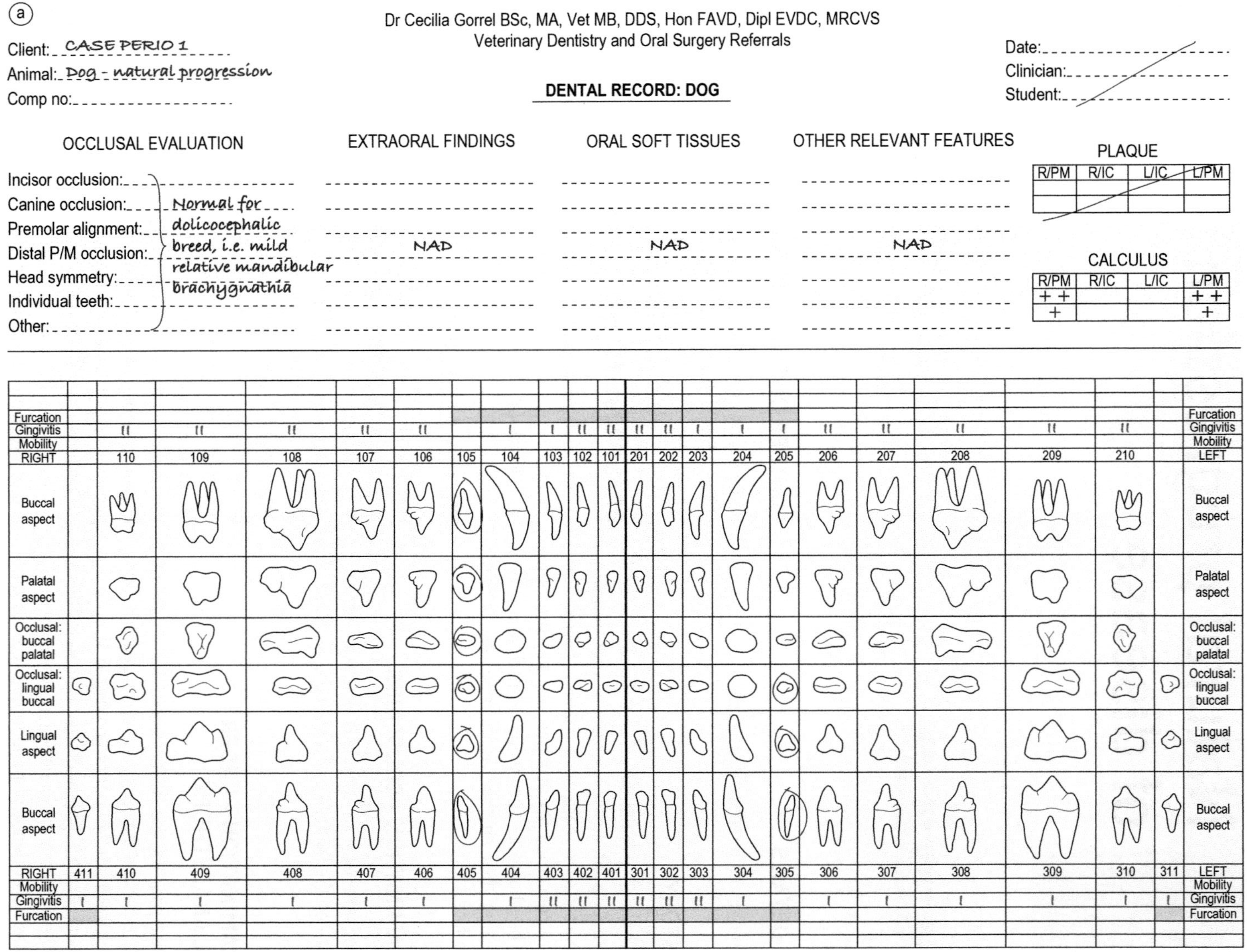

(a)

Dr Cecilia Gorrel BSc, MA, Vet MB, DDS, Hon FAVD, Dipl EVDC, MRCVS
Veterinary Dentistry and Oral Surgery Referrals

DENTAL RECORD: DOG

Client: _CASE PERIO 1_
Animal: _Dog - natural progression_
Comp no: _____

Date: _____
Clinician: _____
Student: _____

OCCLUSAL EVALUATION	EXTRAORAL FINDINGS	ORAL SOFT TISSUES	OTHER RELEVANT FEATURES

Incisor occlusion: _Normal for_
Canine occlusion: _dolicocephalic_
Premolar alignment: _breed i.e. mild_
Distal P/M occlusion: _relative mandibular_
Head symmetry: _brachygnathia_
Individual teeth: _____
Other: _____

EXTRAORAL FINDINGS: NAD

ORAL SOFT TISSUES: NAD

OTHER RELEVANT FEATURES: NAD

PLAQUE	R/PM	R/C	L/C	L/PM

CALCULUS	R/PM	R/C	L/C	L/PM
	+	+	+	+
	+			+

Figure 6.1 Front page (a) and back page (b) of the dental record.

(a) All clinical findings are reported on the front page of the dental record. Normal periodontal probing depth (PPD) is not noted on the dental record to avoid clutter. This dog had no increased periodontal probing sites. Apart from the generalized gingivitis, the only other abnormality detected was absence of 105, 305 and 405. After Gorrel C, Derbyshire S (2005): Veterinary Dentistry for the Nurse and Technician, with permission of Elsevier.

ORAL PROBLEM LIST

1. Moderate generalized gingivitis
2. Missing 105, 305 and 405

PERIODONTICS

☐ Sonic scaling   ☑ Ultrasonic scaling
☑ Subgingival curettage   ☐ Periodontal debridement
☑ Pumice polishing   ☐ Air polishing
☐ Periodontal surgery

OTHER DENTAL PROCEDURES

Radiographs of 105, 305, 405 reveal congenital absence of these teeth

THERAPEUTIC PLAN

→ 1. Periodontal therapy and home care
→ 2. Radiograph

ORAL SURGERY (Note sites on graph - X)

☐ Closed extraction(s):
☐ Open extraction(s):
☐ Incisional biopsy   ☐ Excisional biopsy
☐ Other/comments

COMPLICATIONS/COMMENTS

Give toothbrushing instruction at discharge

Home with brush and paste. Advise daily brushing.

Recheck in one month.

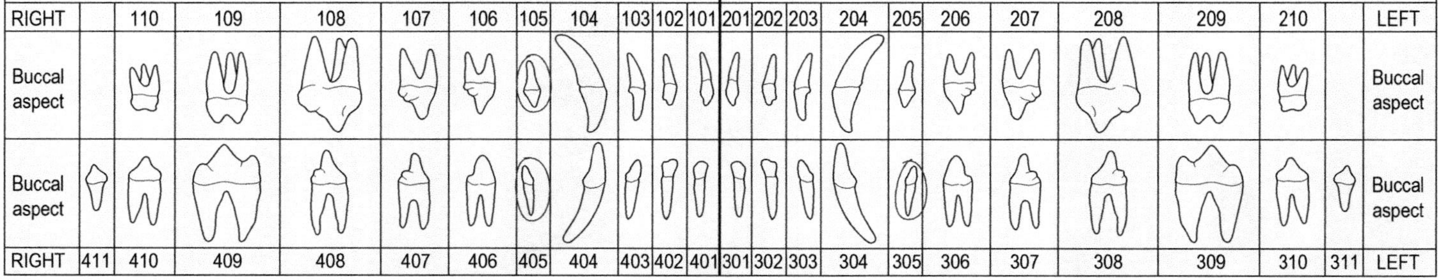

RIGHT	110	109	108	107	106	105	104	103	102	101				201	202	203	204	205	206	207	208	209	210		LEFT
Buccal aspect																									Buccal aspect
Buccal aspect											401	402	403	301	302	303	304	305	306	307	308	309	310	311	Buccal aspect
RIGHT	410	409	408	407	406	405	404	403	402	401															LEFT

Figure 6.1 (continued)

(b) Details of treatment are reported on the back page of the dental record. Treatment consisted of periodontal therapy (supra- and subgingival scaling and crown polishing). Radiographs were taken that confirmed that 105, 305 and 405 were congenitally absent. After Gorrel C, Derbyshire S (2005): Veterinary Dentistry for the Nurse and Technician, with permission of Elsevier.

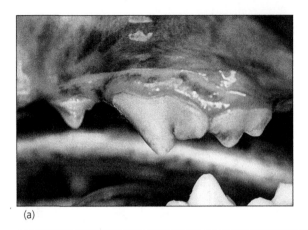
(a)

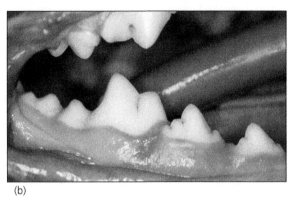
(b)

Figure 6.2 Lateral photographs of the left upper premolar and molar region (a) and of the right lower jaw (b).

(a) Note the swelling and reddening of the gingival margin indicating moderate to severe gingival inflammation in response to the accumulation of plaque. The buccal tooth surfaces are covered in dental deposits (plaque and calculus).

(b) Dental deposits have been removed. The gingival inflammation is evident, especially interproximal 408 and 409.

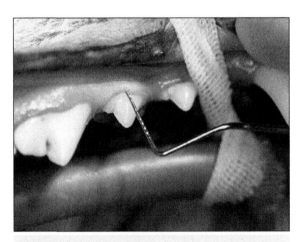

Figure 6.3 Lateral photograph of gingival probing of sulcus of 107. The probe is inserted at several sites around the whole circumference of each tooth to measure periodontal probing depth. In this dog, the probe could not be inserted to a depth greater than 1–2 mm at any site around any tooth, i.e. only normal sulcus depths were recorded. This is a case of gingivitis, with no evidence of periodontitis.

pattern of bone destruction may also proceed in a vertical direction along the root to form angular bony defects. The periodontal pocket is now intra- or subalveolar, i.e. below the level of the crestal bone.

Diagnosis of periodontal disease relies on clinical examination of the periodontium in the anaesthetized animal. In addition, radiography is mandatory if there is

evidence of periodontitis on clinical examination. It is essential to differentiate between gingivitis and periodontitis in order to institute appropriate treatment. In individuals with gingivitis, the aim is to restore the tissues to clinical health; in individuals with established periodontitis, the aim of therapy is to prevent progression of disease.

The following parameters need to be assessed and recorded for *each tooth* in *all patients*:

1. Gingivitis and gingival index
2. Periodontal probing depth (PPD)
3. Gingival recession (GR)
4. Furcation involvement
5. Mobility
6. Periodontal/clinical attachment loss (PAL/CAL).

Periodontal probing depth, gingival recession, furcation involvement and mobility measure the extent of destruction of the periodontium, i.e. they assess the presence and severity of periodontitis.

It is essential to remember that PPD is not necessarily correlated with severity of attachment loss. Gingival hyperplasia may contribute to a deep pocket (or pseudo-pocket if there is no attachment loss), while gingival recession may result in the absence of a pocket but also minimal remaining attachment. Periodontal attachment loss (PAL) records the distance from the cemento-enamel junction (or from a fixed point on the tooth) to the base or apical extension of the pathological pocket. It is thus a more accurate assessment of tissue loss in periodontitis. PAL is either measured directly with a periodontal probe or it is calculated (e.g. PPD + gingival recession).

In this case the inflammation was limited to the gingivae, i.e. gingivitis.

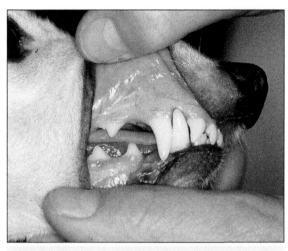

Figure 6.4 Lateral photograph of the right rostral oral cavity. The gingivae show no clinical evidence of inflammation, i.e. they are pale pink and there is no bleeding on brushing or careful probing. Daily toothbrushing for 1 month has resolved the gingivitis.

TREATMENT OPTIONS

A combination of regular professional periodontal therapy (to remove established dental deposits) and daily home care (to minimize plaque accumulation) is the treatment for gingivitis.

TREATMENT PERFORMED

Periodontal therapy (supra- and subgingival scaling and crown polishing), to remove plaque and calculus and provide a clean environment (which the owner can then keep clean with daily toothbrushing), was performed.

The owners and the eldest daughter (15 years old) were instructed in toothbrushing technique. They were given complementary toothbrush and paste, and advised to start daily brushing.

RECHECKS

At recheck 1 month later, the owners reported that there was no halitosis. The dog had readily accepted toothbrushing and the eldest daughter was brushing the dog's teeth every evening. The dog would not eat the dental diet and had shown no interest in dental hygiene chews (in fact, he had buried the dental hygiene chews in the garden). Conscious clinical examination revealed that the gingivae were clinically healthy (Fig. 6.4) and plaque disclosing solution revealed virtually no plaque (the daughter had brushed the teeth just before the appointment).

The dog was rechecked (conscious examination) every 6 months for 3 years. The daughter performed meticulous toothbrushing and the gingivae were clinically healthy. He was placed under general anaesthesia to suture a skin laceration when he was 4 years old and oral examination at the time revealed clinically healthy gingivae with probing depths of 1 mm or less at all sites, i.e. no evidence of periodontitis. It was decided to put him on an annual recall system.

He was brought in to see me 9 months later due to halitosis. The eldest daughter had left home to attend university and the parents had not been brushing his teeth. Conscious clinical exam revealed the presence of dental deposits and generalized gingivitis, complicated by periodontitis (Fig. 6.5a, b). Based on the findings at

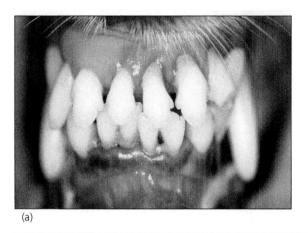 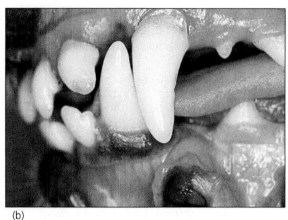

(a)   (b)

Figure 6.5 Anterior (a) and lateral (b) photographs of the rostral oral cavity. There is obvious accumulation of dental deposits and a marked gingival inflammatory response. Note the gingival recession affecting 101, 201, 202, 203, 204 and all lower incisors. There is also an uncomplicated crown fracture (UCF) of 203.

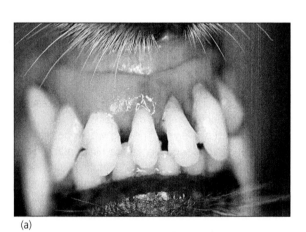 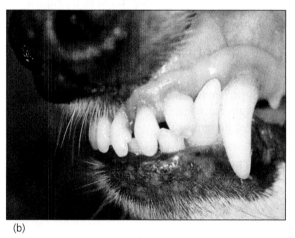

(a)   (b)

Figure 6.6 Anterior (a) and lateral (b) photographs of the rostral oral cavity. Note the reduction in gingival inflammation (gingivae are less oedematous and less red) achieved with 3 weeks of daily toothbrushing without removing dental deposits. Whenever possible, it is useful to institute daily toothbrushing prior to the professional periodontal cleaning. There will be a reduction in gingivitis and the dog will be habituated to the daily toothbrushing, which is important immediately after periodontal therapy.

conscious examination, daily toothbrushing was immediately resumed and the dog was booked for examination under general anaesthesia and periodontal treatment 3 weeks later.

Conscious examination 3 weeks later showed reduction in the severity of the gingivitis (Fig. 6.6a, b). Oral examination under general anaesthesia confirmed periodontitis at several sites. In fact, some of the lower incisors had lost so much periodontal attachment (Fig. 6.7a,

b) that they were extracted. Following the professional periodontal therapy and extractions, the owners resumed daily toothbrushing and the gingivitis resolved. See the front of the dental record for details of findings (Fig. 6.8a) and the back of the dental record for details of treatment (Fig. 6.8b).

After this treatment, the dog was placed on an annual recall system for 5 years. In this time, he was examined under anaesthesia twice. The owners were brushing

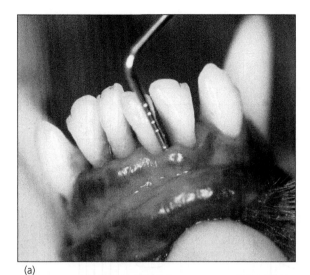

(a)

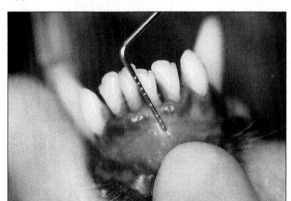

(b)

Figure 6.7 Anterior view of the lower incisors.

(a) The periodontal probe is in situ at the bucco-distal aspect of 301.

(b) The periodontal probe has been removed from the pocket and placed on the surface of the gingiva to demonstrate the recorded probing depth. At this site there was a probing depth of 5 mm and a gingival recession of 3 mm. The periodontal attachment loss is thus 8 mm.

daily and no further intervention was required. The gingivae remained clinically healthy and there was no progression of the periodontitis (affected sites remained static and no new sites developed).

PROGNOSIS

The dog is allowing optimal home care, i.e. daily toothbrushing. The result is maintenance of clinically healthy gingivae and the prevention of periodontitis. As long as the owners carry on with daily toothbrushing, periodontal health will be maintained. If they reduce the frequency of brushing or stop altogether, then periodontitis will rapidly develop.

COMMENTS

The dog is now 10 years old. He maintains healthy gingivae and has not developed further periodontitis. His history is really a textbook description of the natural progression of periodontal disease, i.e. undisturbed plaque accumulation results in gingivitis and untreated gingivitis often results in periodontitis. In a periodontitis-prone individual the development of periodontitis can and often does occur rapidly.

To summarize, when he was 14 months old he presented with gingivitis due to plaque accumulation. For 3 years he maintained clinically healthy gingivae as a consequence of the daughter brushing his teeth daily. Toothbrushing was then stopped and within 9 months of undisturbed plaque accumulation he presented with periodontitis (severe enough to require extraction of several teeth). Daily toothbrushing was then resumed and for 5 years he has maintained gingival health with no further periodontitis.

Client education is of paramount importance in preventing and treating periodontal diseases. They must be fully aware that it is the daily removal of plaque by means of toothbrushing that is the most important step. The effect of professional periodontal therapy lasts at most only 3 months. Feeding of a dental diet or dental hygiene chews will reduce the accumulation of plaque and calculus, but will not result in clinically healthy gingivae and the prevention of periodontitis.

In this case, because the daughter had been brushing the teeth the owners had not quite realized how important the daily toothbrushing was. It wasn't until it was stopped and disease rapidly developed that the vital nature of daily toothbrushing became clear to them.

Plaque disclosing solution is a useful tool to monitor the efficacy of toothbrushing. I advise owners to brush as well as they possibly can and then to apply plaque disclosing solution to identify any remaining plaque which they can then brush away. Optimally, they should check toothbrushing efficacy with a plaque disclosing solution frequently, e.g. initially every day and then once a week.

It must be noted that halitosis is often a sign of periodontal disease, although gingivitis and periodontitis can be present without obvious halitosis.

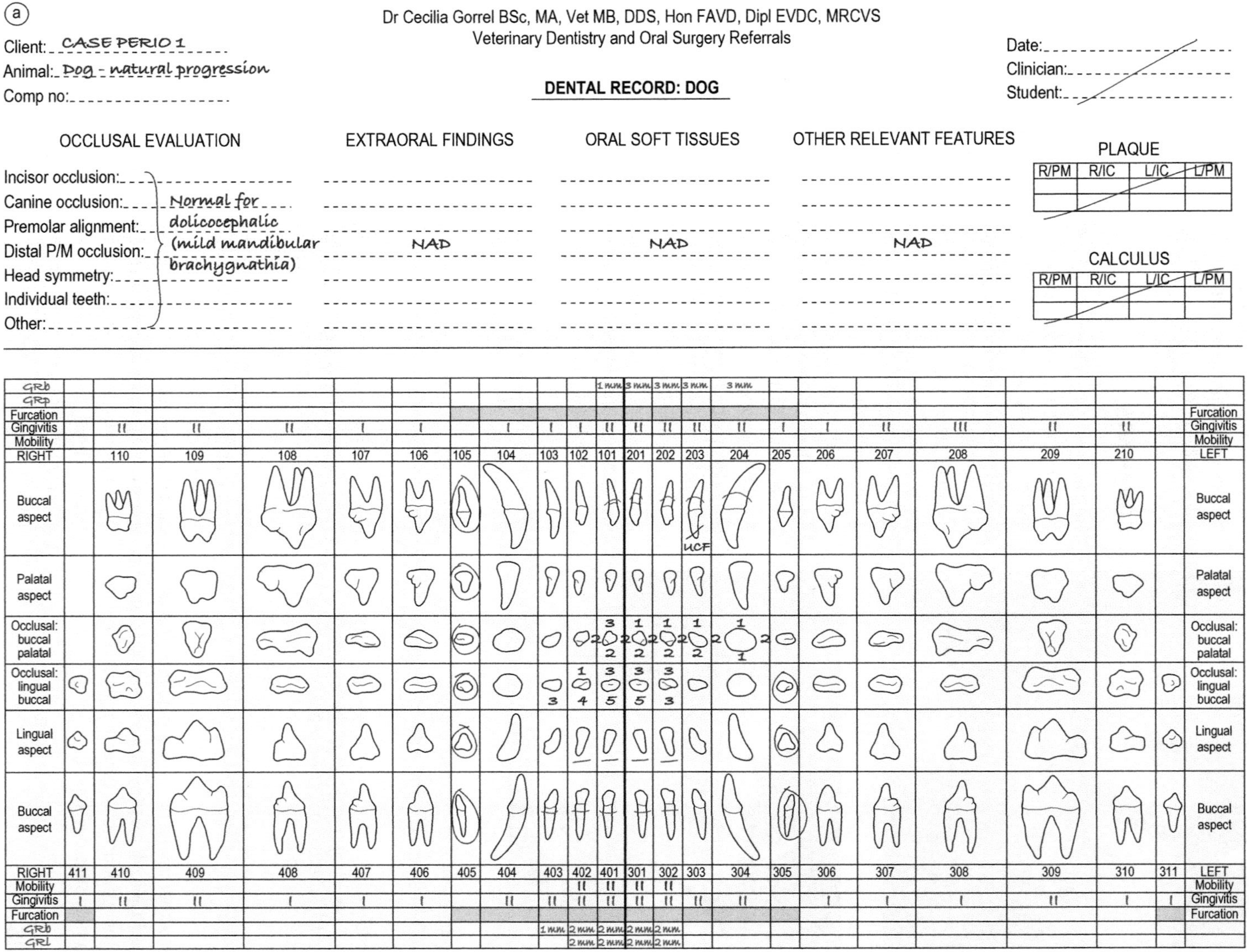

(a)

Dr Cecilia Gorrel BSc, MA, Vet MB, DDS, Hon FAVD, Dipl EVDC, MRCVS
Veterinary Dentistry and Oral Surgery Referrals

DENTAL RECORD: DOG

Client: _CASE PERIO 1_
Animal: _Dog - natural progression_
Comp no: _____

Date: _____
Clinician: _____
Student: _____

OCCLUSAL EVALUATION

Incisor occlusion: _____
Canine occlusion: _Normal for_
Premolar alignment: _dolicocephalic_
Distal P/M occlusion: _(mild mandibular_
Head symmetry: _brachygnathia)_
Individual teeth: _____
Other: _____

EXTRAORAL FINDINGS

ORAL SOFT TISSUES   NAD   NAD

OTHER RELEVANT FEATURES

PLAQUE

	R/PM	R/IC	L/IC	L/PM

CALCULUS

	R/PM	R/IC	L/IC	L/PM

Figure 6.8 Front page (a) and back page (b) of the dental record.

(a) All clinical findings are reported on the front page of the dental record. Remember that periodontitis is a site-specific disease. PPD is recorded on the occlusal view of the tooth on the dental record so that you can easily identify the precise site of disease. Normal periodontal probing depth (PPD) is not noted on the dental record to avoid clutter. However, when gingival recession is present, then PPDs are always recorded so that periodontal attachment loss (PAL) can be calculated (GR + PPD) and entered on the record at its precise site in green ink. PAL is a more accurate assessment of attachment loss. In this case, there was insufficient space

ORAL PROBLEM LIST

1. Generalized gingivitis
2. Periodontitis 101, 201, 202, 203, 204, 301, 302, 401, 402, 403
3. Uncomplicated crown fracture 203

PERIODONTICS

☐ Sonic scaling   ☑ Ultrasonic scaling
☑ Subgingival curettage   ☐ Periodontal debridement
☑ Pumice polishing   ☐ Air polishing
☐ Periodontal surgery

PAL 101 buccal = 4 mm   401 buccal = 7 mm
     201, 202, 203, 204 buccal = 4 mm 401 lingual = 5 mm
     301 buccal = 7 mm
     305 lingual = 5 mm   402 buccal = 6 mm
                                       402 lingual = 5 mm
     302 buccal = 5 mm   403 buccal = 4 mm
     302 lingual = 5 mm

OTHER DENTAL PROCEDURES

Radiographs of all teeth affected by periodontitis (4 films)

Radiograph 203 UCF (1 film)

Postextraction radiographs 301, 302, 401, 402 (1 film)

THERAPEUTIC PLAN

1. Periodontal therapy followed by home care
2. Radiograph followed by periodontal therapy and extraction as needed
3. Radiograph

ORAL SURGERY (Note sites on graph - X)

☐ Closed extraction(s):
☐ Open extraction(s): 301, 302, 401, 402. Flaps closed with 5/0 Monocryl
☐ Incisional biopsy   ☐ Excisional biopsy
☐ Other/comments

COMPLICATIONS/COMMENTS

203 UCF = NAD on radiograph ——> monitor

Home with daily toothbrushing. Recall in one month for conscious exam then in 6 months' time for EVA and radiographs

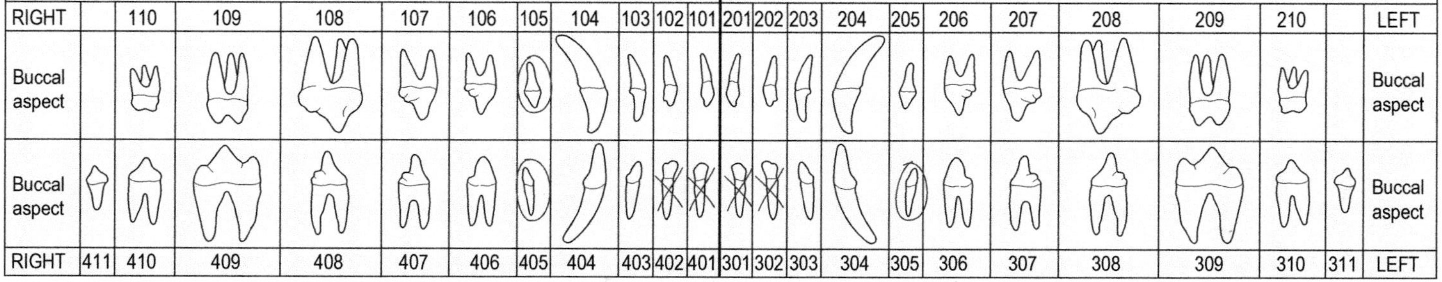

RIGHT	110	109	108	107	106	105	104	103	102	101	201	202	203	204	205	206	207	208	209	210	LEFT
Buccal aspect																					Buccal aspect
Buccal aspect																					Buccal aspect
RIGHT	411	410	409	408	407	406	405	404	403	402	401	301	302	303	304	305	306	307	308	309	310	311	LEFT

Figure 6.8 (continued)

(b) Details of treatment are reported on the back page of the dental record. Treatment consisted of periodontal therapy (supra- and subgingival scaling and crown polishing), and open extraction of 301, 302, 401 and 402. Flaps were closed with 5/0 Monocryl. Radiographs were taken of all teeth affected by periodontitis to assess the full extent of the disease. A baseline radiograph of 203 (uncomplicated crown fracture) was taken to assess pulp and periapical status. Post-extraction radiographs were also taken. After Gorrel C, Derbyshire S (2005): Veterinary Dentistry for the Nurse and Technician, with permission of Elsevier.

It is prudent to take radiographs of sites where teeth are clinically absent to determine whether the tooth is congenitally absent or unerupted. An increased risk of cyst formation has been reported with unerupted teeth. The follicle of the unerupted tooth undergoes cystic transformation. The resultant follicular (dentigerous) cyst may cause extensive alveolar bone resorption as it increases in size. These cysts expand as an osmotic gradient develops between the cyst lumen and the surrounding tissues. The pressure of the expanding cyst stimulates resorption of the bone. Follicular cysts can become large and cause extensive resorption of the surrounding alveolar bone. Consequently, unerupted teeth that are maintained require regular radiographic monitoring to identify development of a follicular cyst at an early stage. Treatment then consists of removing the unerupted tooth and its associated cyst. Some clinicians choose to extract unerupted teeth as a prophylactic measure.

The uncomplicated crown fracture of 203 has been monitored radiographically and no pulp or periapical disease has developed, so no treatment is indicated.

7 Periodontitis in a cat

INITIAL PRESENTATION

Non-healing extraction site and ulcerated lip.

PATIENT DETAILS

A 7-year-old, neutered female, domestic short-haired cat.

CASE HISTORY

The cat had received three episodes of periodontal treatment in the last 4 years. These had consisted of scaling, polishing and extraction (no record of which teeth or reason for extraction). Six months prior to the referral it was noted that the left upper canine extraction socket had not healed. The cat had received several courses of antibiotics with no improvement. Also, the left lower canine was catching the upper lip and causing ulceration.

The cat was referred to us for management of the non-healing extraction socket and the lip lesion.

ORAL EXAMINATION – CONSCIOUS

The cat was relatively amenable to quick conscious oral examination, which revealed the following:
1. Missing teeth (presumably extracted)
2. Generalized moderate to severe gingivitis
3. Non-healed extraction socket of 204
4. Ulcer left upper lip (due to traumatic occlusion from 304).

ORAL EXAMINATION – UNDER GENERAL ANAESTHETIC

See the front page of the dental record (Fig. 7.1) for details of findings.

In summary, examination under general anaesthesia identified the following:
1. Missing teeth (103, 109, 201, 203, 204, 209 and 409)
2. Generalized moderate to severe gingivitis
3. Non-healed extraction socket of 204 (Fig. 7.2)
4. Non-healed extraction socket of 409 (Fig. 7.3)
5. Ulcer left upper lip
6. Gingival recession affecting 104, 107 (Fig. 7.4a, b), 108, 207, 208, 304, 309, 404 and 408
7. Grade I furcation involvement of 207
8. Grade III furcation involvement of 107 (Fig. 7.4a, b), 309 and 408
9. Grade II mobility of 408.

FURTHER INVESTIGATIONS

Full-mouth radiographs (10 views) were taken.

RADIOGRAPHIC FINDINGS

The radiographs revealed a generalized horizontal alveolar bone loss, which was more severe in the upper jaw (Fig. 7.5). There was extensive bone loss at the furcation of 107 (Fig. 7.5), 309 (Fig. 7.6) and 408 (Fig. 7.7). The bone loss at 408 had a vertical (as well as horizontal) component and there was a pathological fracture of the mesial root (Fig. 7.7). In addition, the root of the extracted 204 (Fig. 7.8) and the distal root of the extracted 409 were retained.

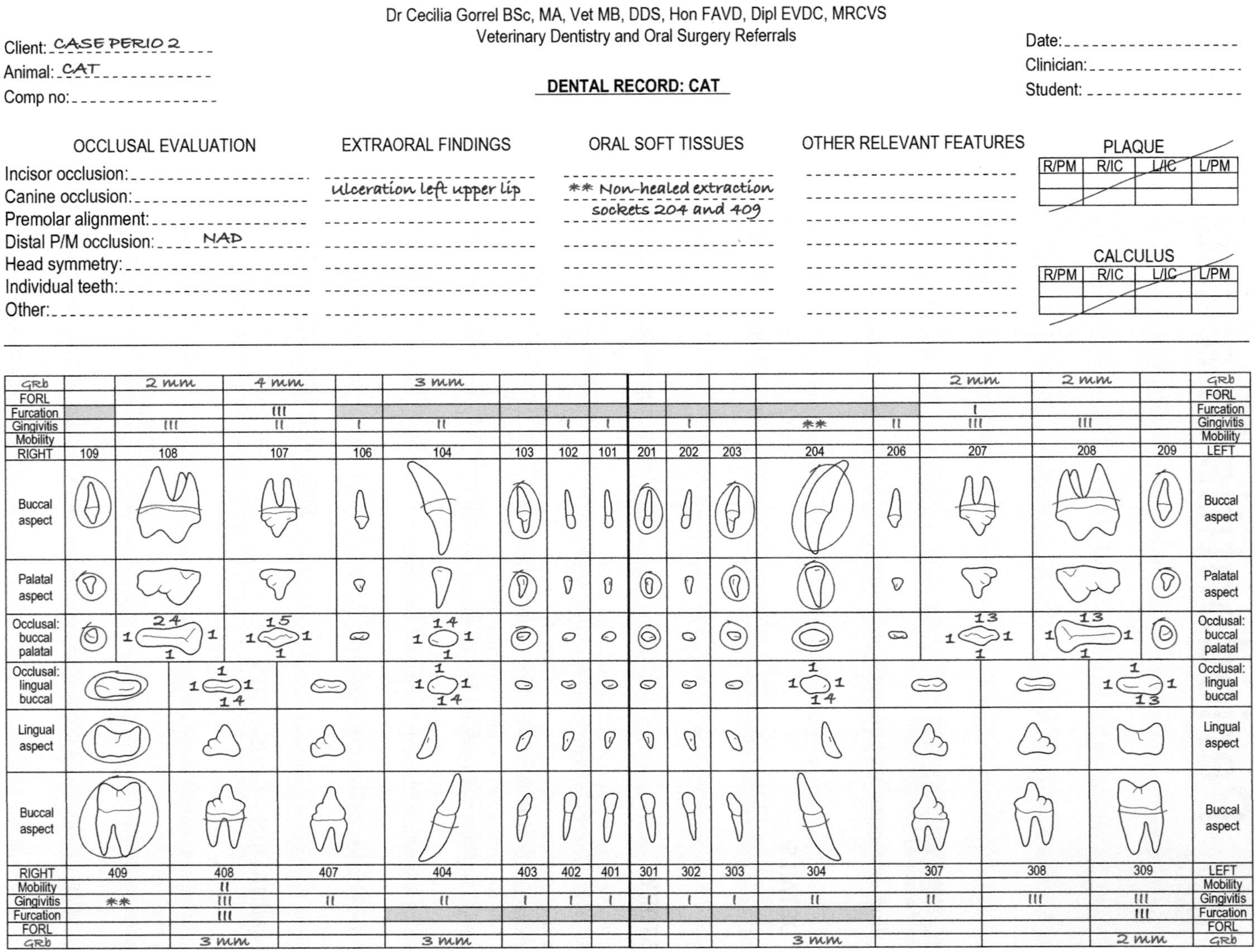

Dr Cecilia Gorrel BSc, MA, Vet MB, DDS, Hon FAVD, Dipl EVDC, MRCVS
Veterinary Dentistry and Oral Surgery Referrals

Client: CASE PERIO 2
Animal: CAT
Comp no:

DENTAL RECORD: CAT

Date:
Clinician:
Student:

OCCLUSAL EVALUATION	EXTRAORAL FINDINGS	ORAL SOFT TISSUES	OTHER RELEVANT FEATURES
Incisor occlusion:		** Non-healed extraction	
Canine occlusion:	ulceration left upper lip	sockets 204 and 409	
Premolar alignment:			
Distal P/M occlusion: NAD			
Head symmetry:			
Individual teeth:			
Other:			

PLAQUE

R/PM	R/IC	L/IC	L/PM

CALCULUS

R/PM	R/IC	L/IC	L/PM

GRb		2 mm	4 mm		3 mm									2 mm	2 mm		GRb
FORL																	FORL
Furcation			III											I			Furcation
Gingivitis		III	II	I	II		I	I		I		**	II	III	III		Gingivitis
Mobility																	Mobility
RIGHT	109	108	107	106	104	103	102	101	201	202	203	204	206	207	208	209	LEFT
Buccal aspect																	Buccal aspect
Palatal aspect																	Palatal aspect
Occlusal: buccal palatal		24 / 1 / 1 / 1	15 / 1 / 1 / 1		14 / 1 / 1 / 1									13 / 1 / 1 / 1	13 / 1 / 1 / 1		Occlusal: buccal palatal

Occlusal: lingual buccal	409	408	407	404	403	402	401	301	302	303	304	307	308	309	Occlusal: lingual buccal
Occlusal: lingual buccal		1 / 1 / 1 / 14		1 / 1 / 1 / 14							1 / 1 / 1 / 14			1 / 1 / 1 / 13	Occlusal: lingual buccal
Lingual aspect															Lingual aspect
Buccal aspect															Buccal aspect
RIGHT	409	408	407	404	403	402	401	301	302	303	304	307	308	309	LEFT
Mobility		II													Mobility
Gingivitis	**	III	II	II	I	I	I	I	I	I	II	II	III	III	Gingivitis
Furcation		III												III	Furcation
FORL															FORL
GRb		3 mm		3 mm							3 mm			2 mm	GRb

Figure 7.1 Dental record. All clinical findings are reported on the front page of the dental record. Remember that periodontitis is a site-specific disease. PPD is recorded on the occlusal view of the tooth on the dental record so that you can easily identify the precise site of disease. Normal periodontal probing depth (PPD) is not noted on the dental record to avoid clutter. However, when gingival recession is present, then PPDs are always recorded so that periodontal attachment loss (PAL) can be calculated (GR + PPD) and entered on the record at its precise site in green ink. PAL is a more accurate assessment of attachment loss.

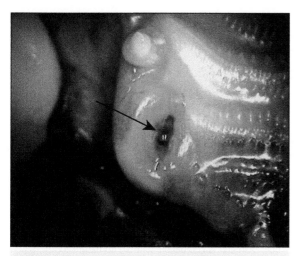

Figure 7.2 Occlusal view of the non-healed extraction socket of 204.

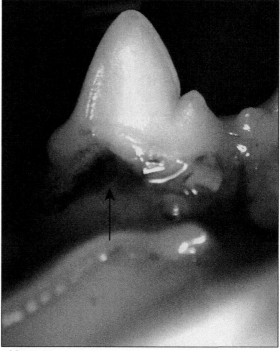

(a)

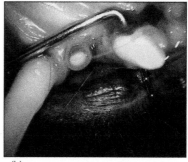

(b)

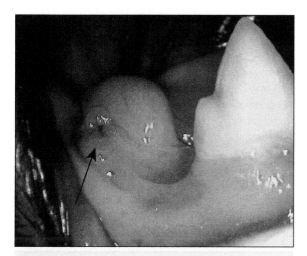

Figure 7.3 Lateral photo of the non-healed extraction socket of 409.

Figure 7.4 Advanced periodontitis.

(a) Bone loss and gingival recession have resulted in exposure of the furcation on the palatal aspect of 107.

(b) Tooth 107 has a grade III furcation lesion, i.e. the probe can be passed through the furcation.

ORAL PROBLEM LIST

1. Generalized gingivitis
2. Moderate periodontitis in 104, 108, 207, 208, 304 and 404
3. Advanced periodontitis in 107, 309 and 408 (pathological fracture of the mesial root)
4. Root remnants from previous extractions (204 and the distal root of 409)
5. Ulcer left upper lip (due to traumatic occlusion from 304).

THEORY REFRESHER

Periodontal disease is a collective term for plaque-induced inflammatory lesions that affect the periodontium.

In gingivitis, the plaque-induced inflammation is limited to the soft tissue of the gingiva. Sulcus depths are normal (i.e. periodontal probing depths are 1–3 mm

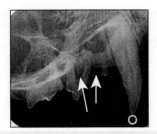

Figure 7.5 Advanced periodontitis. Radiograph reveals generalized horizontal bone loss and extensive loss of furcation bone of 107.

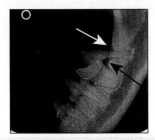

Figure 7.6 Advanced periodontitis. Radiograph demonstrates horizontal bone loss and furcation involvement of 309.

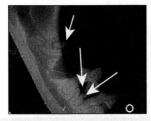

Figure 7.7 Advanced periodontitis, pathological root fracture and retained root from previous extraction. Radiograph demonstrates horizontal bone loss and external root resorption of 408. Remember that inflammatory root resorption is a feature of periodontitis and needs to be differentiated from idiopathic root resorption. The bone loss at the furcation of 408 is severe. Note the pathological fracture of the mesial root of 408, which explains the grade II mobility recorded for this tooth. Note also the retained distal root from extraction of 409, which prevented healing of the socket.

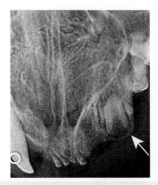

Figure 7.8 Partial extraction. Note the retained root from extraction of 204. This explains why the socket was not healing. The pulp diameter of the retained root is much larger than that of the contralateral tooth. In fact, the pulp diameter is compatible with an immature tooth. Consequently, the injury that caused pulp necrosis and cessation of tooth development probably occurred before the cat was a year old.

depths increase). If the inflammatory disease is permitted to progress, the crestal portion of the alveolar process begins to resorb. Alveolar bone destruction type and extent are diagnosed radiographically. The bone resorption may proceed apically on a horizontal level. Horizontal bone destruction is often accompanied by gingival recession (as in this case), so periodontal pockets may not form. If there is no gingival recession, the periodontal pocket is supra-alveolar, i.e. above the level of the alveolar margin. The pattern of bone destruction may also proceed in a vertical direction along the root to form angular bony defects. The periodontal pocket is now intra- or subalveolar, i.e. below the level of the crestal bone. Inflammatory root resorption may also occur in periodontitis. This type of external root resorption needs to be differentiated from idiopathic root resorption (see Chapter 17).

Diagnosis of periodontal disease relies on clinical examination of the periodontium in the anaesthetized animal. In addition, radiography to assess the type and extent of alveolar bone destruction is mandatory if there is evidence of periodontitis on clinical examination. It is essential to differentiate between gingivitis and periodontitis in order to institute appropriate treatment. In individuals with gingivitis, the aim is to restore the tissues to clinical health; in individuals with established periodontitis, the aim of therapy is to prevent progression of disease.

The following parameters need to be assessed and recorded for *each tooth* in *all patients*:

in the dog and 0.5–1 mm in the cat). As periodontitis occurs, the inflammatory destruction of the coronal part of the periodontal ligament allows apical migration of the epithelial attachment and the formation of a pathological periodontal pocket (i.e. periodontal probing

1. Gingivitis and gingival index
2. Periodontal probing depth (PPD)
3. Gingival recession (GR)
4. Furcation involvement
5. Mobility
6. Periodontal/clinical attachment loss (PAL/CAL).

Periodontal probing depth, gingival recession, furcation involvement and mobility measure the extent of destruction of the periodontium, i.e. they assess the presence and severity of periodontitis.

It is essential to remember that PPD is not necessarily correlated with severity of attachment loss. Gingival hyperplasia may contribute to a deep pocket (or pseudo-pocket if there is no attachment loss), while gingival recession may result in the absence of a pocket but also minimal remaining attachment. PAL records the distance from the cemento-enamel junction (or from a fixed point on the tooth) to the base or apical extension of the pathological pocket. It is thus a more accurate assessment of tissue loss in periodontitis. PAL is either measured directly with a periodontal probe or it is calculated (e.g. PPD + gingival recession).

A detailed examination of the periodontal ligament space and interproximal alveolar margin requires the use of an intra-oral radiographic technique. The radiographic changes associated with periodontal disease include resorption of the alveolar margin, widening of the periodontal space, a break in the path or loss of the radiopacity of the lamina dura and destruction of alveolar bone, resulting in supra- or infra-bony pockets. Radiographs using a parallel technique will demonstrate more accurately the features of periodontitis because this technique provides a better view of the alveolar margin and reveals more accurately the actual extent or depth of the periodontal lesion in relation to the root of the tooth. Radiographs produced with a bisecting angle technique may appear to indicate greater destruction of the alveolar bone than is actually present, because the central ray is directed obliquely to the long axis of the teeth and jaw, which produces dimensional distortion. Moreover, with the bisecting angle technique, subgingival calculus may be superimposed on alveolar bone and would thus not be detected. The film taken using a parallel technique will demonstrate deposits of subgingival calculus and defects of the cementum, but may not cover a sufficient area to demonstrate extensive periodontitis lesions adequately. In the maxilla and anterior mandible, bisecting angle and parallel views of the same region may be required to visualize the extent of the tissue destruction more accurately.

> ### CLINICAL TIPS
>
> - Horizontal bone destruction is often accompanied by gingival recession and periodontal pockets may not form.
> - Try to differentiate inflammatory root resorption from idiopathic root resorption.
> - Therapy for established periodontitis is intended to prevent progression of disease.
> - Periodontal probing depth does not always correlate with loss of attachment.
> - Radiographs using a parallel technique will demonstrate periodontitis more accurately.
> - If home care is not tolerated, or certain teeth are not accessible to cleaning, further extractions may be required.
> - Extractions should be confirmed radiographically.

TREATMENT OPTIONS

1. Extraction of all teeth affected by periodontitis. In the absence of frequent (daily) plaque control, periodontitis will progress. The great majority of adult cats are not amenable to toothbrushing and extraction of all teeth showing evidence of loss of attachment is often the treatment of choice.
2. Extraction of teeth most severely affected and then home care to try to prevent further periodontal destruction. The owner was keen to maintain as many teeth as possible. Also, the cat was docile and friendly, and the owner was sure that she would allow toothbrushing.

TREATMENT PERFORMED

See the back page of the dental record (Fig. 7.9) for details of the treatment performed.
1. Periodontal therapy to remove plaque and calculus and provide a clean environment.
2. Open extraction of root remnants (204, distal root of 409). Successful extraction was confirmed radiographically.
3. Open extraction of 107, 309 and 408. Successful extraction was confirmed radiographically.

ORAL PROBLEM LIST

1. Generalized gingivitis
2. Moderate periodontitis 104, 108, 207, 208, 304, 404
3. Advanced periodontitis 309, 408, 107
4. Root remnants 204, 409 (distal root)
5. Traumatic occlusion 304 ⟶ Lip ulceration

PERIODONTICS

- ☐ Sonic scaling   ☑ Ultrasonic scaling
- ☐ Subgingival curettage   ☐ Periodontal debridement
- ☑ Pumice polishing   ☐ Air polishing
- ☐ Periodontal surgery

OTHER DENTAL PROCEDURES

1. Full-mouth radiographs (10 films)
2. Post-extraction radiographs (4 films)
3. Shortening and endodontic treatment and restoration of 304 (3 films)

THERAPEUTIC PLAN

1. Periodontal debridement and home care
2. Periodontal debridement and home care
3. Extract 309 and 408
4. Extract root remnants 204 and 409 (distal)
5. Shortening and endodontic treatment and restoration of 304

ORAL SURGERY (Note sites on graph - X)

- ☐ Closed extraction(s):
- ☑ Open extraction(s): 204 RR, 409 RR, 309, 408
- ☐ Incisional biopsy   ☐ Excisional biopsy
- ☑ Other comments   Flaps replaced with 5/0 Monocryl®

COMPLICATIONS/COMMENTS

1. Institute home care and
   Book for conscious recheck in 3 weeks to evaluate
2. Book for GA/radiographs of 304 in 6 months

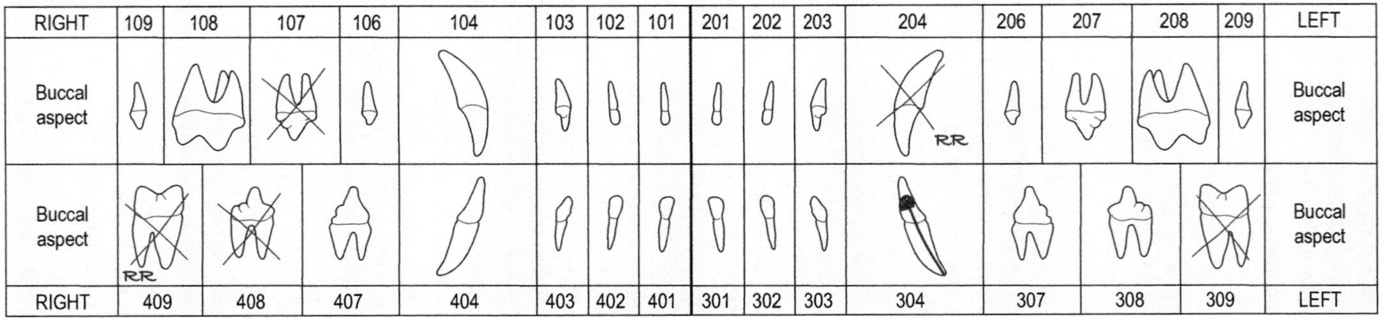

RIGHT	109	108	107	106	104	103	102	101	201	202	203	204	206	207	208	209	LEFT
Buccal aspect																	Buccal aspect
Buccal aspect																	Buccal aspect
RIGHT	409	408	407		404	403	402	401	301	302	303	304	307	308	309		LEFT

Figure 7.9 Dental record. Details of treatment are reported on the back page of the dental record.

4. Shortening and endodontic treatment and restoration of 304 to remove traumatic occlusion and thus allow the lip ulcer to heal.

POSTOPERATIVE CARE

- Daily chlorhexidine rinse for 3 weeks
- Booked for conscious examination in 3 weeks.

RECHECKS

At recheck 3 weeks later, the owner reported that there had been no problems in administering chlorhexidine. The extraction sites had all healed uneventfully. The owner was shown how to brush the teeth. They were given complementary toothbrush and paste and booked for check-up in 1 month.

At recheck 1 month later, the owner reported that she was brushing the cat's teeth daily. However, she found it difficult to access the posterior teeth in the upper jaw. The gingivae of all teeth except 108, 207 and 208 appeared clinically healthy. There was gingival inflammation at 108, 207 and 208. The owner was keen to persevere with the toothbrushing.

The cat was seen 6 months later for examination under anaesthesia and radiographic assessment of the endodontic therapy of 304. Examination showed clinically healthy gingivae of most teeth except 108, 207 and 208, which had moderate gingivitis and further gingival recession (i.e. periodontitis was progressing). Radiographs confirmed successful outcome of the endodontic therapy of 304. Further treatment consisted of open extraction of 108, 207 and 208. It was decided to put the cat on an annual recall, i.e. examination under general anaesthesia and radiographs once a year.

At recheck 1 year later, the cat had clinically healthy gingivae and no evidence of progression of periodontitis (gingival recession remained unchanged).

PROGNOSIS

This cat is allowing optimal home care, i.e. daily toothbrushing. She will still require professional treatment at regular intervals, which need to be decided based on efficacy of home care. Annual recall may be sufficient for this particular cat.

COMMENTS

In my experience, most adult cats are not amenable to toothbrushing. However, in situations where the owner is confident that they can do it I will give them the benefit of the doubt. If home care is successful, as in this case, then the prognosis is excellent. Sites that are affected by periodontitis will not regenerate, but the disease can be halted. If home care is not tolerated, or certain teeth are not accessible to cleaning, then further extractions are required.

8 Importance of periodontal probing depth (PPD)

INITIAL PRESENTATION

Recurrent gingivitis and halitosis.

PATIENT DETAILS

An 8-year-old, neutered female, golden retriever.

CASE HISTORY

There were no oral or dental problems until around 8 months ago, when severe gingivitis localized to the upper canine teeth was noted. Three episodes of professional periodontal therapy (scaling and polishing and extraction of 'some' teeth) under general anaesthesia had been performed in the last 6 months and the dog had received a short course of antibiotics following each dental cleaning. The gingivae had appeared healthy for approximately 3 weeks after each cleaning and antibiotic course, and then the gingival inflammation had flared up again.

The dog was referred to us for management of recurrent gingivitis affecting the upper canine teeth. The owner did not feel that the oral inflammation was affecting the general well-being of the dog (i.e. interested in walks and eating well), but he did not appreciate the halitosis.

ORAL EXAMINATION – CONSCIOUS

The dog was relatively amenable to quick conscious oral examination, which revealed the following:
1. Missing teeth (presumably extracted)
2. Generalized moderate gingivitis
3. More severe gingivitis around upper canines
4. Gingival recession of the buccal aspect of 104 and 204
5. Gingival draining tracts of the buccal aspect of 204
6. Halitosis.

ORAL EXAMINATION – UNDER GENERAL ANAESTHETIC

See the front page of the dental record (Fig. 8.1) for details of findings.

In summary, examination under general anaesthesia identified the following:
1. Missing teeth (101, 102, 110, 202, 205, 210, 311 and 411)
2. Generalized mild to moderate gingivitis (Fig. 8.2a, b)
3. Severe gingivitis at upper canines (Fig. 8.3a, b)
4. Gingival recession of the buccal (Fig. 8.3a, b) and palatal aspects of 104 and 204
5. Gingival draining tracts buccally of 204 (Figs 8.2b and 8.3b)
6. Gingival recession of the buccal and lingual aspects of 304 and 404
7. Gingival recession and furcation involvement (grade III) of 206 (Figs 8.2b and 8.3b)
8. Gingival recession buccally over the distal root of 109 (Fig. 8.4) and 209
9. Increased periodontal probing depth of 104, 204, 109, 209, 304 and 404 (see dental record for precise location)
10. Uncomplicated crown fracture of 208 (Fig. 8.2b).

FURTHER INVESTIGATIONS

Radiographs were taken of 104, 204, 206, 109 and 209 to assess the extent and severity of the periodontitis. A baseline radiograph of 208 (UCF) was also taken to assess pulp and periapical status.

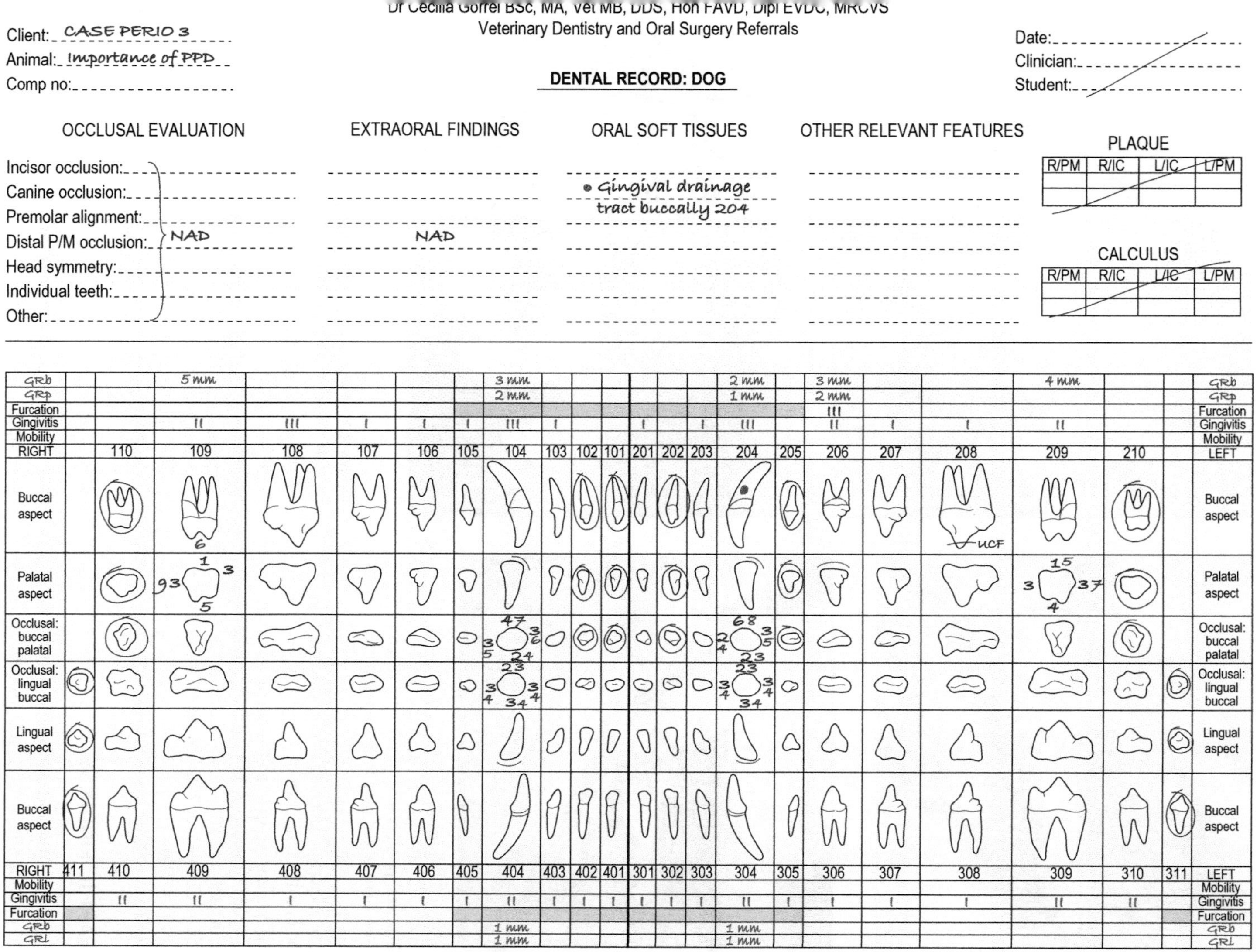

Dr Cecilia Gorrel BSc, MA, vet MB, DDS, Hon FAVD, Dipl EVDC, MRCVS
Veterinary Dentistry and Oral Surgery Referrals

DENTAL RECORD: DOG

Client: _CASE PERIO 3_
Animal: _Importance of PPD_
Comp no: _____

Date: _____
Clinician: _____
Student: _____

OCCLUSAL EVALUATION

Incisor occlusion: _____
Canine occlusion: _____
Premolar alignment: _____
Distal P/M occlusion: _NAD_
Head symmetry: _____
Individual teeth: _____
Other: _____

EXTRAORAL FINDINGS

NAD

ORAL SOFT TISSUES

• _Gingival drainage_
  tract buccally 204

OTHER RELEVANT FEATURES

PLAQUE

	R/PM	R/IC	L/IC	L/PM

CALCULUS

	R/PM	R/IC	L/IC	L/PM

Figure 8.1 Dental record. All clinical findings are reported on the front page of the dental record. Remember that periodontitis is a site-specific disease. PPD is recorded on the occlusal view of the tooth on the dental record so that you can easily identify the precise site of disease. Normal periodontal probing depth (PPD) is not noted on the dental record to avoid clutter. However, when gingival recession is present, then PPDs are always recorded, so that periodontal attachment loss (PAL) can be calculated (GR + PPD) and entered on the record at its precise site in green ink. PAL is a more accurate assessment of attachment loss.

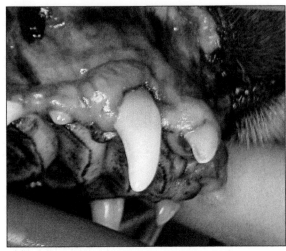

(a)

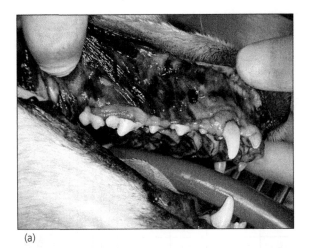

(a)

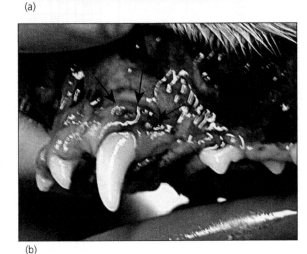

(b)

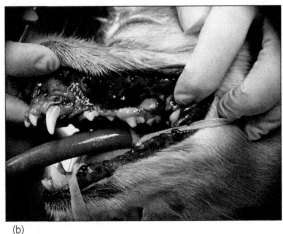

(b)

Figure 8.2 Lateral photographs of the right (a) and left (b) upper jaw. Generalized mild to moderate gingivitis is evident.

(a) Note the gingival recession on the buccal aspect of 104 and over the distal root of 109.

(b) Note the gingival recession on the buccal aspect of 204 and 206. The gingival draining tracts located to the buccal aspect of 204 are obvious, as is the furcation involvement at 206. The crown fracture of 208 is also obvious.

Figure 8.3 Lateral photographs centred on the right (a) and left (b) upper canine teeth.

(a) The gingiva of 104 is inflamed and there is a buccal gingival recession.

(b) The gingivae of 204 and 206 are inflamed and the gingival margin has receded apically. Three gingival drainage tracts are evident in the buccal gingiva of 204. The furcation of 206 is clearly involved in the disease process.

RADIOGRAPHIC FINDINGS

The radiographs of 104 and 204 confirmed the clinical diagnosis of periodontitis. There was resorption of the alveolar margin and widening of the periodontal space. The radiograph of 104 showed extensive bone loss extending beyond the apex (Fig. 8.5).

The radiograph of 206 showed horizontal bone loss and obvious furcation involvement (Fig. 8.6),

again confirming the clinical diagnosis of advanced periodontitis.

The radiographs of 109 (Fig. 8.7a) and 209 (Fig. 8.7b) demonstrated marked periapical destruction at the palatal root.

The radiograph of 208 (UCF) showed no evidence of pulp or periapical pathology.

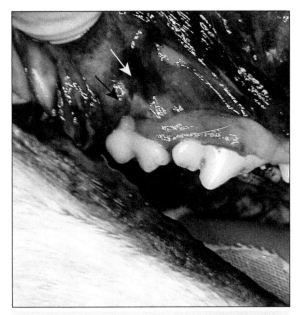

Figure 8.4 Lateral photograph of the right caudal maxilla. The gingiva has receded to expose most of the buccal aspect of the distal root of 108. Note the location of the zygomatic and parotid papillae.

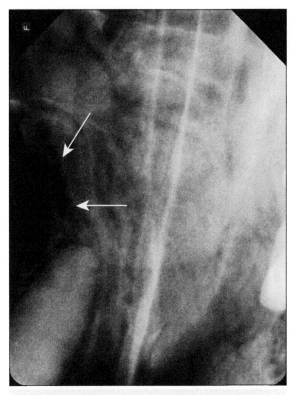

Figure 8.5 Radiograph of 104. Note the extensive bone loss on the buccal aspect that extends beyond the apex.

ORAL PROBLEM LIST

1. Generalized gingivitis
2. Periodontitis in 104, 204, 206, 109, 209, 304 and 404
3. Lateral periodontal abscess in 204
4. Class II (periodontic–endodontic) lesions of 109 and 209.

THEORY REFRESHER

In gingivitis, the plaque-induced inflammation is limited to the soft tissue of the gingiva. Sulcus depths are normal (i.e. periodontal probing depths are 1–3 mm in the dog and 0.5–1 mm in the cat). As periodontitis occurs, the inflammatory destruction of the coronal part of the periodontal ligament allows apical migration of the epithelial attachment and the formation of a pathological periodontal pocket (i.e. periodontal probing depths increase). If the inflammatory disease is permitted to progress, the crestal portion of the alveolar process begins to resorb. The extent and type of alveolar bone destruction are diagnosed radiographically. The resorption may proceed apically on a horizontal level. Horizontal bone destruction is often accompanied by gingival recession, so

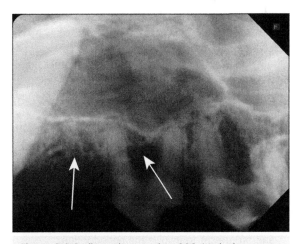

Figure 8.6 Radiograph centred on 206. Marked horizontal bone loss and furcation involvement of 206 is evident.

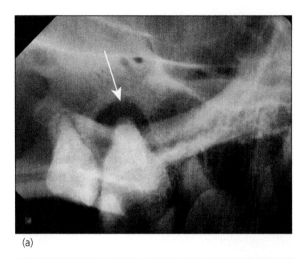
(a)

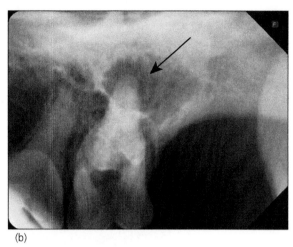
(b)

Figure 8.7 Radiographs centred on 109 (a) and 209 (b). Note the periapical bone destruction (of periodontal origin) around the palatal root of both teeth.

periodontal pockets may not form. If there is no gingival recession, the periodontal pocket is supra-alveolar, i.e. above the level of the alveolar margin. The pattern of bone destruction may also proceed in a vertical direction along the root to form angular bony defects. The periodontal pocket is now intra- or subalveolar, i.e. below the level of the crestal bone.

There are possible pathways of communication between the pulp and the periodontium: via denuded dentine tubules, via lateral and/or accessory pulp canals, and at the apical foramen. Consequently, a periapical lesion may have a periodontal origin and a periodontal-type lesion may originate from the pulp. Another possibility is that a lesion is the result of a combination of endodontic and periodontal pathology. In this case, the periapical lesions are the consequence of spread of the periodontal infection to involve the pulp tissue, with the development of secondary endodontic disease as a complication.

The lesions are classified according to aetiology as follows:

- A Class I lesion, or endodontic–periodontic lesion, is endodontic in origin, i.e. pathology begins in the pulp and progresses to involve the periodontium.
- A Class II lesion, or periodontic–endodontic lesion, is periodontic in origin, i.e. pathology begins in the periodontium and progresses to involve the pulp.
- A Class III lesion, or true combined lesion, is a fusion of independent periodontic and endodontic lesions.

The prognosis for long-term retention of the tooth is based on the above classification. Class I lesions have a better prognosis, as endodontic treatment may lead to resolution of the periodontal extension of the inflammation. In contrast, Class II and III lesions require endodontic treatment as well as extensive periodontal therapy, and the periodontal destruction is often too extensive to be amenable to treatment, with extraction of the tooth usually being required.

A periodontal abscess is an acute exacerbation of the process occurring in a chronic periodontal pocket. It usually occurs from partial or complete obstruction of the orifice of the pocket. The acute periodontal abscess may produce rapid and extensive bone loss. In some instances, the bone loss will extend beyond the apices of the roots of the teeth.

Diagnosis of periodontal disease relies on clinical examination of the periodontium in the anaesthetized animal. In addition, radiography is mandatory if there is evidence of periodontitis on clinical examination. It is essential to differentiate between gingivitis and periodontitis in order to institute appropriate treatment. In individuals with gingivitis, the aim is to restore the tissues to clinical health; in individuals with established periodontitis, the aim of therapy is to prevent progression of disease.

The following parameters need to be assessed and recorded for *each tooth* in *all patients*:

1. Gingivitis and gingival index
2. Periodontal probing depth (PPD)

3. Gingival recession (GR)
4. Furcation involvement
5. Mobility
6. Periodontal/clinical attachment loss (PAL/CAL).

Periodontal probing depth, gingival recession, furcation involvement and mobility measure the extent of destruction of the periodontium, i.e. they assess the presence and severity of periodontitis.

It is essential to remember that PPD is not necessarily correlated with severity of attachment loss. Gingival hyperplasia may contribute to a deep pocket (or pseudo-pocket if there is no attachment loss), while gingival recession may result in the absence of a pocket but also minimal remaining attachment. PAL records the distance from the cemento-enamel junction (or from a fixed point on the tooth) to the base or apical extension of the pathological pocket. It is thus a more accurate assessment of tissue loss in periodontitis. PAL is either measured directly with a periodontal probe or it is calculated (e.g. PPD + gingival recession).

As already mentioned, radiography to assess the type and extent of alveolar bone destruction is mandatory for periodontitis patients. The radiographic changes associated with periodontal disease include resorption of the alveolar margin, widening of the periodontal space, a break in the path or loss of the radiopacity of the lamina dura, and destruction of alveolar bone resulting in supra- or infra-bony pockets.

TREATMENT OPTIONS

Extraction of 104, 204, 206, 109 and 209 is the only treatment option. This needs to be followed by daily home care to prevent progression of periodontitis (304 and 404) and development of new lesions at other sites.

TREATMENT PERFORMED

The dog received the following treatment (see back page of the dental record depicted in Fig. 8.8):
1. Periodontal therapy to remove plaque and calculus and provide a clean environment.
2. Open extraction of 104, 204, 206, 109 and 209. Successful extraction was confirmed radiographically before replacing the flaps (Fig. 8.9a, b). Figures 8.10, 8.11, 8.12, 8.13 and 8.14 show the full extent of periodontitis of these teeth.

POSTOPERATIVE CARE

- Daily chlorhexidine rinse for 1 week
- Start daily toothbrushing
- Booked for conscious examination in 1 month.

RECHECK

At recheck 1 month later, the owner reported that he was brushing the dog's teeth almost daily and that they both enjoyed the interaction. He also reported that she was much brighter and more playful than before the extractions.

All extraction sites were healed and there was no halitosis. Plaque disclosing solution revealed virtually no plaque (the owner had brushed the teeth an hour before the appointment). The gingivae were clinically healthy.

A recall in 3 months' time was advised (examination under anaesthesia) to assess efficacy of home care and recheck radiographs of 208 to assess pulp and periapical status.

PROGNOSIS

The dog is allowing optimal home care, i.e. daily toothbrushing. It is also being fed a dental diet and given dental hygiene chews. The dog will still require professional treatment at regular intervals, which need to be decided based on efficacy of home care. As long as

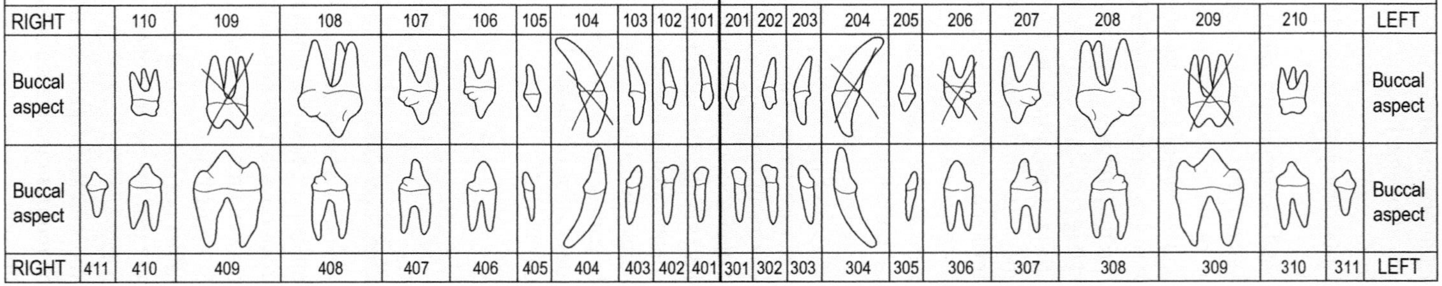

ORAL PROBLEM LIST
1. Generalized gingivitis
2. Periodontitis 104, 204, 206, 109, 209, 304 and 404
3. Lateral periodontal abscess 204
4. Class II (perio-endo) lesions 109 and 209
5. UCF 208

PERIODONTICS
- [ ] Sonic scaling
- [x] Subgingival curettage
- [x] Pumice polishing
- [ ] Periodontal surgery
- [x] Ultrasonic scaling
- [ ] Periodontal debridement
- [ ] Air polishing

OTHER DENTAL PROCEDURES
Radiographs of 104, 206, 109 and 209 (5 films)

Radiograph of 208 (2 films)

Post-extraction radiographs (5 films)

THERAPEUTIC PLAN
1. Periodontal therapy and homecare
2. Extract 104, 204, 206, 109 and 209
3. Extract 204
4. Extract 109 and 209 and periodontal therapy and homecare for 304 and 404
5. Radiograph

ORAL SURGERY (Note sites on graph - X)
- [ ] Closed extraction(s):
- [x] Open extraction(s): 104, 109, 204, 206, 209
- [ ] Incisional biopsy
- [ ] Other/comments
- [ ] Excisional biopsy

Flaps closed with 5/0 Monocryl

COMPLICATIONS/COMMENTS
Home with chlorhex rinse. Give toothbrushing instruction at discharge.
Advise immediate start with brushing.
Rebook for conscious exam in one month.

UCF 28 = NAD on rad → monitor/recall 3 months

RIGHT	110	109	108	107	106	105	104	103	102	101	201	202	203	204	205	206	207	208	209	210	211	LEFT
Buccal aspect																						Buccal aspect

Buccal aspect																						Buccal aspect
RIGHT	410	409	408	407	406	405	404	403	402	401	301	302	303	304	305	306	307	308	309	310	311	LEFT

Figure 8.8 Dental record. Details of treatment are reported on the back page of the dental record.

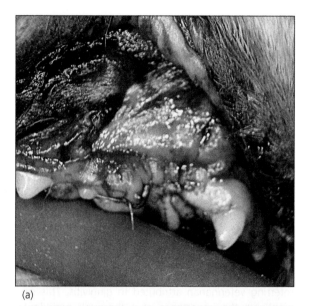

(a)

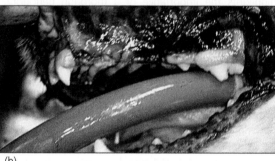

(b)

Figure 8.9 Lateral photographs of extraction sites of 104 (a), and 204 and 206 (b). Successful extraction was confirmed radiographically before closing. The buccal flap was sutured to the palatal gingiva (a simple interrupted suture pattern) using 5/0 Monocryl. The closure was without tension.

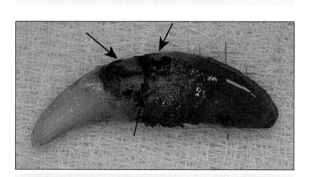

Figure 8.10 Photograph of extracted 104. Note the extensive loss of periodontal ligament and accumulation of subgingival calculus at the mesiopalatal aspect of the tooth.

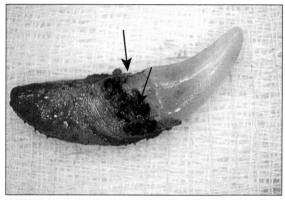

Figure 8.11 Photograph of extracted 204. Note the extensive loss of periodontal ligament and accumulation of subgingival calculus at the mesiopalatal aspect of the tooth.

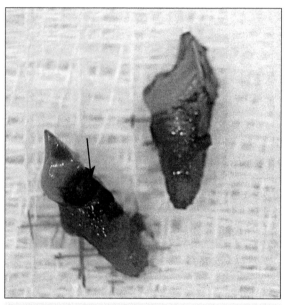

Figure 8.12 Photograph of extracted 106. The tooth was sectioned into two single-rooted units prior to extraction. Note the loss of attachment and accumulation of subgingival calculus at the furcation.

effective home care is maintained, the prognosis for this dog is excellent!

COMMENTS

Uncomplicated gingivitis is generally not associated with discomfort or pain in humans. In fact, it is an insidious

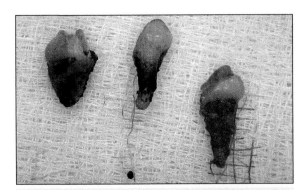

Figure 8.13 Photograph of extracted 109. The tooth was sectioned into three single-rooted units prior to extraction. The distal and palatal roots have lost virtually all their support and are covered with calculus. In contrast, the mesial root has lost very little attachment and is covered by healthy periodontal ligament. Remember, periodontitis is a site-specific disease!

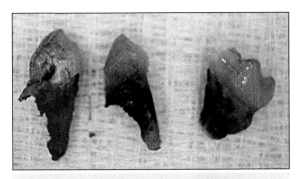

Figure 8.14 Photograph of extracted 209. The tooth was sectioned into three single-rooted units prior to extraction. The distal and palatal roots have lost virtually all their support and are covered with calculus. In contrast, the mesial root has lost very little attachment and is covered by healthy periodontal ligament. Remember, periodontitis is a site-specific disease!

process and the patient may be unaware of its existence. The significance of gingivitis is that, if untreated, periodontitis may develop.

Based on feedback from human patients, uncomplicated periodontitis is also not associated with severe pain or discomfort. In contrast, complications such as the development of a lateral periodontal abscess or ulcers in the mucous membranes are very painful.

At initial examination, the owner did not feel that the oral condition was causing any discomfort or pain. However, at check-up 1 month after extraction of the teeth he remarked on how much brighter and more playful the dog was. In fact, he described her as 'being like a puppy again'. In my experience, it is often not until an oral condition has been treated that the owner notices a difference in behaviour.

The owner was concerned about halitosis, which the referring veterinarian attributed to gingivitis. This case highlights the importance of a thorough periodontal examination to diagnose periodontal disease. Periodontal probing at several sites around each tooth is essential. In this case, periodontal probing was not performed by the referring veterinarian and the cause of the halitosis was thus misdiagnosed as gingivitis of two teeth (104 and 204), when it was in fact advanced periodontitis of five teeth (104, 204, 206, 109 and 209) and moderate periodontitis of two teeth (304 and 404). Once periodontitis has been diagnosed, radiographs are mandatory. In this case, radiographs revealed periodontic–endodontic lesions (109 and 209) that were not detectable on clinical periodontal examination.

It is essential to differentiate between gingivitis and periodontitis in order to institute appropriate treatment. Supragingival scaling and antibiotics do not address the inflammation below the gingival margin and will have no effect on periodontitis.

9 Systemic effects of periodontitis

INITIAL PRESENTATION

Ten-month history of a progressively worsening cough.

PATIENT DETAILS

A 12-year-old, neutered male, Yorkshire terrier.

CASE HISTORY

The dog was being treated for septic pneumonia, with consolidation of the left cranial lung lobe likely to be secondary to his periodontal disease. He also had tracheitis and collapsing trachea. He was referred to us to manage the periodontal disease. No history of any previous oral or dental disease or treatment was available to us.

ORAL EXAMINATION – CONSCIOUS

The dog was amenable to conscious facial and oral examination, which revealed the following:
1. Missing teeth (presumably extracted, but some may have been congenitally absent); no teeth at all in the upper jaw, with lower incisors, canines and some premolars missing.
2. Oronasal communication at sites of 104, 108 and 204.
3. Severe accumulation of dental deposits in lower premolars and molars (suspect advanced periodontitis).
4. Marked rostral bone loss of both upper and lower jaw.
5. Separation of mandibular symphysis; the right and left mandibles were freely movable.

In addition, there was moderate ocular discharge, a right-sided nasal discharge and right mandibular lymph node enlargement.

ORAL EXAMINATION – UNDER GENERAL ANAESTHESIA

See the front page of the dental record (Fig. 9.1) for details of findings.

In summary, examination under general anaesthesia identified the following:
1. Missing teeth (all teeth in the upper jaw, all lower incisors, canines, 306, 310, 311, 405, 406, 410).
2. Advanced periodontitis in 305, 307, 308, 309, 407, 408, 409 and 411. The loss of attachment was manifested clinically as gingival recession and furcation exposure.
3. Marked bone loss in the rostral lower jaw with symphyseal separation; the right and left mandibles were freely movable (Fig. 9.2).
4. Oronasal communication at sites of 104, 108 (Fig. 9.3) and 204. Root remnants are present in oronasal communication at the site of 108.

FURTHER INVESTIGATIONS

1. A series of full-mouth radiographs (14 films) was taken.
2. In lieu of the extreme rostral bone loss in both the upper and lower jaw, a biopsy (gingiva, underlying connective tissue and bone) was harvested from the rostral mandible and sent for histopathological examination.

RADIOGRAPHIC FINDINGS

The radiographs showed the following:
1. Severe loss of alveolar bone in the rostral upper (Fig. 9.4) and lower jaw (Fig. 9.5)

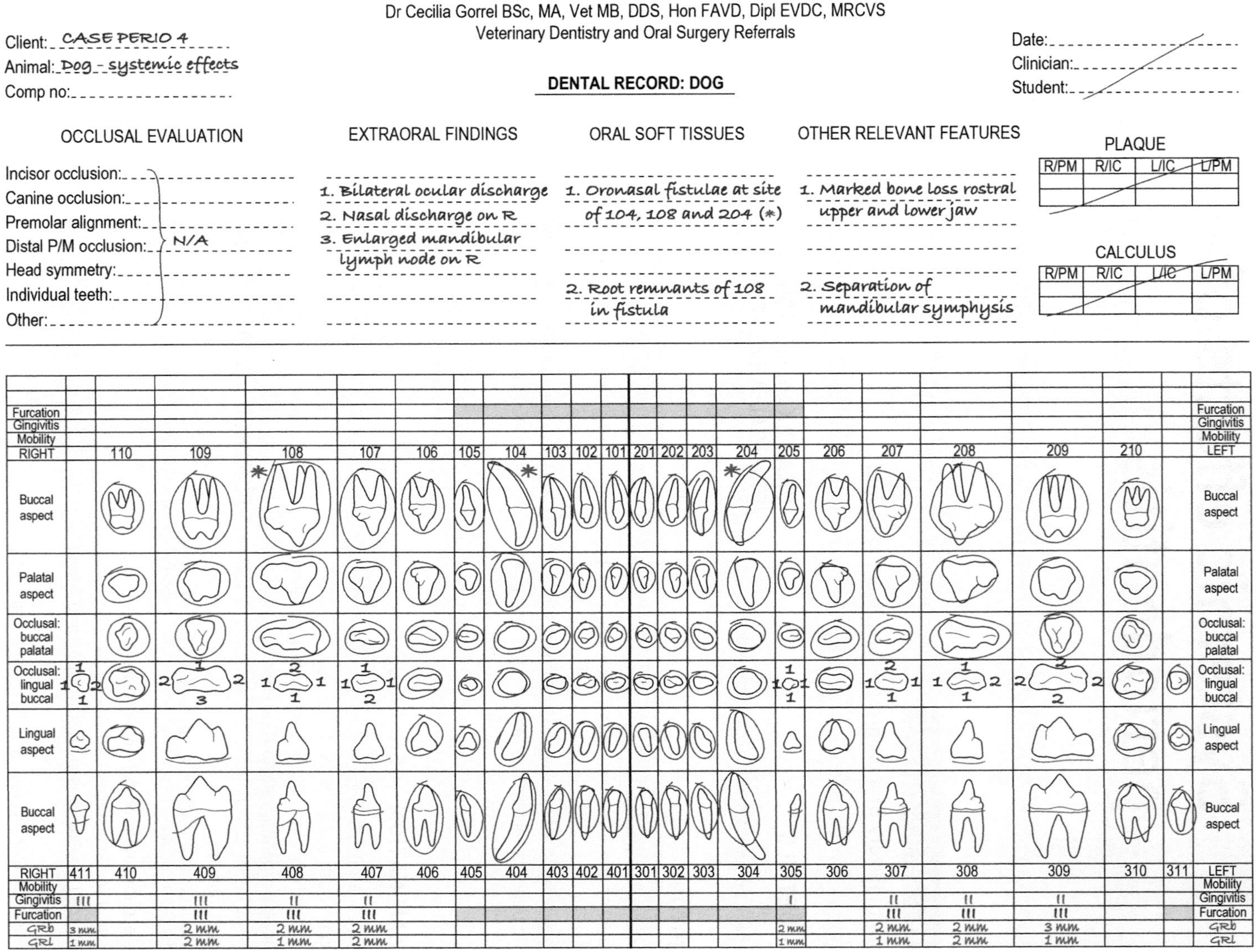
Dr Cecilia Gorrel BSc, MA, Vet MB, DDS, Hon FAVD, Dipl EVDC, MRCVS
Veterinary Dentistry and Oral Surgery Referrals
Client: CASE PERIO 4
Animal: Dog - systemic effects
Comp no:
DENTAL RECORD: DOG
Date:
Clinician:
Student:
OCCLUSAL EVALUATION
Incisor occlusion:
Canine occlusion:
Premolar alignment:
Distal P/M occlusion:
Head symmetry:
Individual teeth:
Other:
N/A
EXTRAORAL FINDINGS
1. Bilateral ocular discharge
2. Nasal discharge on R
3. Enlarged mandibular lymph node on R
ORAL SOFT TISSUES
1. Oronasal fistulae at site of 104, 108 and 204 (*)
2. Root remnants of 108 in fistula
OTHER RELEVANT FEATURES
1. Marked bone loss rostral upper and lower jaw
2. Separation of mandibular symphysis
PLAQUE
R/PM R/IC L/IC L/PM
CALCULUS
R/PM R/IC L/IC L/PM
Furcation
Gingivitis
Mobility
RIGHT 110 109 108 107 106 105 104 103 102 101 201 202 203 204 205 206 207 208 209 210 LEFT
Buccal aspect
Palatal aspect
Occlusal: buccal palatal
Occlusal: lingual buccal
Lingual aspect
Buccal aspect
RIGHT 411 410 409 408 407 406 405 404 403 402 401 301 302 303 304 305 306 307 308 309 310 311 LEFT
Mobility
Gingivitis
Furcation
GRb
GRl
2 mm
1 mm
3 mm

Figure 9.1 Dental record. All clinical findings are reported on the front page of the dental record. Normal periodontal probing depth (PPD) is not noted on the dental record to avoid clutter. However, when gingival recession is present, then PPDs are always recorded. True attachment loss is the sum of the recession and probing depth. Remember that periodontitis is a site-specific disease. PPD is recorded on the occlusal view of the tooth on the dental record so that you can easily identify the precise site of the disease.

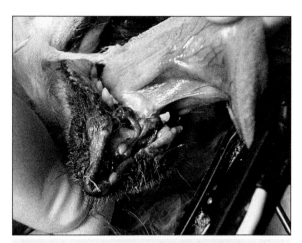

Figure 9.2 Extensive alveolar bone loss. The lower incisor and canine teeth were absent and there had been extensive bone loss. In fact, the bone loss had resulted in destruction and separation of the mandibular symphysis, and the left and right mandibles were freely movable.

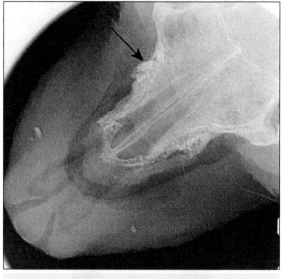

Figure 9.4 Radiograph of the upper jaw. The only remaining tooth is a root remnant of 108. Note the atrophy of the alveolar bone as a result of tooth loss.

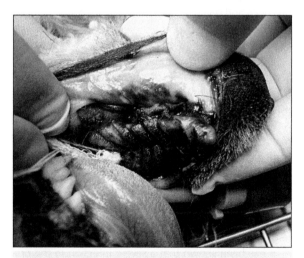

Figure 9.3 Occlusal photograph showing the oronasal communication (as a result of the severe periodontitis) at the sites of 104 and 108.

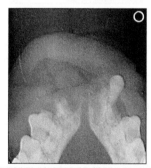

Figure 9.5 Radiograph of the rostral lower jaw. The alveolar bone associated with incisors and canines has been resorbed. The mandibular symphysis is virtually destroyed by the inflammatory process. Tooth 305 has lost most of its supportive bone.

2. Root remnant of 108 (Fig. 9.4)
3. Advanced periodontitis in 305, 307, 308, 309, 407, 408, 409 and 411 (Figs 9.6 and 9.7).

ORAL PROBLEM LIST

1. Oronasal communication at 104, 108 (with retained root remnants in fistula) and 204

2. Periodontitis in 305, 307, 308, 309, 407, 408, 409 and 411
3. Mandibular symphyseal separation.

THEORY REFRESHER

Periodontal disease is a collective term for a number of plaque-induced inflammatory lesions that affect the periodontium.

In gingivitis, the plaque-induced inflammation is limited to the soft tissue of the gingiva. Sulcus depths

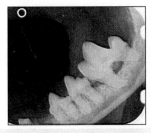

Figure 9.6 Radiograph of the left mandible. Advanced periodontitis is manifested by horizontal bone loss and furcation exposure of the remaining teeth. Note the thin cortical plate at the ventral border of the mandible.

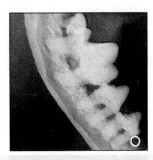

Figure 9.7 Radiograph of the right mandible. Advanced periodontitis is manifested by horizontal bone loss and furcation exposure of the remaining teeth. Note the thin cortical plate at the ventral border of the mandible.

are normal (i.e. periodontal probing depths are 1–3 mm in the dog and 0.5–1 mm in the cat). As periodontitis occurs, the inflammatory destruction of the coronal part of the periodontal ligament allows apical migration of the epithelial attachment and the formation of a pathological periodontal pocket (i.e. periodontal probing depths increase). If the inflammatory disease is permitted to progress, the crestal portion of the alveolar process begins to resorb. The type and extent of alveolar bone destruction are diagnosed radiographically. The resorption may proceed apically on a horizontal level. Horizontal bone destruction is often accompanied by gingival recession, so periodontal pockets may not form. If there is no gingival recession the periodontal pocket is supra-alveolar, i.e. above the level of the alveolar margin. The pattern of bone destruction may also proceed in a vertical direction along the root to form angular bony defects. The periodontal pocket is now intra- or subalveolar, i.e. below the level of the crestal bone. The end result of periodontitis is loss of the tooth. The crestal portion of the alveolar bone will undergo atrophy once the tooth is lost.

Diagnosis of periodontal disease relies on clinical examination of the periodontium in the anaesthetized animal. Radiographs are mandatory if there is evidence of periodontitis on clinical examination. It is essential to differentiate between gingivitis and periodontitis in order to institute appropriate treatment. In individuals with gingivitis, the aim is to restore the tissues to clinical health; in individuals with established periodontitis, the aim of therapy is to prevent progression of disease.

The following parameters need to be assessed and recorded for *each tooth* in *all patients*:
1. Gingivitis and gingival index
2. Periodontal probing depth (PPD)
3. Gingival recession (GR)
4. Furcation involvement
5. Mobility
6. Periodontal/clinical attachment loss (PAL/CAL).

Periodontal probing depth, gingival recession, furcation involvement and mobility measure the extent of destruction of the periodontium, i.e. they assess the presence and severity of periodontitis. Radiographs must be taken of any tooth showing clinical signs of periodontitis.

It is essential to remember that PPD is not necessarily correlated with severity of attachment loss. Gingival hyperplasia may contribute to a deep pocket (or pseudo-pocket if there is no attachment loss), while gingival recession may result in the absence of a pocket but also minimal remaining attachment. PAL records the distance from the cemento-enamel junction (or from a fixed point on the tooth) to the base or apical extension of the pathological pocket. It is thus a more accurate assessment of tissue loss in periodontitis. PAL is either measured directly with a periodontal probe or it is calculated (e.g. PPD + gingival recession).

It has been shown that a severe infection in the oral cavity, such as extensive periodontitis, will lead to a transient bacteraemia on chewing. In fact, an association has been demonstrated between periodontal disease and histopathological changes in the kidney, myocardium and liver. The association between severe periodontal disease and respiratory disease is accepted in human dentistry. While it cannot be proven that the tracheitis, collapsing trachea, septic bronchopneumonia and consolidated left lung lobe diagnosed in this dog were directly caused by the periodontitis, at the very least the presence of communication between the oral cavity and nasal passages would complicate resolution of the respiratory disease. It was deemed essential to

ORAL PROBLEM LIST

1. Oronasal communication at extraction sites of 104, 108, 204.
2. Advanced periodontitis 305, 307, 308, 309, 407, 408, 409, 411.
3. Root remnants 108.
4. Mandibular symphyseal separation.

PERIODONTICS

☐ Sonic scaling ☑ Ultrasonic scaling
☐ Subgingival curettage ☐ Periodontal debridement
☐ Pumice polishing ☐ Air polishing
☐ Periodontal surgery

OTHER DENTAL PROCEDURES

Full-mouth radiographs (14 films)

Post-extraction radiographs (3 films)

THERAPEUTIC PLAN

→ 1. Single layer repair
→ 2. Open extraction
→ 3. Open extraction
→ 4. No treatment required

ORAL SURGERY (Note sites on graph - X)
☐ Closed extraction(s):
☑ Open extraction(s): 305, 307, 308, 309, 407, 408, 409, 411, 108 RR
☐ Incisional biopsy ☑ Excisional biopsy
☑ Other/comments

1. Debride and single layer closure of oronasal fistulae at 104, 108 and 204. 5/0 Monocryl closure.
2. Biopsy (gingiva, connective tissue, bone) rostral mandible. 5/0 Monocryl closure.

COMPLICATIONS/COMMENTS

Home with soft food and analgesics. Continue treatment for respiratory disease. Daily chlorhexidine oral rinse.
Recheck in 3 weeks.

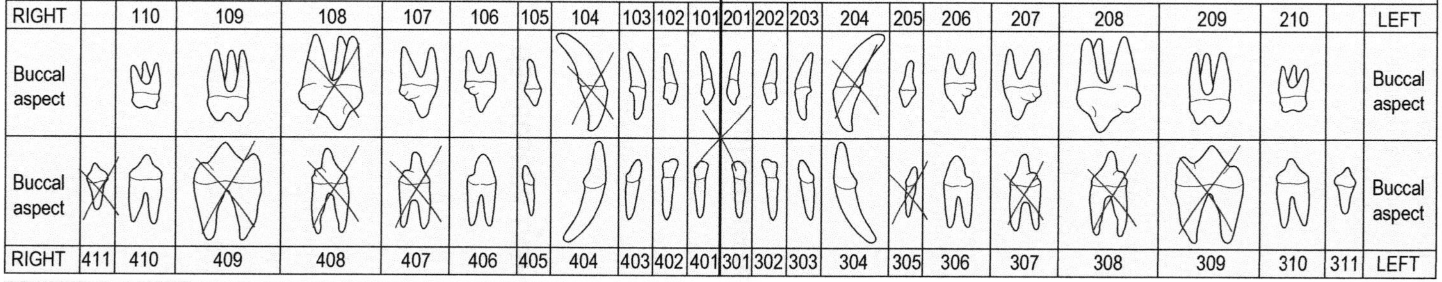

RIGHT	110	109	108	107	106	105	104	103	102	101	201	202	203	204	205	206	207	208	209	210	LEFT
Buccal aspect																					Buccal aspect
Buccal aspect																					Buccal aspect
RIGHT	410	409	408	407	406	405	404	403	402	401	301	302	303	304	305	306	307	308	309	310	311	LEFT

Figure 9.8 Dental record. Details of treatment are reported on the back page of the dental record.

repair the oronasal communications and remove the focus of infection (periodontitis) for there to be any chance of resolution of the respiratory problems.

TREATMENT OPTIONS

Repair of oronasal communications and extraction of all remaining teeth is the required treatment for this dog. The mandibular symphyseal separation is causing no discomfort and requires no treatment.

TREATMENT PERFORMED

See also the dental record (Fig. 9.8) for details of the treatment performed.

1. Open extraction of all remaining teeth. Successful extraction was confirmed radiographically (Figs 9.9 and 9.10).
2. Open extraction of root remnants of 108. Successful extraction was confirmed radiographically.
3. Repair of oronasal communications at sites of 104, 108 and 204. Single-layer repair was used (Fig. 9.11).

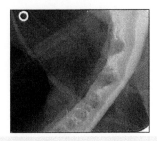

Figure 9.9 Radiograph of the left mandible. The post-extraction radiograph confirms successful extraction of all teeth.

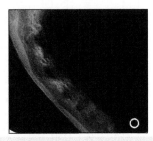

Figure 9.10 Radiograph of the right mandible. The post-extraction radiograph confirms successful extraction of all teeth.

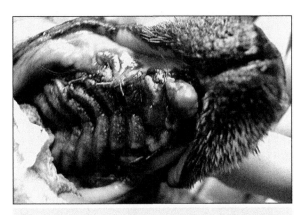

Figure 9.11 Oronasal fistulae repair. Occlusal photograph demonstrating the single-layer oronasal communication repair utilized. The flaps were closed with 5/0 Monocryl.

RECHECK

At recheck 3 weeks later, the oronasal communication repair and extraction sites were healing nicely. The histopathology report on the biopsy from the rostral mandible was compatible with periodontitis, i.e. bone with reactive features and no evidence of neoplasia. The dog was coughing less and seemed brighter. He was eating well and had gained some weight. He was still on antibiotics and steroids for the respiratory disease.

The dog was rebooked for conscious exam 1 month later. At this time, all surgical sites were fully healed. The dog was bright and alert, and while he still coughed, it was mainly on excitement. The referring veterinarian reported that the septic bronchopneumonia was resolved.

PROGNOSIS

There should be no further problems in the oral cavity (edentulous and no oronasal communications). He will always require soft food. The mandibular symphyseal separation is not causing any discomfort or worsening of remaining function and thus requires no intervention.

The septic bronchopneumonia was resolved, but the dog is likely to still have signs associated with the collapsing trachea and consolidated lung lobe.

COMMENTS

Periodontitis can result in dramatic bone loss. In this dog, the anterior portion of both the upper and lower jaw had been lost. It was one of the most dramatic cases of bone loss due to periodontitis that I have ever seen! Consequently, I took the biopsy for histopathological examination, which is not routine for periodontitis.

Early detection (periodontal probing and radiographs) and treatment of the periodontal disease (periodontal therapy and extraction) would have prevented the severe bone loss and establishment of oronasal communications, and may well have prevented the development of the severe respiratory disease.

10 Iatrogenic injuries

Mandibular fracture.

PATIENT DETAILS

A 10-year-old, neutered male, shih-tzu.

CASE HISTORY

The dog was referred to us for management of an iatrogenic jaw fracture that had occurred the previous day during extraction of the left lower canine tooth. The referring veterinarian also indicated that he may have left a few root remnants from other extractions.

The dog had been discharged with analgesics overnight. He was extremely uncomfortable and the owners were most distressed. They had not been aware that there could be any complications associated with what they thought was a 'simple dental cleaning and possibly a few teeth pulled'. The dog had received periodontal therapy and extraction (in fact, only a few teeth were remaining) several times during its life, with no complications. The dog had been discharged by one of the nurses and not by the veterinarian; in fact, the referring veterinarian had apparently refused to speak to the owners. In short, an unpleasant miscommunication had occurred.

ORAL EXAMINATION – CONSCIOUS

The dog was too uncomfortable for conscious oral examination to even be attempted.

ORAL EXAMINATION – UNDER GENERAL ANAESTHETIC

See the front page of the dental record (Fig. 10.1) for details of findings.

In summary, examination under general anaesthesia identified the following:
1. Fracture of the left mandible level with the apex of extracted 304.
2. Advanced periodontitis of 404 (gingival recession, increased PPD) and 409 (gingival recession, increased PPD, grade III furcation). Teeth 404 and 409 were the only ones remaining.
3. Extraction sockets (from surgery the day before) filled with coagulum (Fig. 10.2).
4. The mesial root of 309 still in the socket.
5. Lacerations of oral soft tissues, especially the ventral tongue (Fig. 10.2).

FURTHER INVESTIGATIONS

Radiographs were taken of the right and left mandible. The upper jaw contained no teeth and the bone was covered by healthy mucosa, so radiographs were not indicated.

RADIOGRAPHIC FINDINGS

Eight films were required to visualize the left and right mandible.

The radiographs showed the following:
1. A fractured left mandible, with the fracture lines extending from the apical region of the extracted 304 to the ventral border of the mandible (Fig. 10.3).
2. A crown remnant of 305 (Fig. 10.3).
3. Partial extraction of 309; the mesial root was still in place in the socket (Fig. 10.4).
4. Partial extraction of 408; there were both mesial and distal root remnants (Fig. 10.5a, b).

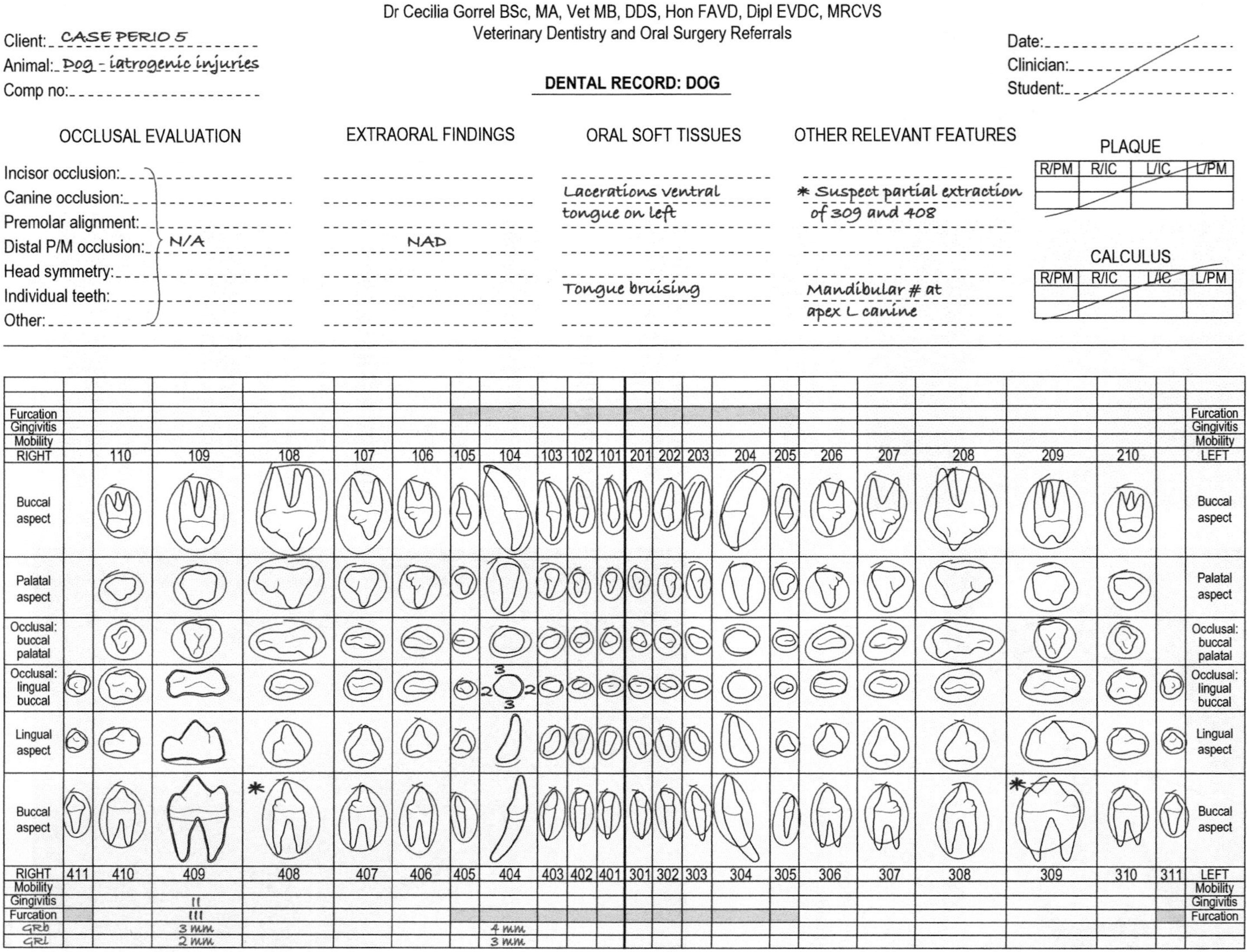
Dr Cecilia Gorrel BSc, MA, Vet MB, DDS, Hon FAVD, Dipl EVDC, MRCVS
Veterinary Dentistry and Oral Surgery Referrals
DENTAL RECORD: DOG
Client: CASE PERIO 5
Animal: Dog - iatrogenic injuries
Comp no:
Date:
Clinician:
Student:
OCCLUSAL EVALUATION
Incisor occlusion:
Canine occlusion:
Premolar alignment:
Distal P/M occlusion:
Head symmetry:
Individual teeth:
Other:
N/A
EXTRAORAL FINDINGS
NAD
ORAL SOFT TISSUES
Lacerations ventral tongue on left
Tongue bruising
OTHER RELEVANT FEATURES
* Suspect partial extraction of 309 and 408
Mandibular # at apex L canine
PLAQUE
R/PM R/IC L/IC L/PM
CALCULUS
R/PM R/IC L/IC L/PM
Furcation
Gingivitis
Mobility
RIGHT
110 109 108 107 106 105 104 103 102 101 201 202 203 204 205 206 207 208 209 210
LEFT
Buccal aspect
Palatal aspect
Occlusal: buccal palatal
Occlusal: lingual buccal
Lingual aspect
Buccal aspect
411 410 409 408 407 406 405 404 403 402 401 301 302 303 304 305 306 307 308 309 310 311
Mobility
Gingivitis
Furcation
GRb
GRl
II
III
3 mm
2 mm
4 mm
3 mm
3 2 2 3
*
*

Figure 10.1 Dental record. All clinical findings are reported on the front page of the dental record. Normal periodontal probing depth (PPD) is not noted on the dental record to avoid clutter. However, when gingival recession is present, then PPDs are always recorded. True attachment loss is the sum of the recession and probing depth. Remember that periodontitis is a site-specific disease. PPD is recorded on the occlusal view of the tooth on the dental record so that you can easily identify the precise site of disease.

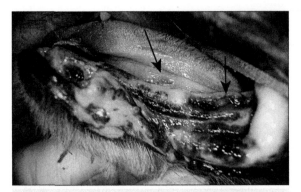

Figure 10.2 Occlusal photograph of the left mandible. The extraction sockets of 304, 308 and 309 are filled with coagulum, but the retained mesial root of 309 is evident. Note the lacerations on the tongue. These are likely to have been caused by slippage with a dental luxator or elevator.

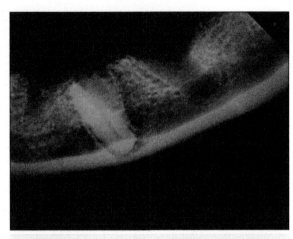

Figure 10.4 Radiograph of the retained mesial root of 309. The retained mesial root was also evident on clinical examination.

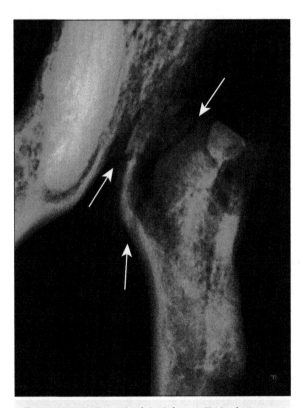

Figure 10.3 Radiograph of the left mandibular fracture. The fracture originates level with the apex of the extracted 304. There is one fracture line through the alveolar bone and two fracture lines extending to the ventral border of the mandible. Note the retained crown portion of 305.

5. Periodontitis (alveolar bone loss, furcation exposure) of 409 (Fig. 10.5b).

ORAL PROBLEM LIST

1. Iatrogenic fracture of the left mandible
2. Advanced periodontitis in 404 and 409
3. Root remnants of 309 (mesial root) and 408 (mesial and distal roots)
4. Crown remnant of 305.

THEORY REFRESHER

Teeth affected by advanced periodontitis require extraction. Many extractions due to periodontitis are relatively easy to perform as most of the attachment apparatus has been lost by the disease process. Remember that periodontitis is a site-specific disease (loss of periodontal attachment may only affect one or a few sites around the circumference of the tooth, with other sites unaffected by bone loss) and thus some extractions may be really difficult despite advanced disease.

Possible complications to extraction of teeth include the following:

Thermal bone injury: Adequate water-cooling of the bur (whether used in a high- or slow-speed handpiece) is mandatory. Overheating will result in damage to both the soft tissue and bone. Thermal necrosis of bone usually results in the development of a bone sequestrum

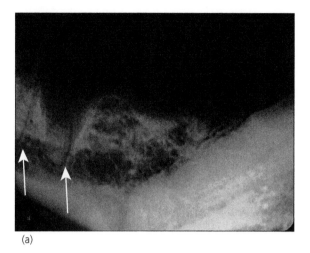
(a)

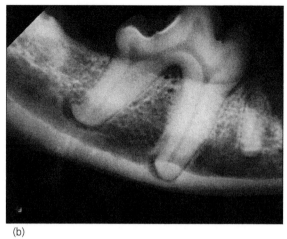
(b)

Figure 10.5 Radiographs of partially extracted 408. While both mesial and distal root remnants are obvious in the view in (a), a second view (b) was taken to fully visualize the retained distal root. This view clearly depicts the retained distal root of 408 as well as tooth 409. Note the horizontal bone loss and furcation exposure of 409.

that needs to be surgically retrieved as a second procedure.

Tooth fracture: Extraction may result in fracture of the tooth, either the crown or the root. Fracture of the crown is usually due to excessive force with elevators or using dental forceps. If the root is in one piece and can be visualized, it is removed using small luxators and elevators to cut the remaining periodontal ligament fibres. This is where a small (2 mm) luxator or root tip pick come in handy. Visibility is essential to be able to place instruments in the periodontal ligament space. Use the water spray to remove blood. If the root fractures, a radiograph is required to assess how much root is still in place and its position. Based on the radiographic findings, the extraction can be planned. An open extraction may be required to access the root remnant. If the root tip cannot be removed, the client must be informed and the affected jaw monitored clinically and radiographically for evidence of pathology.

Oronasal communication: A communication between a maxillary tooth alveolus and the nasal chamber may occur. Established fistulae are lined by epithelium and will therefore not heal spontaneously. The three most common causes of oronasal fistula formation involving the maxillary alveolus area are:
• Advanced periodontal disease
• Periapical lesions
• Iatrogenic.

An oronasal fistula in the region of the canine tooth is usually the result of advanced periodontal disease, where the process caused destruction of the medial bony wall of the alveolus. Periapical pathology of the maxillary canine teeth and premolars can also cause perforation of the medial bony wall of the alveolus. Extraction of a maxillary canine tooth may also cause perforation of the medial bony wall when an incorrect technique is used. A small iatrogenic perforation will probably heal if the gingival flap is replaced and sutured. Large fresh defects or long-standing defects causing clinical signs, such as nasal discharge, food impaction and chronic infection, should be surgically repaired.

Emphysema: Emphysema can occur if the high-speed handpiece is angled in such a way that air is blown into the bone and soft tissues. Continuous air-drying, especially if the air is directed into the alveolus, can also lead to emphysema. Cats seem particularly prone, and on recovery have swelling across the base of the nose and forehead. There is obvious crepitus on palpation of the swelling. Alternatively, the floor of the mouth is swollen. The condition usually resolves over a few hours/days. The owners are often concerned and it is best avoided.

Sublingual oedema: Traumatizing the lingual mucosa may result in sublingual oedema. If severe, it may require medical management with anti-inflammatory drugs and sometimes diuretics. It is easily avoided by using a gentle technique.

Jaw fracture: Advanced periodontal disease around mandibular teeth will weaken the mandible itself, and jaw fractures can and do happen. Extreme caution should be used in elderly toy and small breeds that seem most prone to this. Preoperative radiographs prior to all extractions are strongly recommended.

Some mandibular fractures do not need surgical fixation, particularly those where the fracture lines are contained within the areas of attachment of the masticatory muscles, as the muscles will effectively splint the fracture during healing. Mandibular fractures will need repair if they cause:

- Malocclusion
- Instability.

Stable fractures, if causing malocclusion, need repair to recreate a normal occlusion.

In many situations, a tape muzzle for 3–4 weeks may provide sufficient stability for the fracture to heal. It can also be used as temporary support or as an adjunct to other methods of fixation.

Haemorrhage: Clotting defects may not be apparent until after you have extracted a tooth, when the associated haemorrhage does not stop after a few minutes, but continues copiously, and can become life threatening. Suturing the gingiva with a haemostatic gauze or plug in the alveolus can help.

CLINICAL TIPS

- Use adequate water to cool both high- and low-speed burs. Thermal necrosis of bone usually results in the development of a bone sequestrum that needs to be surgically retrieved as a second procedure.
- Some extractions may be really difficult despite advanced periodontal disease.
- If the root fractures, a radiograph is required to assess how much root is still in place and its position.
- Extraction sites should be radiographed postoperatively.
- If the root tip cannot be removed, the client must be informed and the affected jaw monitored clinically and radiographically for evidence of pathology.

- Established oronasal fistulae are lined by epithelium and will not heal spontaneously.
- A small iatrogenic perforation will probably heal if the gingival flap is replaced and sutured.
- Caution should be used when extracting teeth in elderly toy and small breeds. Preoperative radiographs prior to all extractions are strongly recommended.
- Mandibular fractures will need repair if they cause malocclusion or are unstable.
- Suturing the gingiva with a haemostatic gauze or plug in the alveolus can help control haemorrhage.
- Jaw fracture is not an uncommon complication to extraction of mandibular canines. The owners should always be made aware of this risk.

TREATMENT OPTIONS

The remaining root remnants and remaining diseased teeth need to be extracted. Management of the mandibular fracture would require surgical fixation only if the fracture was unstable after reduction. The dog is edentulous so occlusion is not an issue.

TREATMENT PERFORMED

The dog received the following treatment (see the back page of the dental record depicted in Fig. 10.6):

1. A large buccal and lingual mucoperiosteal flap was raised extending from the midline to distal 309. The crown remnant of 305 and 309 (mesial root) were removed. Uneven bone was smoothed using a diamond round bur in a high-speed handpiece. The fracture was reduced and the buccal flap was sutured to the lingual flap. The replaced flap maintained the fracture in a stable reduced position. Consequently, surgical fixation of the fracture was not required.
2. Open extraction of 404 and of the mesial and distal root remnants of 408.

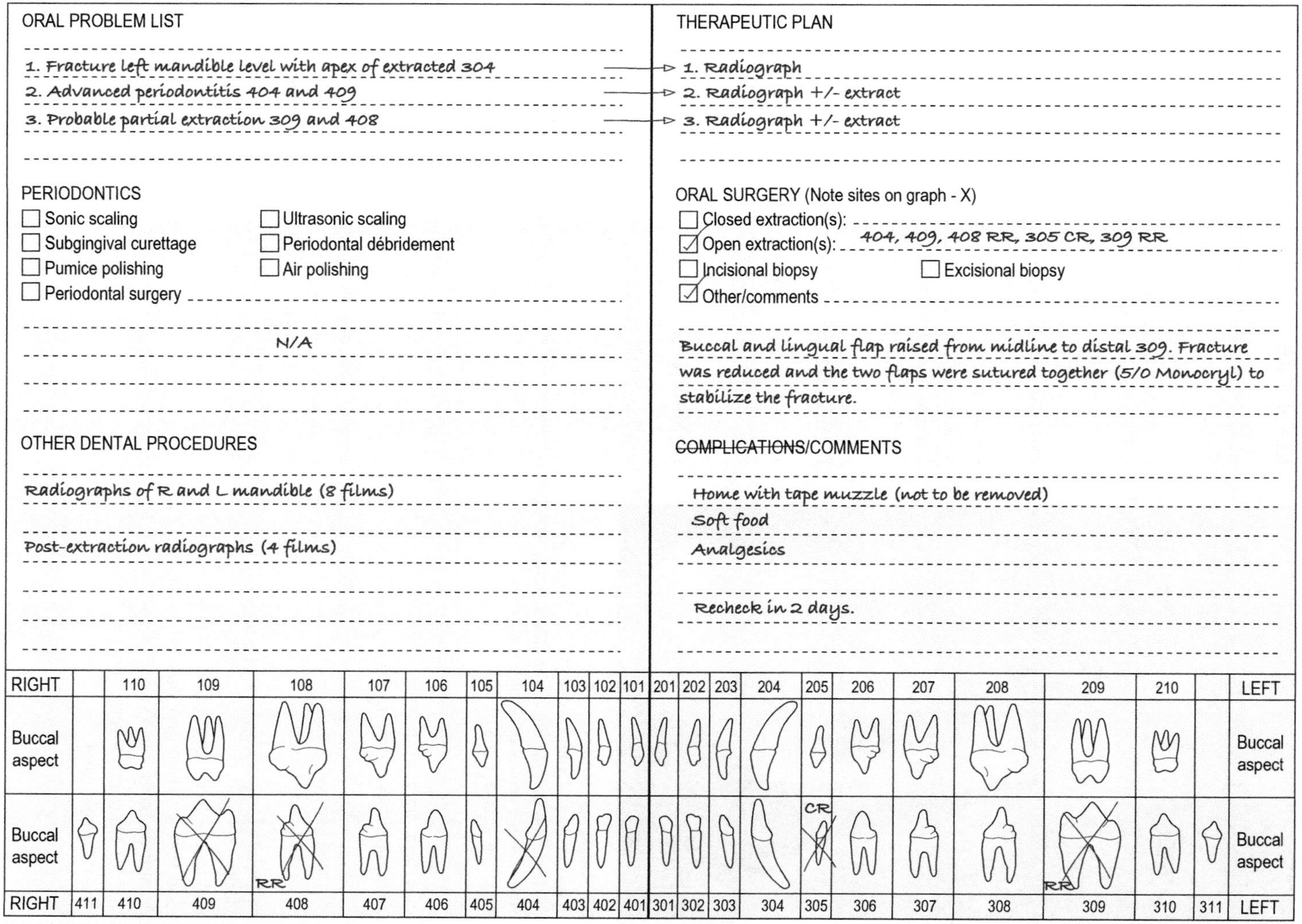

ORAL PROBLEM LIST

1. Fracture left mandible level with apex of extracted 304
2. Advanced periodontitis 404 and 409
3. Probable partial extraction 309 and 408

PERIODONTICS

- [ ] Sonic scaling
- [ ] Subgingival curettage
- [ ] Pumice polishing
- [ ] Periodontal surgery

- [ ] Ultrasonic scaling
- [ ] Periodontal débridement
- [ ] Air polishing

N/A

OTHER DENTAL PROCEDURES

Radiographs of R and L mandible (8 films)

Post-extraction radiographs (4 films)

THERAPEUTIC PLAN

1. Radiograph
2. Radiograph +/- extract
3. Radiograph +/- extract

ORAL SURGERY (Note sites on graph - X)

- [ ] Closed extraction(s):
- [x] Open extraction(s): 404, 409, 408 RR, 305 CR, 309 RR
- [ ] Incisional biopsy
- [x] Other/comments

- [ ] Excisional biopsy

Buccal and lingual flap raised from midline to distal 309. Fracture was reduced and the two flaps were sutured together (5/0 Monocryl) to stabilize the fracture.

COMPLICATIONS/COMMENTS

Home with tape muzzle (not to be removed)
soft food
Analgesics

Recheck in 2 days.

RIGHT	110	109	108	107	106	105	104	103	102	101	201	202	203	204	205	206	207	208	209	210	211	LEFT
Buccal aspect																						Buccal aspect
Buccal aspect															CR							Buccal aspect
RIGHT	410	409	408	407	406	405	404	403	402	401	301	302	303	304	305	306	307	308	309	310	311	LEFT

Figure 10.6 Dental record. Details of treatment are reported on the back page of the dental record.

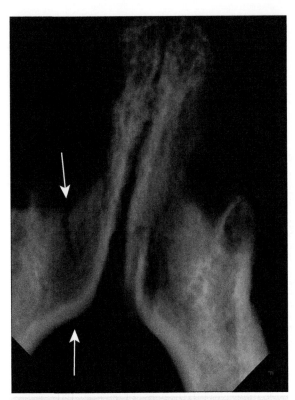

Figure 10.7 Radiograph of the rostral mandible. The radiograph was taken to confirm successful extraction of 404 and to check that the fracture at the site of 304 was reduced. Note the thin ventral bone and the incipient fracture line in the alveolar bone of 404.

Extractions and fracture fixation (Fig. 10.7) were checked radiographically before replacing the flaps.

POSTOPERATIVE CARE

- Analgesics
- Soft food
- Tape muzzle – to be kept on at all times – fitted so that a 1.0 cm gap was left to allow eating and drinking
- Booked for conscious examination in 2 days and then 4 weeks later.

RECHECKS

At recheck 2 days after surgery, the dog seemed comfortable. It was eating well and did not mind the tape muzzle. The fracture was reduced and seemed stable. Analgesics were supplied for a total of 10 days, and the owner was advised to feed only soft food and to keep the tape muzzle in place for 3 weeks.

The dog was seen again a month later. The owners reported that he was back to his normal self. He was eating well and had in fact put on some weight. A callus was palpable along the ventral border of the left mandible and there was no evidence of any instability in the fracture line. The owners were advised that he would need soft food as there were no remaining teeth.

PROGNOSIS

The dog has no remaining teeth and the fracture has healed. No further treatment is anticipated.

COMMENTS

Jaw fracture is not an uncommon complication to extraction of mandibular canines. The owners should always be made aware of this risk.

Preoperative radiographs will provide information about the extent of the periodontitis and the integrity of the remaining alveolar bone, and will allow planning of the extraction procedure to avoid fracture, e.g. a larger flap is raised and more alveolar bone is removed in cases where the ventral mandibular border is only a thin shell. In my opinion, extraction of mandibular canines with advanced periodontitis is the most difficult of all extractions. In fact, I have plans for fracture repair already outlined in my mind before I start the extraction. A gentle technique and the removal of buccal and lingual alveolar bone are essential.

CHRONIC GINGIVOSTOMATITIS

SECTION

CHRONIC GINGIVOSTOMATITIS

11 Chronic gingivostomatitis – an introduction

Chronic gingivostomatitis (CGS) describes a clinical syndrome characterized by focal or diffuse inflammation of the gingivae and oral mucosa. It occurs in dogs but is predominantly seen in cats.

CATS

Commonly described clinical findings in cats with CGS include elevated serum immunoglobulins (immunoglobulin (Ig) G, IgM and IgA are all raised). They also tend to have raised salivary concentrations of IgG and IgM, but reduced concentration of salivary IgA. It is unclear if the Ig pattern described is a cause or result of the inflammatory disease. Histological examination of affected oral mucosa shows a submucosal inflammatory infiltrate consisting of plasma cells, lymphocytes, macrophages and neutrophils.

The elevated serum globulins in affected cats and the nature of the submucosal inflammatory infiltrate have lead a number of authors to suggest that there may be an immunological basis for the condition. To date, no underlying intrinsic immunological abnormality in cats affected by CGS has been identified; however, the condition may still be immune mediated. Clinical studies have implicated the potential involvement of various viral agents, feline calici virus (FCV) in particular, as well as Gram-negative anaerobic bacterial species. However, attempts to reproduce the disease using these putative infective aetiological agents have been unsuccessful.

The most common sign of feline immunodeficiency virus (FIV) infection is oral inflammation. However, most cats with CGS test negative for FIV, but it needs to be excluded. Feline leukaemia virus (FeLV) also needs to be excluded in the initial work-up. The role of FCV in the development of CGS is unclear. FCV has been isolated from up to 100% of CGS cases, compared with up to 25% of cats in a healthy population, indicating that the carrier state may be a prerequisite for the induction of chronic stomatitis. However, FCV isolated from cats with CGS and then inoculated into specific pathogen-free cats produced signs of acute calici virus infection but not CGS, suggesting that other factors contribute towards the development of the oral inflammation. The fact that CGS often resolves in FCV-positive cats after extraction of all or most teeth and the subsequent reduction in dental plaque suggests that other antigenic stimuli are involved in the pathogenesis of the condition. It is possible that it is the sum of the total antigenic stimulation from plaque bacteria and viruses that is significant in the development of CGS.

Historically, the intractable nature of the disease, in combination with a poor understanding of the aetiopathogenesis of feline CGS, has resulted in the widespread use of empirical symptomatic treatment regimens.

The current treatment recommendations for cats with CGS include a combination of periodontal therapy and a home care regimen whereby plaque accumulation is kept to a minimum. In some cats, this may result in a reduction in inflammation. Unfortunately, most cats will not cooperate adequately with home care measures and plaque reforms beyond a critical level. These cats need extraction of premolar and molar teeth. In some cats, all teeth may require removal. The extraction of all premolar and molar teeth has given the most dependable results, with up to 80% of cats being clinically cured or significantly improved. The 20% that are non-responsive to extraction can be treated with antiseptics, intermittent antibiotics or interferon.

FCV isolation should always be performed prior to using interferon and also to monitor viral status as a consequence of treatment. Interferon should only be used in FCV-positive cats where extraction of at least all premolar and molar teeth has not led to cure. Using interferon without surgical treatment (extraction) has not been shown to have any benefit.

Cats with CGS require a thorough work-up prior to any treatment. The purpose of the work-up is not to reach a diagnosis per se, but rather an attempt to identify possible underlying causes. The minimal work-up includes: testing for FIV and FeLV; routine haematology and blood biochemistry; and a thorough oral and dental examination (including full-mouth radiographs to identify the presence of periodontitis, resorptive lesions, retained root remnants or other lesions). Systemic diseases, e.g. chronic renal failure and diabetes mellitus, which may predispose to the development of severe gingival inflammation in the presence of plaque, must be excluded before any treatment is initiated. Additional investigations include testing for FCV and/or biopsy and microscopic examination of the affected tissues. We do not routinely test for FCV. It is only if the cat does not respond to extraction of all or most teeth that we determine FCV status. Only cats that test positive (virtually 100%) will be treated with interferon therapy. Biopsy and histopathological examination of affected tissue are only performed if the lesions are asymmetrical. There have been recent reports of squamous cell carcinoma developing in cats with GCS. We have seen one case where surgical management lead to cure of the CGS. Two years after the curative treatment, localized intense inflammation of the right glossopalatine mucosa developed (the rest of the oral mucosa was healthy). Biopsy and histopathological examination of the affected mucosa revealed squamous cell carcinoma.

DOGS

CGS is less common in dogs than it is in cats. It is thought to be an inappropriate response to oral antigens, namely bacterial plaque present on the tooth surfaces. While underlying vesiculo-bullous disease, e.g. pemphigus and pemphigoid or discoid lupus erythematosus (DLE) cannot be excluded, it is essential to have plaque control before these can be investigated.

In the dog, I approach CGS as follows:
1. Haematology and biochemistry screens to exclude systemic diseases, e.g. endocrine or renal disorders, which may predispose to the development of severe gingival inflammation in the presence of plaque.
2. Meticulous oral examination to identify a possible reason for the intense inflammatory response, e.g. retained root remnants, periodontitis, other dental pathology.
3. Periodontal therapy (scaling and polishing) and treatment of pathological lesions, i.e. extract root remnants, extract teeth affected by periodontitis.
4. Daily home care (mechanical and chemical plaque control) is instituted.
5. Assess the response to treatment.

In the great majority of cases, the above approach results in complete cure. In some cases, the owner is not able to maintain adequate plaque control and selective extraction (removal of teeth that the owner cannot keep clean, usually the posterior teeth) is then performed. This is usually sufficient. In one aggressive dog that would not allow home care, all teeth were extracted. This resulted in healthy oral mucosa.

Healthy oral mucosa are maintained with daily toothbrushing and adjunctive chlorhexidine rinsing as required. As long as adequate plaque control is maintained, the prognosis is excellent. However, if the owners become lax with plaque removal the gingivostomatitis will return within a few weeks. It is crucial that the owner understands this.

Chronic gingivostomatitis as a consequence of periodontitis and iatrogenic injuries

INITIAL PRESENTATION

Inappetance, drooling associated with gingivostomatitis.

PATIENT DETAILS

A 9-year-old, neutered female, domestic long-haired cat.

CASE HISTORY

There was no history of any oral disease or dental/periodontal therapy until 2 years ago, when the cat received 'dental with extractions due to heavy accumulation of plaque and calculus'. Within 2 weeks of treatment the cat presented with inappetance and drooling, and gingivostomatitis was diagnosed by the referring veterinary surgeon.

In the last 2 years the cat had undergone five episodes of periodontal treatment. These had consisted of scaling, polishing and extraction (there was no record of which teeth had been extracted). There had been some improvement immediately following each treatment (the cat would start eating), but the inflammatory reaction had flared up again within weeks (the cat would stop eating). Several courses of antibiotics and the administration of long-acting steroid had shown initial improvement and then deterioration within a few weeks. The latest long-acting steroid injection had not had any beneficial effect at all. The cat was referred to us for management of the chronic gingivostomatitis. Prior to referral we requested haematology and biochemistry screen and FeLV and FIV testing to be performed by the referring veterinary surgeon. The cat was found to be negative to both FIV and FeLV and the only blood abnormality was elevated plasma globulins.

ORAL EXAMINATION – CONSCIOUS

This was an intensely uncomfortable cat that would not allow conscious examination of its face or oral cavity.

ORAL EXAMINATION – UNDER GENERAL ANAESTHETIC

See the front of the dental record sheet (Fig. 12.1) for details of findings.

In summary, examination under general anaesthesia identified the following:
1. Moderate to severe gingivitis of incisors and canines
2. Missing all premolars and molars
3. Severe gingivostomatitis of the alveolar, buccal and glossopalatine mucosae
4. Marked hyperplasia of the inflamed glossopalatine mucosa (Fig. 12.2)
5. Complicated crown fracture (CCF) of 204
6. Gingival recession of 104, 204, 304 and 404
7. Increased periodontal probing depth of 104, 204, 304 and 404.

FURTHER INVESTIGATIONS

A series of full-mouth radiographs (10 views) was taken.

RADIOGRAPHIC FINDINGS

Radiographs identified retained root remnants (presumably from previous extractions) of 108 (Fig. 12.3), 208,

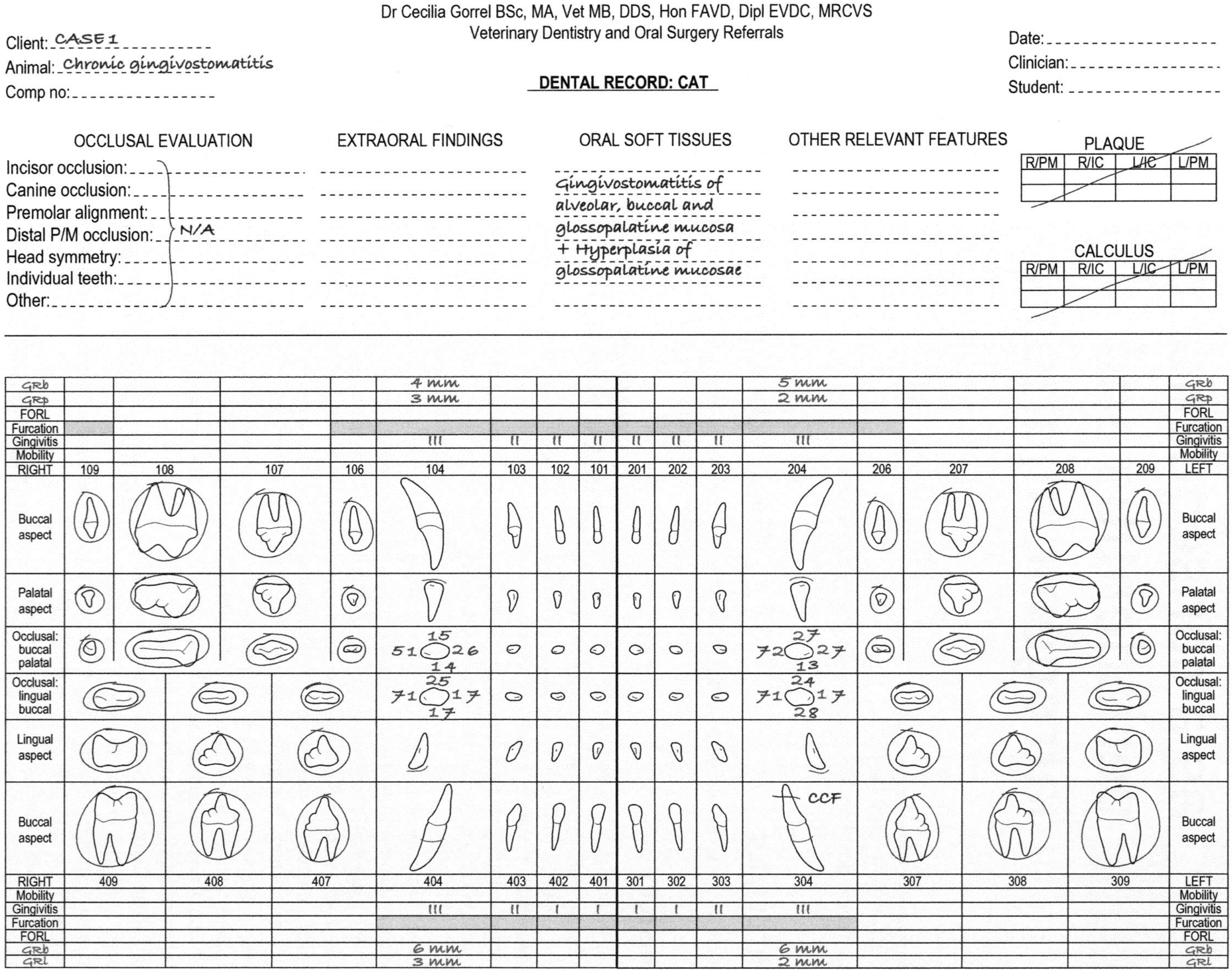
Dr Cecilia Gorrel BSc, MA, Vet MB, DDS, Hon FAVD, Dipl EVDC, MRCVS
Veterinary Dentistry and Oral Surgery Referrals
Client: CASE 1
Animal: Chronic gingivostomatitis
Comp no:
DENTAL RECORD: CAT
Date:
Clinician:
Student:
OCCLUSAL EVALUATION
Incisor occlusion:
Canine occlusion:
Premolar alignment:
Distal P/M occlusion:
Head symmetry:
Individual teeth:
Other:
N/A
EXTRAORAL FINDINGS
ORAL SOFT TISSUES
Gingivostomatitis of alveolar, buccal and glossopalatine mucosa + Hyperplasia of glossopalatine mucosae
OTHER RELEVANT FEATURES
PLAQUE
R/PM R/IC L/IC L/PM
CALCULUS
R/PM R/IC L/IC L/PM
GRb
GRp
FORL
Furcation
Gingivitis
Mobility
RIGHT
LEFT
109 108 107 106 104 103 102 101 201 202 203 204 206 207 208 209
4 mm
3 mm
5 mm
2 mm
Buccal aspect
Palatal aspect
Occlusal: buccal palatal
15 51 26 14
27 72 27 13
Occlusal: lingual buccal
25 71 17 17
24 71 17 28
Lingual aspect
CCF
409 408 407 404 403 402 401 301 302 303 304 307 308 309
GRl
6 mm
3 mm
6 mm
2 mm

Figure 12.1 The front page of the dental record sheet is used to record all clinical findings. Remember that periodontitis is a site-specific disease. PPD is recorded on the occlusal view of the tooth on the dental record so that you can easily identify the precise site of disease. Normal periodontal probing depth (PPD) is not noted on the dental record to avoid clutter. However, when gingival recession is present, then PPDs are always recorded so that periodontal attachment level (PAL) can be calculated (GR + PPD) and entered on the record at its precise site in green ink. PAL is a more accurate assessment of attachment loss.

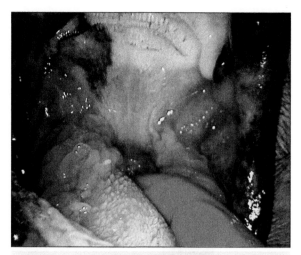

Figure 12.2 Rostrocaudal photograph of the oropharynx. Note the hyperplastic and intensely inflamed glossopalatine folds.

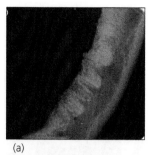

(a)

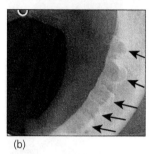

(b)

Figure 12.4

(a) Preoperative radiograph of the left mandibular premolar and molar region. The roots of all the teeth in this quadrant (307, 308 and 309) are retained from previous surgery. This could, at best, be called partial extraction.

(b) Postoperative radiograph of the left mandibular premolar and molar region. The postoperative view shows empty extraction sockets and confirms complete removal of all root remnants. Note the intact lamina dura of all sockets, confirming that the integrity of the mandibular canal (carrying the neurovascular supply to teeth and soft tissue) was not broached during the extraction procedure.

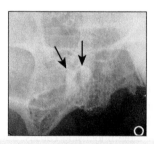

Figure 12.3 Lateral radiograph of the right upper premolar and molar region. Note the retained root remnants of 108.

307 (Fig. 12.4a), 308 (Fig. 12.4a), 309 (Fig. 12.4a), the mesial root of 408, and 409.

Periodontal bone loss affecting the canines was also evident (Figs 12.5a, b, 12.6a and 12.7a).

ORAL PROBLEM LIST

1. Moderate to severe gingivitis of incisors and canines
2. Gingivostomatitis of alveolar, buccal and glossopalatine mucosae
3. Marked hyperplasia of inflamed glossopalatine mucosa
4. Complicated crown fracture of 204
5. Root remnants of 108, 208, 307, 308, 309, 408 (mesial root) and 409
6. Advanced periodontitis of 104, 204, 304 and 404.

THEORY REFRESHER

Chronic gingivostomatitis (CGS) describes a clinical syndrome characterized by focal or diffuse inflammation of the gingivae and oral mucosa. It occurs in dogs but is predominantly seen in cats.

Commonly described clinical findings in cats with CGS include elevated serum globulins, predominantly hypergammaglobulinaemia, and a submucosal inflammatory infiltrate consisting of plasma cells, lymphocytes, macrophages and neutrophils. The elevated serum globulins in affected cats and the nature of the submucosal inflammatory infiltrate have lead a number of authors to suggest that there may be an immunological basis for the condition. To date, no underlying intrinsic immunological abnormality in cats affected by CGS has been identified;

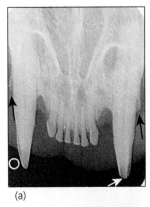

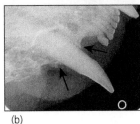

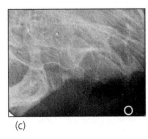

(a)

(b)

(c)

Figure 12.5

(a) Rostrocaudal radiograph of the rostral upper jaw. Note the loss of alveolar bone height associated with the canines. The proliferation of the buccal bone plate is also an indicator of periodontitis. The crown fracture of 204 is also obvious. The pulp system diameter of 204 is wider than in 104, indicating pulp necrosis of 204.

(b) Lateral radiograph of 104. Note the loss of alveolar bone height surrounding 104.

(c) Lateral radiograph of extraction site of 104. The socket of 104 is empty and the lamina dura is intact. The successful removal of the retained root remnant of 108 is also confirmed by this view.

however, the condition may still be immune mediated. Clinical studies have implicated the potential involvement of various viral agents, calicivirus in particular, as well as Gram-negative anaerobic bacterial species. However, attempts to reproduce the disease using these putative infective aetiological agents have been unsuccessful.

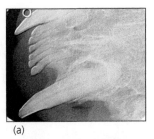

(a)

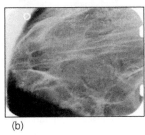

(b)

Figure 12.6

(a) Lateral radiograph of 204. The loss of alveolar bone height surrounding 204 is obvious in this view. Note also the complicated crown fracture of 204.

(b) Lateral radiograph of extraction site of 204. The socket of 204 is empty and the lamina dura is intact.

Cats with chronic stomatitis require a thorough work-up prior to any treatment. The purpose of the work-up is not to reach a diagnosis per se, but rather an attempt to identify possible underlying causes. Such a work-up includes: testing for FIV and FeLV; routine haematology and blood biochemistry; and sometimes biopsy and microscopic examination of the affected tissues. A meticulous oral and dental examination, including full-mouth radiographs to identify the presence of periodontitis, resorptive lesions, retained root remnants or other lesions, is mandatory. Systemic diseases, e.g. chronic renal failure and diabetes mellitus, which may predispose to the development of severe gingival inflammation in the presence of plaque, must also be excluded before any treatment is initiated.

In this case, a probable underlying cause for the inflammatory reaction in the oral mucous membranes was identified, namely root remnants from previous extractions and periodontitis of the canine teeth. Extraction of diseased teeth and root remnants is likely to result in a complete cure.

In summary, cats with chronic gingivostomatitis are usually extremely uncomfortable. Every attempt should be made to identify and eliminate or treat any underlying cause for the intense oral inflammation. Full-mouth

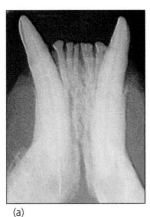

(a)

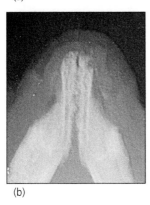

(b)

Figure 12.7 Rostrocaudal radiographs of the rostral mandible pre-extraction (a) and post-extraction (b).

(a) Note the loss of alveolar margin associated with periodontitis of both canine teeth.

(b) The sockets are empty and the lamina dura intact, confirming successful extraction of the mandibular incisors and canines.

radiographs are a mandatory component of the diagnostic work-up.

CLINICAL TIPS

- Cats with chronic stomatitis require a thorough work-up, including FeLV and FIV testing, prior to any treatment to try to identify any underlying cause for the condition.
- Full-mouth radiographs are a mandatory component of the diagnostic work-up.
- The success of tooth extraction should be confirmed radiographically.
- Cats without any teeth may require assistance with grooming.

TREATMENT OPTIONS

Extraction of all teeth affected by periodontitis and removal of all root remnants are necessary.

TREATMENT PERFORMED

1. Extraction of root remnants (108, 208, 307, 308, 309, 408 mesial root, and 409) with an open technique; flaps were replaced with 5/0 Monocryl. Successful removal was confirmed radiographically at all sites.
2. Extraction of 104, 204, 304 and 404 with an open technique; flaps were replaced with 5/0 Monocryl. Successful extraction was confirmed by radiographs.

See Figs 12.4b, 12.5c, 12.6b and 12.7b for some of the postoperative radiographs taken.

POSTOPERATIVE CARE

- A 10-day course of antibiotics (given as daily injection by referring veterinary surgeon for the first 3 days postoperatively, then as palatable drops in food)
- Analgesics for 3 days (vetergesic by syringe)
- Booked for conscious examination 1 month later.

RECHECK

At recheck 1 month later, the extraction sites had all healed uneventfully and there was no evidence of gingivostomatitis.

PROGNOSIS

The cause of the inflammation (periodontitis and retained root remnants from previous extractions) has been removed and there should be no need for any further dental treatment.

COMMENTS

The chronic gingivostomatitis in this case was caused by the presence of numerous root remnants from dental extraction, i.e. it was iatrogenic. Careful extraction with radiographic facilities could have prevented the problem. The cat also had periodontitis of the canines but there was no evidence of gingivostomatitis in the incisor or canine regions. The gingivostomatitis was localized to the alveolar gingivae (overlying the retained root remnants), and extended laterally to involve the buccal mucosa and distally to affect the glossopalatine folds. In fact, the glossopalatine folds were inflamed and hyperplastic.

The success of tooth extraction should be confirmed radiographically. Ideally, the whole tooth should be extracted. If this cannot be achieved, the owner needs to be aware that there are root remnants which may need to be removed as a second procedure.

In a significant number of cats referred to us we can identify an underlying cause for inflammation, often retained root remnants from previous extractions. In my opinion, any cat anaesthetized for a dental procedure should receive a series of full-mouth radiographs to identify pathology and allow optimal treatments. Also, extractions must be evaluated radiographically, especially in the cat.

Cats without any teeth may require assistance with grooming. This long-haired cat required daily brushing.

13 Chronic gingivostomatitis associated with FeLV and FIV

INITIAL PRESENTATION

Inappetance, drooling, sockets from previous extractions not healing.

PATIENT DETAILS

An adult (estimated 7 years), neutered male, domestic short-haired cat.

CASE HISTORY

The cat was an adopted stray cat that had been with the owners for 6 years and was at least a year old when they adopted him. He lived in a multi-cat household (eight other cats). All cats were indoor/outdoor cats.

The cat had received 'routine dental' treatment 10 weeks prior to referral. At this time several teeth were extracted, but no record of which teeth was made. It was noted on the record that some teeth had fractured during extraction and had been 'drilled out'. Within a week of treatment the cat started drooling and stopped eating. Non-healing sockets were identified and several courses of antibiotics had been administered with no improvement. The cat was referred to us 10 weeks after the initial treatment.

ORAL EXAMINATION – CONSCIOUS

The cat allowed general physical examination but would not allow conscious examination of the face or oral cavity.

Blood was drawn for haematology and biochemistry screen and FeLV/FIV testing. It was decided not to wait for these results before inducing anaesthesia, as the cat was deemed safe for anaesthesia based on the general clinical examination. The owner was made aware that FeLV and/or FIV infection was a possibility.

ORAL EXAMINATION – UNDER GENERAL ANAESTHETIC

A thorough oral examination, including investigating periodontal parameters, was performed and all findings were noted on the dental record.

In summary, examination under general anaesthesia identified the following:
1. Teeth 204, 208, 209, 107, 108, 109, 309 and 409 were missing (presumably extracted 10 weeks earlier)
2. Non-healing extraction sockets of 204 (Fig. 13.1a), 309 and 409 (Fig. 13.2a)
3. Gingivostomatitis associated with the extraction socket of 204 (Fig. 13.1a)
4. Gingivostomatitis of alveolar and buccal mucosa bilaterally in the edentulous upper premolar and molar regions (Fig. 13.3).

FURTHER INVESTIGATIONS

A series of full-mouth radiographs (10 views) was taken.

RADIOGRAPHIC FINDINGS

The radiographs revealed no evidence of any retained root remnants in the upper jaw (Fig. 13.1b). In the lower jaw, it was found that the roots of 309 (Fig. 13.4) and 409 (Fig. 13.2b) were retained.

ORAL PROBLEM LIST

1. Gingivostomatitis bilaterally in the edentulous upper premolar and molar regions (not associated with retained roots from previous extractions)

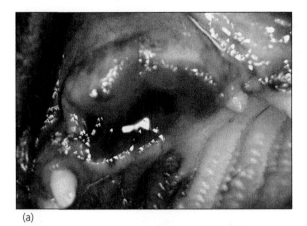

(a)

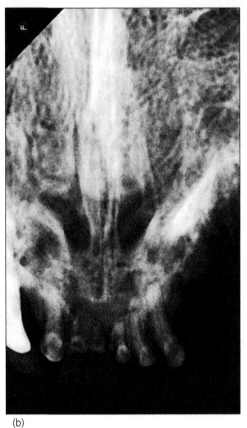

(b)

Figure 13.1 Occlusal photograph (a) and rostrocaudal radiograph (b) of the non-healing extraction socket of 204.

(a) The socket has not healed after extraction of 204 10 weeks earlier. In fact, the owner reported that the defect was larger than it was immediately after the extraction.

(b) The radiograph shows an empty socket with no evidence of any retained root material.

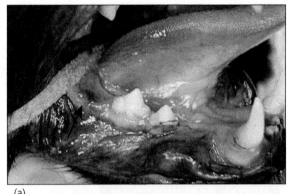

(a)

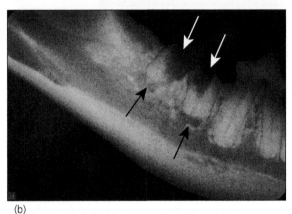

(b)

Figure 13.2 Lateral photograph (a) and radiograph (b) of the right mandibular quadrant.

(a) Note the non-healing extraction socket of 409.

(b) The radiograph reveals that both the mesial and distal roots of 409 have not been extracted. Note the radiolucent areas where atomization (drilling away root substance) was attempted.

2. Gingivostomatitis and non-healing socket of 204 (not associated with a retained root remnant)
3. Gingivostomatitis and non-healing socket of 309 with retained root remnants
4. Gingivostomatitis and non-healing socket of 409 with retained root remnants.

At this time the blood results were available. The only blood abnormality was elevated plasma globulins and a left shift in the neutrogram. However, the cat tested positive for both FeLV and FIV.

THEORY REFRESHER

Chronic gingivostomatitis (CGS) describes a clinical syndrome characterized by focal or diffuse inflammation of

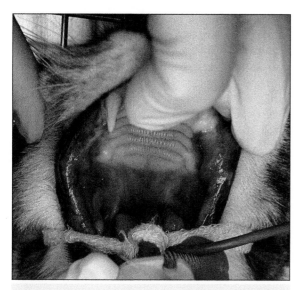

Figure 13.3 Occlusal photograph of the upper jaw. Note the gingivostomatitis affecting the alveolar and buccal mucosa over the edentulous premolar and molar regions bilaterally.

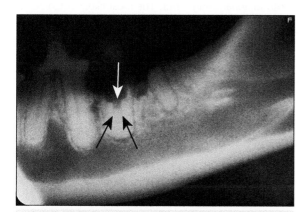

Figure 13.4 Lateral radiograph of the left caudal premolar and molar region. The radiograph reveals retention of both roots of 309. Note the radiolucent region in the mesial root as a consequence of atomization.

the gingivae and oral mucosa. It occurs in dogs but is predominantly seen in cats.

Cats with chronic stomatitis require a thorough work-up prior to any treatment. The purpose of the work-up is not to reach a diagnosis per se, but rather an attempt to identify possible underlying causes. Such a work-up includes: testing for FIV and FeLV, possibly also for FCV; routine haematology and blood biochemistry; and sometimes biopsy and microscopic examination of the affected

tissues. A meticulous oral and dental examination, including full-mouth radiographs to identify the presence of periodontitis, resorptive lesions, retained root remnants or other lesions, is mandatory. Systemic diseases, e.g. chronic renal failure and diabetes mellitus, which may predispose to the development of severe gingival inflammation in the presence of plaque, must also be excluded before any treatment is initiated.

In this case, a probable underlying cause for the inflammatory reaction in the oral mucous membranes and non-healing of the extraction sockets was identified, namely FeLV and FIV infection. The presence of root remnants from previous extractions at 309 and 409 would further contribute to the non-healing of these sockets.

The fact that this cat tested positive for both FeLV and FIV creates a complicated situation. The cat is part of a multi-cat household and the risk of infection of the other cats needs to be taken into account. This cat would need to be restricted to an indoor lifestyle to prevent spreading infection.

CLINICAL TIPS

- Cats with chronic stomatitis require a thorough work-up, including FeLV and FIV testing, prior to any treatment to try to identify any underlying cause for the condition.
- The best way to remove root remnants is to raise a mucoperiosteal flap and carefully bur away some buccal bone plate to allow insertion of a luxator or elevator into the periodontal ligament space and then loosen the root in the conventional way.
- FeLV- and FIV-infected cats need to be restricted to an indoor-only lifestyle to prevent spread of infection.

TREATMENT OPTIONS

1. Euthanasia – the cat is infective and part of a multi-cat household.
2. Symptomatic treatment (remove retained root remnants 309 and 409, debride socket of 204, antibiotics and anti-inflammatory agents as required). Biopsy from the non-healing socket of 204 would also be prudent. Following symptomatic treatment, the cat would need to be restricted to an indoor lifestyle

only to prevent potential spread of FeLV and FIV. The FeLV and FIV status of the other cats in the household needs to be ascertained and appropriate action taken.

TREATMENT PERFORMED

The implications of an FeLV- and FIV-positive cat in a multi-cat household were discussed at length with the owner over the telephone. The owner requested symptomatic treatment while they thought about the implications of the viral status. They arranged with their own veterinary surgeon to have the other eight cats tested.

Treatment performed consisted of:

1. Periodontal therapy.
2. Open extraction of root remnants of 309 and 409. The access flaps for the extractions were closed with 5/0 Monocryl. Postoperative radiographs were taken to confirm successful extraction.
3. Curettage of the socket of 204.
4. Biopsy of the non-healing socket of 204.

On reflection, the owner decided to opt for euthanasia, which was performed immediately.

COMMENTS

Cats with FeLV and/or FIV have an altered immune response. Severe oral inflammation may be one mani-festation of this. It is good practice to test for FeLV and FIV early on in cats that manifest with oral inflammation. Most cats with inflammatory oral disease will test negative, but it needs to be excluded.

The identification of FeLV and/or FIV infection is in itself not an indication for euthanasia. Many cats do well with symptomatic management, i.e. strict plaque control, usually by means of radical extraction, and medical management (antibiotics, anti-inflammatory drugs) if acute phases develop. However, infected cats need to be restricted to an indoor-only lifestyle to prevent spread of infection.

The decision to take a biopsy from the non-healing extraction socket of 204 was taken in lieu of recent reports of squamous cell carcinoma developing in chronic gingivostomatitis cats. The histopathological findings in this case were chronic inflammation, with no evidence of neoplasia.

Atomization of root remnants as attempted in this case is unlikely to achieve the goal of removing the retained roots. It is impossible to differentiate between tooth and bone, and to selectively remove tooth material using a bur. The most likely outcome, as in this case, is to drill canals into the roots. The best way to remove root remnants is to raise a mucoperiosteal flap and carefully bur away some buccal bone plate to allow insertion of a luxator or elevator into the periodontal ligament space, then loosen the root in the conventional way.

14 Idiopathic chronic gingivostomatitis with extraction leading to cure

INITIAL PRESENTATION

Inappetance and drooling.

PATIENT DETAILS

A 6-year-old, neutered male, domestic short-haired cat.

CASE HISTORY

There was no history of any oral disease until 1 year ago, when the cat presented with inappetance and drooling. The owner reported that he would start to eat and then back off his food as if he was in pain. The oral mucous membranes were intensely inflamed. He had been treated with antibiotics and corticosteroids intermittently (six treatments in total) during the last year. Initially, the combination of a short course of antibiotics and long-acting steroid had resulted in clinical improvement in that the cat had resumed eating. The effect had only lasted for 4–6 weeks and become shorter for each course. The last course of antibiotics and long-acting steroid had been ineffective. There was no history of oral/dental examination under general anaesthesia or periodontal therapy. The referring veterinarian reported that the cat was FeLV and FIV negative. The only blood abnormality was elevated plasma globulins and a left shift in the neutrogram.

The cat was referred to us for management of the chronic gingivostomatitis.

ORAL EXAMINATION – CONSCIOUS

The cat would not allow conscious examination of the face or oral cavity.

ORAL EXAMINATION – UNDER GENERAL ANAESTHETIC

A thorough oral examination, including investigating periodontal parameters, was performed and all findings were noted on the dental record.

In summary, examination under general anaesthesia identified a severe generalized oral inflammation. The gingivae as well as the buccal mucosa and the glossopalatine folds were intensely inflamed (Fig. 14.1a–c). Moderate amounts of plaque and calculus were present on the buccal aspects of the upper premolars. All teeth were present and showed no evidence of periodontitis.

FURTHER INVESTIGATIONS

A series of full-mouth radiographs (10 views) was taken.

An oropharyngeal swab from the glossopalatine mucosa was taken and submitted for feline calici virus (FCV) isolation.

RADIOGRAPHIC FINDINGS

No obvious pathology (Fig. 14.2a, b) could be identified on any of the 10 views.

ORAL PROBLEM LIST

Idiopathic chronic gingivostomatitis.

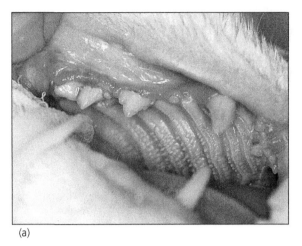

(a)

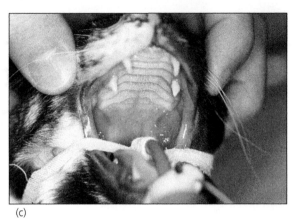

(c)

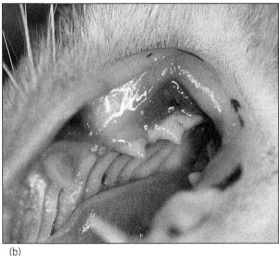

(b)

Figure 14.1 Right lateral (a), left lateral (b) and rostrocaudal (c) photographs of the oral cavity.

(a) The inflammation affects free and attached gingivae, and extends into the buccal mucosa distally.

(b) Note the extension of the inflammation to involve the buccal mucosa.

(c) The inflammatory reaction extends caudally to involve the glossopalatine folds.

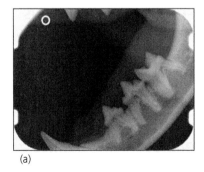

(a)

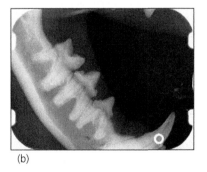

(b)

Figure 14.2 Left (a) and right (b) lateral radiographs of mandibular premolars and molars. All teeth are present and there is no evidence of any dental or periodontal disease. This applied to all 10 views taken.

THEORY REFRESHER

Chronic gingivostomatitis (CGS) describes a clinical syndrome characterized by focal or diffuse inflammation of the gingivae and oral mucosa. It occurs in dogs but is predominantly seen in cats. It is thought to be an inappropriate response to oral antigens, namely bacterial plaque present on the tooth surfaces.

It is useful to view CGS as being subdivided into three different types, which may overlap. In one type, an underlying cause that explains the inflammatory response (albeit not the intensity) can be identified. Common causes are retained root remnants from previous extraction, periodontitis or other dental pathology. In the second type, concurrent disease that alters the animal's ability to mount an appropriate inflammatory response can be identified. Systemic diseases, e.g. chronic renal failure and diabetes mellitus, will alter the immune response and may predispose to the development of severe gingival inflammation in the presence of plaque. Cats infected with FeLV and/or FIV are also unable to mount an appropriate immune response to the presence of plaque on the tooth surfaces. Cats infected with FCV are also likely to have an altered immune response. In the third type, no obvious dental pathology or underlying immune incompetence can be identified, i.e. idiopathic.

Cats with CGS require a thorough work-up prior to any treatment. The purpose of the work-up is not to reach a diagnosis per se, but rather an attempt to identify possible underlying causes. Such a work-up includes: testing for FIV and FeLV infection; sometimes testing for FCV infection; routine haematology and blood biochemistry; and sometimes biopsy and microscopic examination of the affected tissues. A meticulous oral and dental examination, including full-mouth radiographs to identify the presence of periodontitis, resorptive lesions, retained root remnants or other lesions, is mandatory. Systemic diseases, e.g. chronic renal failure and diabetes mellitus, which may predispose to the development of severe gingival inflammation in the presence of plaque, must also be excluded before any treatment is initiated.

In this case, no underlying cause for the inflammatory reaction in the oral mucous membranes was identified. The cat appeared otherwise healthy based on clinical examination and blood results. It tested negative to FeLV and FIV, and FCV could not be cultured from oral swabs. All teeth were present, with no evidence of periodontitis or resorptive lesions.

CLINICAL TIPS

- Cats with chronic stomatitis require a thorough work-up, including FeLV (perhaps FCV) and FIV testing, prior to any treatment to try to identify any underlying cause for the condition.
- Chlorhexidine is the gold standard antiplaque agent.
- Extraction of all premolars and molars results in cure in roughly 80% of cats.
- Radiographic assessment of all extraction sites is mandatory.
- Following extensive extraction procedures, cats should be hospitalized for controlled administration of analgesics and antibiotics until they are eating.
- If intra-oral sutures induce inflammation, they should be removed under anaesthesia after the wound has healed.
- In assessing the outcome of treatment, the oral inflammatory reaction needs to be linked to clinical behaviour. In some cases, the cats show no evidence of any oral discomfort in spite of having some residual oral inflammation.

TREATMENT OPTIONS

1. Conservative management, i.e. meticulous periodontal therapy followed by daily home care (daily chlorhexidine rinse and toothbrushing). Theoretically, once dental deposits have been removed, if the owner controls plaque accumulation then the inflammatory reaction should subside. Plaque control by the owner would consist of daily removal using a toothbrush (mechanical plaque removal), augmented by daily rinsing of the oral cavity with the gold standard antiplaque agent, namely chlorhexidine (chemical plaque control). This regime would need to be followed daily for the rest of the animal's life to maintain healthy gingivae and oral mucosae. In practical terms, it is difficult to convince an adult cat with inflamed oral soft tissues to accept any sort of home care. In a few selected cats, we have been able to control plaque with twice-daily chlorhexidine rinsing and postoperative antibiotics for 3 weeks immediately after professional periodontal therapy. This achieved a level of gingival and oral mucosal health which allowed brushing to be instituted without causing discomfort. The health of the gingival and

oral mucosa was then maintained by daily brushing and chlorhexidine rinsing as required, i.e. the owners would notice when the gums started to look more inflamed and use chlorhexidine for a few days. This cat did not allow conscious examination of the oral cavity and the owner was absolutely sure that he would not be able to perform any home care. Consequently, conservative management was not considered suitable for this cat.

2. Extraction of all premolars and molars, which results in cure in roughly 80% of cats. This is the option of choice for this cat. It was emphasized to the owner that it may not result in complete cure, and that further extraction (all teeth) and adjunctive medical management (intermittent antibiotics or interferon) may be required.

TREATMENT PERFORMED

1. Periodontal therapy of the incisors and canines.
2. Open extraction of all premolars and molars; flaps were replaced with 5/0 Monocryl. Postoperative radiographs were taken to confirm successful extraction at all sites.

POSTOPERATIVE CARE

- It was planned to hospitalize the cat for 3 days to provide antibiotics and analgesia by injection until he started eating. He was tempted with soft palatable food.
- He started eating the day after surgery and was discharged with no medication.
- The cat was rebooked for conscious examination a month later.

RECHECKS

At recheck 1 month later, the owner reported that the cat was bright, alert and eating well. He was being fed soft food but had started to steal kibbles from the other cat. Conscious oral examination was permitted and revealed that the extraction sites were healing nicely, but there was a reaction to the suture material. The cat was anaesthetized and the remaining sutures removed.

At recheck 3 weeks after removing the remaining sutures, all extraction sites were healed and there was no evidence of inflammation of the gingivae or oral mucosae (Fig. 14.3a, b).

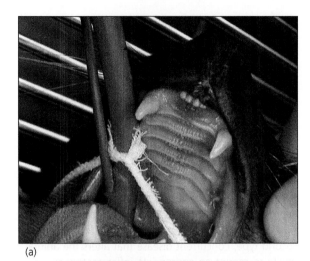

(a)

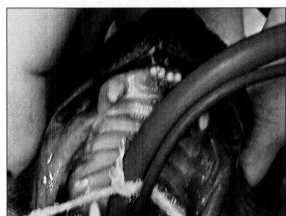

(b)

Figure 14.3 Oblique occlusal (a) and occlusal (b) photographs of the upper jaw.

(a) At recheck 1 month after extraction, all the extraction sites were healing nicely, but there was a reaction to the suture material.

(b) The remaining sutures have been removed.

At recheck 6 months after the extractions, the owner reported that the cat was doing very well and conscious examination revealed a healthy oral cavity (Fig. 14.4). The cat did not resent handling and oral examination, and it was recommended that the owner try to brush the remaining incisors and canines to keep plaque at a minimum. It was also recommended that the cat be examined under general anaesthesia at regular intervals, e.g. annually, to monitor the status of the remaining teeth.

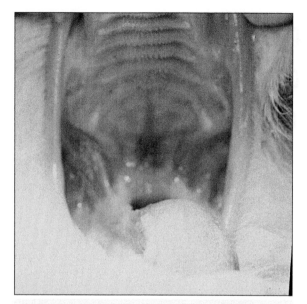

Figure 14.4 Rostrocaudal photograph of the oral cavity. Note the healthy oral cavity 6 months after extraction of all premolars and molars.

PROGNOSIS

The fact that there is no evidence of gingivostomatitis 6 months after extraction is promising. If the owner manages to brush the remaining teeth and maintain clinically healthy gingivae, this cat may never require further extractions. However, if plaque is allowed to accumulate and gingivitis/periodontitis or gingivostomatitis develops, then the remaining teeth will need removal. Frequent professional checks and intervention as required is recommended.

COMMENTS

The idiopathic type of CGS is treated by extracting premolars and molars. It is essential that the whole tooth is removed, as retained root fragments will sustain the inflammatory response. Radiographic assessment of all extraction sites is mandatory.

Even with successful extraction, the outcome is difficult to predict. In roughly 80% of cases removal of the premolars and molars results in reduction of the inflammation, if not cure. In the remaining 20% of cases further treatment is required, i.e. extraction of remaining teeth, intermittent antibiotics, interferon. It is essential that the owner is aware of this from the outset.

In assessing outcome of treatment, the oral inflammatory reaction needs to be linked to clinical behaviour. In some cases, the cats show no evidence of any oral discomfort, i.e. they eat, drink and groom themselves, yet on oral examination there is evidence of inflammation, although not as severe as before extraction. I view these as successful and do not interfere unless clinical signs of discomfort develop.

I would strongly recommend hospitalization for controlled administration of analgesics and antibiotics following extensive extraction procedures. We normally hospitalize such patients until they are eating and drinking. This generally means 1–3 days in hospital.

It is not uncommon to find that, 3–4 weeks after surgery, the extraction sites are healing nicely but the sutures have become plaque-retentive surfaces and are causing an inflammatory response. If this occurs, the animal should be placed under anaesthesia and the remaining sutures removed.

15 Chronic gingivostomatitis with extraction leading to partial cure

INITIAL PRESENTATION

Reluctance to eat, progressive apathy and weight loss.

PATIENT DETAILS

An 8-year-old, neutered female, domestic short-haired cat.

CASE HISTORY

The cat was referred to us for management of chronic oral inflammation of 2 years' duration. Presenting signs had been a progressive reluctance to eat, apathy and weight loss. During the first year, she had been treated with antibiotics and corticosteroids intermittently (five treatments in total). Initially, the combination of a short course of antibiotics and a long-acting steroid had resulted in clinical improvement in that the cat had resumed eating. The effect had only lasted for 3–6 weeks and become shorter for each course. In the last year, the cat had received professional periodontal therapy with extractions twice, as well as four courses of antibiotics and long-acting steroid. There had been short periods of improvement after each episode of therapy. At the second episode of periodontal therapy, it was recorded which teeth had been removed (108, 208, 309, 409 and root remnants from previous extraction) and the extractions had been confirmed radiographically. The procedure had been performed by a veterinarian with a special interest and training in dentistry. She arranged referral to us and did preoperative blood and viral testing. The cat was FeLV and FIV negative, but FCV positive.

ORAL EXAMINATION – CONSCIOUS

The cat allowed conscious oral examination, which revealed the absence of all premolars and molars, and gingivostomatitis of the mucosa overlying the alveolar bone as well as the buccal mucosa and glossopalatine folds.

ORAL EXAMINATION – UNDER GENERAL ANAESTHETIC

A thorough oral examination, including investigating periodontal parameters, was performed and all findings were noted on the dental record.

In summary, examination under general anaesthesia identified the following:
1. All premolars and molars were missing
2. Gingivostomatitis (alveolar, buccal and glossopalatine mucosae) affecting the premolar and molar regions in all four quadrants (Fig. 15.1)
3. Mild gingivitis associated with the canines (Fig. 15.1)
4. No gingivitis associated with incisor teeth (Fig. 15.1).

FURTHER INVESTIGATIONS

A series of full-mouth radiographs (10 views) was taken.

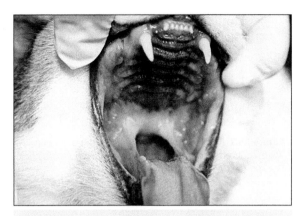

Figure 15.1 Rostrocaudal photograph of the oral cavity. This was the clinical appearance of the oral mucosa immediately before treatment with feline omega interferon. Note that the upper incisors have no clinical evidence of gingivitis and the upper canines only show mild gingival inflammation.

RADIOGRAPHIC FINDINGS

No obvious pathology could be identified. There was no evidence of any retained roots from previous extractions.

ORAL PROBLEM LIST

1. Mild gingivitis (canines)
2. Refractory chronic gingivostomatitis (premolar and molar regions all four quadrants).

THEORY REFRESHER

Chronic gingivostomatitis (CGS) is a common condition of the cat characterized by intense inflammation of gingival and non-gingival oral mucosa. It is thought to be an inappropriate response to oral antigens, namely bacterial plaque present on the tooth surfaces. Affected cats may show mild to severe dysphagia, with slight to absolute reluctance to eat. The decline in food intake leads to progressive apathy and weight loss.

I find it useful in the clinical situation to view CGS as three different types, with some degree of overlap. In one type, an underlying cause that explains the inflammatory response (albeit not the intensity) can be identified, e.g. retained root remnants from previous extraction, periodontitis or other dental pathology. In the second type, concurrent disease that alters the animal's ability to mount an appropriate inflammatory response can be identified, e.g. chronic renal failure, diabetes mellitus or viral infection (FeLV, FIV, FCV). In the third type, no obvious dental pathology or underlying immune incompetence can be identified, i.e. it is idiopathic.

Cats with chronic stomatitis require a thorough work-up prior to any treatment. The purpose of the work-up is not to reach a diagnosis per se, but rather an attempt to identify possible underlying causes. As a minimum, such a work-up includes testing for FIV and FeLV, and routine haematology and blood biochemistry. A meticulous oral and dental examination, including full-mouth radiographs to identify the presence of periodontitis, resorptive lesions, retained root remnants or other lesions, is mandatory. Systemic diseases, e.g. chronic renal failure and diabetes mellitus, which may predispose to the development of severe gingival inflammation in the presence of plaque, must also be excluded before any treatment is initiated.

The idiopathic type of CGS is refractory to medical management. The extraction of all premolar and molar teeth has given the most dependable results, with up to 80% of cats being clinically cured or significantly improved.

In this case, no underlying cause for the inflammatory reaction in the oral mucous membranes was identified, i.e. it is classified as an idiopathic CGS, but an oropharyngeal swab taken from the glossopalatine mucosa for FCV isolation was positive. The role of FCV in the development of CGS is unclear. FCV has been isolated from up to 100% of CGS cases compared with up to 25% of cats in a healthy population, indicating that the carrier state may be a prerequisite for the induction of chronic stomatitis. However, FCV isolated from cats with CGS and then inoculated into specific pathogen-free cats produced signs of acute calici virus infection but not CGS, suggesting that other factors contribute towards the development of the oral inflammation. The fact that CGS often resolves in FCV-positive cats after extraction of all or most teeth and the subsequent reduction in dental plaque suggests that other antigenic stimuli are involved in the pathogenesis of the condition. It is possible that it is the sum of the total antigenic stimulation from plaque bacteria and viruses that is significant in the development of CGS.

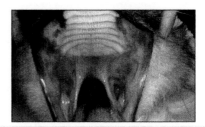

Figure 15.2 Rostrocaudal photograph of the oral cavity. Much reduced oral inflammation is observed 6 weeks after starting treatment with feline omega interferon.

TREATMENT PERFORMED

One mega unit/kg of feline recombinant interferon omega (Virbagen; Virbac) was given by subcutaneous injection on alternative days for five doses. After the fifth dose, 10 000 IU feline recombinant interferon omega (FeIFN) in 2 ml of isotonic saline was given orally by the owner once daily for 2 months and then on alternate days for the third month. No other medication was given.

TREATMENT OPTIONS

1. Conservative management, i.e. meticulous periodontal therapy followed by daily home care (daily chlorhexidine rinse and toothbrushing). The cat only had incisors and canines, and there was only mild gingivitis associated with these teeth. Conservative management was thus deemed inappropriate.
2. Extraction of the remaining teeth. The incisor and canine teeth were not affected by periodontitis, and there was no evidence of oral inflammation in the rostral portion of the mouth. Extracting these teeth was deemed unlikely to have much beneficial effect on the caudal inflammation.
3. Medical management. The cat had already received nine courses of antibiotics and long-acting steroid over the last 2 years. The effect of each treatment had become shorter every time.
4. Interferon. Interferons are cytokines that have antiviral, antiproliferative and immunomodulatory effects through direct and indirect effects on target cells. Studies have shown that interferon shortens the duration of acute calici virus infection in experimentally infected cats. It may thus also be effective in treating cats with CGS in which infection with FCV is a contributory factor.

RECHECKS

The cat was re-examined, and oral swabs were taken for FCV isolation after 6, 10 and 14 weeks. There was a significant reduction in oral inflammation (Fig. 15.2) and no FCV was isolated.

Six months later, the cat was re-examined under general anaesthesia. There was no inflammation of the oral mucosa (Fig. 15.3). Swabs were taken from the tonsils and tonsillar crypts for FCV isolation. The result was negative.

PROGNOSIS

The use of interferon therapy for CGS is still being evaluated. We have treated more than half a dozen cases (all of which were FCV positive, FeLV and FIV negative and had had complete extraction of at least all premolar and molar teeth) and seen improvement in all but one case. The exact treatment regimen is under development. We have treated some cases using the same protocol as described for this case; other cases have been treated using a slightly different protocol in that, following the initial 1 mega unit/kg subcutaneous injection on alternate days for five doses, the same injection regimen was repeated 30 days after the first injection and no oral

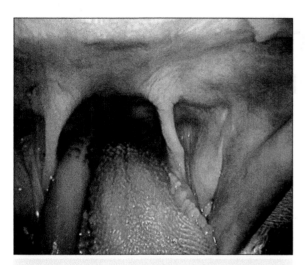

Figure 15.3 Rostrocaudal photograph of the caudal oral cavity. The oral mucosa is not inflamed. This photograph was taken 6 months after treatment with feline omega interferon.

FeIFN was given. We are also evaluating intralesional injection as a possible protocol.

The clinical improvement seen in these cases would suggest that interferon therapy may be useful in cases that are refractory to surgical management.

COMMENTS

CGS resolves in many FCV-positive cases following radical or full-mouth extraction without any specific antiviral treatment. In roughly 80% of cases removal of the premolars and molars results in reduction of the inflammation, if not cure. In the remaining 20% of cases further treatment is required, i.e. extraction of remaining teeth, antiseptics (daily chlorhexidine flushing), intermittent antibiotics, interferon. It is essential that the owner is aware that their cat may fall into the 20% of cases that are refractory to surgical management alone.

In assessing outcome of treatment, the oral inflammatory reaction needs to be linked to clinical behaviour. In some cases, the cats show no evidence of any oral discomfort, i.e. they eat, drink and groom themselves, yet on oral examination there is evidence of inflammation, although not as severe as before extraction. I view these as successful and do not interfere unless clinical signs of discomfort develop.

It should be noted that antiseptics or intermittent antibiotics after surgical treatment (extraction of at least all premolar and molar teeth) may work well for some patients.

In this case, extraction of the remaining teeth was not appropriate and intermittent antibiotics had been tried. Consequently, immune modulation using interferon was chosen. FCV isolation should always be performed prior to using interferon and also to monitor viral status as a consequence of treatment. Interferon should only be used in FCV-positive cats where extraction of at least all premolar and molar teeth has not led to cure. Using interferon without surgical treatment (extraction) has not been shown to have any benefit.

16 Canine chronic gingivostomatitis

INITIAL PRESENTATION

Halitosis and selective feeding.

PATIENT DETAILS

A 6-year-old, neutered male, greyhound.

CASE HISTORY

The dog was a retired racing greyhound. He had been with the owners for 3 months at the time of presentation to the referring veterinarian. The owners were concerned about halitosis and his eating habits. He was on a mixed dry kibble and moist canned food diet, but would only eat the moist food and would not eat every day, and never any large amounts. He had lost 2 kg in 3 months. The referring veterinarian diagnosed 'severe periodontal disease' and the dog received periodontal therapy (scaling and polishing), followed by a short course of antibiotics. This resulted in a reduction of the oral inflammation and increased appetite for a few weeks, after which both the halitosis and eating problems returned. The dog was then referred to us for investigation and treatment. Haematology and biochemistry screens were normal.

ORAL EXAMINATION – CONSCIOUS

Conscious oral examination was allowed, which revealed intense halitosis and gingivostomatitis (Fig. 16.1a). The mandibular lymph nodes were enlarged and seemed painful on palpation.

ORAL EXAMINATION – UNDER GENERAL ANAESTHETIC

A thorough oral examination, including investigating periodontal parameters, was performed and all findings were noted on the dental record.

In summary, examination under general anaesthesia identified the following:

1. Severe inflammation of free and attached gingivae (Fig. 16.1a, b)
2. Inflammation of the buccal mucosa (Fig. 16.2)
3. Inflammation of the lingual mucosa
4. Moderate amounts of plaque and calculus were present on the buccal aspects of the upper premolars and molars (Fig. 16.2)
5. No evidence of periodontitis (loss of periodontal attachment), i.e. no increased PPD or GR.

FURTHER INVESTIGATIONS

All teeth were present and there were no clinical signs of periodontitis, so radiographs were not indicated at this stage.

ORAL PROBLEM LIST

Chronic gingivostomatitis.

THEORY REFRESHER

Chronic gingivostomatitis (CGS) describes a clinical syndrome characterized by focal or diffuse inflammation of the gingivae and oral mucosa. While it is more common in cats, it also occurs in dogs.

It is thought to be an inappropriate response to oral antigens, namely bacterial plaque present on the tooth surfaces. While underlying vesiculo-bullous disease, e.g. pemphigus and pemphigoid or discoid lupus erythema-

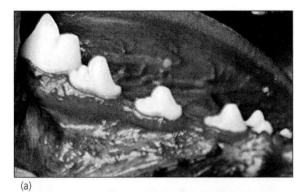

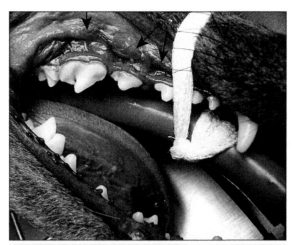

Figure 16.2 Oblique lateral photograph of the right maxilla. There is only a moderate amount of calculus and plaque present. Note the inflammation of the buccal mucosa as well as the gingivae.

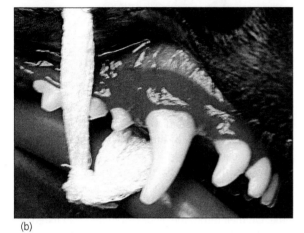

(b)

Figure 16.1 Lateral photograph of the right mandibular premolar region (a) and oblique lateral photograph of the right rostral upper jaw (b). The free and attached gingivae are intensely inflamed. Note the clear demarcation of gingiva from oral mucosa.

tosus (DLE), cannot be excluded, it is essential to have plaque control before these can be investigated.

In the dog, I approach CGS as follows:

1. Haematology and biochemistry screens to exclude systemic diseases, e.g. endocrine or renal disorders, which may predispose to the development of severe gingival inflammation in the presence of plaque
2. Meticulous oral examination with radiographs as necessary to identify a possible reason for the intense inflammatory response, e.g. retained root remnants, periodontitis, other dental pathology
3. Periodontal therapy (scaling and polishing) and treatment of pathological lesions, i.e. extract root remnants, extract teeth affected by periodontitis

4. Daily home care (mechanical and chemical plaque control) is instituted
5. Assess response to treatment.

In the great majority of cases, the above approach results in complete cure. In some cases, the owner is not able to maintain adequate plaque control and selective extraction (removal of teeth that the owner cannot keep clean, usually the posterior teeth) is then performed. This is usually sufficient. In one aggressive dog that would not allow home care, all teeth were extracted. This resulted in healthy oral mucosa.

In this dog, there was no evidence of any underlying systemic disease predisposing to oral inflammation, and all the teeth were present and periodontally sound, i.e. there was no clinical loss of attachment.

CLINICAL TIPS

- It is essential to have plaque control before underlying vesiculo-bullous disease can be investigated.
- Control of this condition relies more on what the owner does at home to keep the plaque burden to a minimum than it does on professional periodontal therapy.

TREATMENT OPTIONS

The treatment of choice for this case was conservative management, i.e. meticulous periodontal therapy followed by daily home care (daily chlorhexidine rinse and toothbrushing). Theoretically, once dental deposits have been removed, if the owner controls plaque accumulation then the inflammatory reaction should subside. Plaque control by the owner would consist of daily removal using a toothbrush (mechanical plaque removal), augmented by daily rinsing of the oral cavity with the gold standard antiplaque agent, namely chlorhexidine (chemical plaque control). This regime would need to be followed daily for the rest of the animal's life to maintain healthy gingivae and oral mucosae.

TREATMENT PERFORMED

Periodontal therapy, i.e. meticulous supra- and subgingival scaling and tooth polishing.

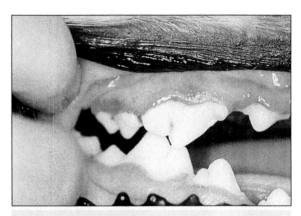

Figure 16.3 Right-side lateral photograph 1 month after initial treatment. The inflammation of the free and attached gingivae is much reduced. The teeth were polished and the owners resumed daily toothbrushing.

POSTOPERATIVE CARE

- Daily toothbrushing
- Daily chlorhexidine rinse
- Ten-day course of antibiotics.
- The dog was booked for conscious examination in 1 month.

The owner was given instructions how to brush the teeth and apply chlorhexidine rinse. Complementary toothbrush and toothpaste were supplied, as well as plaque disclosing swabs, so that he could check the adequacy of the plaque removal.

RECHECKS

At recheck 1 month later, the owners reported that the dog was bright, alert and eating well (kibble as well as the moist food). There had been no problems with the toothbrushing. In fact, they were able to open his mouth and brush palatal and lingual tooth surfaces, as well as the buccal. There was no halitosis. Oral examination under general anaesthesia revealed no dental deposits and relatively healthy gingivae (Fig. 16.3). The teeth were polished. The chlorhexidine rinse was discontinued and the owner advised to carry on with meticulous daily toothbrushing using toothpaste.

At recheck 3 and 6 months after periodontal debridement, conscious examination revealed no dental deposits and clinically healthy gingivae as a result of the continued daily brushing.

Nine months after initial therapy, the owners went on holiday for 2 weeks, and the dog was placed in kennels and did not have its teeth brushed for that period of time. On their return the gingivostomatitis had flared up. They started daily toothbrushing and daily chlorhexidine rinsing, and within 10 days the oral mucosae were no longer inflamed.

One year after initially therapy, the dog was placed under general anaesthesia for oral examination and periodontal therapy as required. A thorough oral examination revealed no clinical evidence of periodontitis, i.e. no increased probing depths and no gingival recession. There was minimal plaque accumulation and virtually no calculus. Mild gingivitis was evident at some sites (Fig. 16.4). The teeth were scaled and polished.

The owners were advised to carry on with daily toothbrushing. They were also reminded that professional periodontal therapy would be required. The dog was booked for re-evaluation in 1 year's time.

PROGNOSIS

As long as the owners carry on with the daily home care, the prognosis for this dog is excellent. However, if the owners become lax with plaque removal the gingivostomatitis will return within a few weeks. This occurred when they went on holiday for 2 weeks. Resuming daily toothbrushing returned the oral mucosa to health.

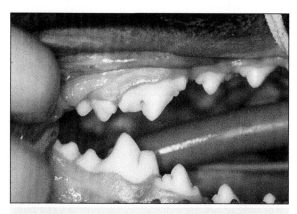

Figure 16.4 Right-side lateral photograph 1 year after initial treatment. After 1 year of daily toothbrushing there is minimal accumulation of dental deposits and only a mild marginal gingivitis. The oral mucosae are not inflamed.

COMMENTS

We have seen many similar cases over the years, and they have all responded to meticulous plaque control and selective extraction in some cases (i.e. extracting posterior teeth that the owner cannot keep clean). I have not identified an underlying autoimmune disorder in any of these cases.

The control of this condition relies more on what the owner does at home to keep the plaque burden to a minimum than it does on professional periodontal therapy. The owner must understand this and be prepared to perform the home care from the outset. In my experience, most owners are prepared to take on this responsibility and, given the right instructions and motivation, they do a very good job. It does require continuous reinforcement!

SECTION 5

ROOT RESORPTION

17 Root resorption – an introduction

Hard tissues are protected from resorption by their surface layers of blast cells. It appears that as long as these layers are intact, resorption cannot occur. Although bone, dentine and cementum are mesenchymal, mineralized tissues composed mainly of collagen and hydroxyapatite, they differ markedly in their susceptibility to resorption.

Two mechanisms are involved in resorption of hard tissue:

1. The trigger
2. A reason for the resorption to continue.

The trigger mechanism in root resorption is a root surface detached from its protective blast cell layer. Detachment may follow any damage to the protective blast layer. For the resorption to continue, a stimulus is required, e.g. infection or a continuous mechanical force.

Root resorption always starts at a surface, and is termed internal if emanating from the root canal wall and as external if emanating from the root surface.

Internal resorption is rare in permanent teeth. Radiographically, it is characterized by an oval-shaped enlargement of the root canal space. Histological examination reveals resorption of the internal aspect of the root by multinucleated giant cells adjacent to granulation tissue in the pulp. There are different theories regarding the origin of the pulpal granulation tissue involved in internal resorption. The most logical explanation is that it is pulp tissue that is inflamed because of an infected coronal pulp space. In addition to the requirement of the presence of granulation tissue, root resorption takes place only if the odontoblast layer and predentine are lost or altered.

Traditionally, a pink tooth has been thought pathognomonic of internal root resorption; the pink colour is caused by granulation tissue in the coronal dentine undermining the crown enamel. However, a pink tooth can also be a feature of a specific type of external root resorption, namely peripheral inflammatory external root resorption (detailed later in this chapter), which must be ruled out before a diagnosis of internal root resorption is made. A pink tooth can also be due to pulpal haemorrhage.

There are different forms of external root resorption described in man. The underlying mechanism is understood for some of these, whereas other forms are still unexplained and therefore termed idiopathic. A classification system for external root resorptions that have a known mechanism has been proposed in man and is as follows:

1. Surface resorption
2. Replacement resorption associated with ankylosis
3. Inflammatory resorption.

This classification system works for external root resorption in cats and dogs as well.

SURFACE RESORPTION

A surface resorption is initiated subsequent to injury of the cementoblast layer. The denuded root surface attracts clast cells, which will resorb the cementum for as long as osteoclast-activating factors are released at the site of injury, usually a few days. When the resorption stops, cells from the periodontal ligament will proliferate and populate the resorbed area, resulting in deposition of reparative dental tissue (new cementum).

It is thought that minor traumas caused by unintentional biting on hard objects, bruxism, etc. can cause localized damage to the periodontal ligament and trigger this type of resorption. The process is self-limiting and reversible.

REPLACEMENT RESORPTION

Replacement resorption results in replacement of the dental hard tissue by bone. When a surface resorption stops, cells from the periodontal ligament will proliferate and populate the resorbed area. If the resorption is large it will take some time for these cells to cover the entire surface. Cells from the nearby bone may then arrive first and establish themselves on the resorbed surface. Bone will thus be formed directly upon the dental hard tissue. This results in fusion between bone and tooth, i.e. ankylosis. This can be seen as a form of healing; the bone has accepted the dental hard tissue as part of itself and the tooth becomes involved in the normal skeletal turnover. So, during consequent remodelling of bone, both dental hard tissue and bone will be resorbed. When the resorptive process is over, the osteoblasts will form bone in the resorbed area. In this way the dental tissues will gradually be replaced by bone. In short, ankylosis is a form of healing of root surface resorption, which from a clinical standpoint may be undesirable.

INFLAMMATORY RESORPTION

In addition to apical root resorption caused by apical periodontitis as a consequence of pulpal necrosis, there are two main forms of external resorption associated with inflammation in the periodontal tissues, namely:

1. Peripheral inflammatory root resorption (PIRR)
2. External inflammatory root resorption (EIRR).

Both forms are triggered by destruction of the cementoblasts. In PIRR, the osteoclast-activating factors, which perpetuate the resorptive process, are provided by an inflammatory lesion in the adjacent periodontal tissues. EIRR, on the other hand, receives its stimulus for continued resorption from an infected necrotic pulp. In other words, the common factor for these two types of resorption is inflammation in the adjacent tissues. As far as PIRR is concerned, the periradicular inflammation per se keeps the resorptive process going, while the stimulus for EIRR is periradicular inflammation caused by products released from the necrotic pulp by way of the dentinal tubules exposed by the resorption.

Peripheral inflammatory root resorption (PIRR): A damaged cervical root surface (e.g. due to excessive scaling or other trauma) is usually covered by junctional epithelium. Sometimes this does not occur; instead, the damaged area will be repopulated by connective tissue. In the presence of a periodontal lesion the onset of a resorptive process is triggered. It is conceivable that the inflammatory cells in the lesion recognize the osteoclast-activating factors of the denuded root surface, and thus

initiate and maintain clastic activity. This type of resorption is found immediately apical to the marginal tissues and thus is often situated cervically, and has therefore been termed cervical root resorption. However, the location is related to the level of the marginal tissues and the pocket depth, and may thus not always be cervical in position.

External inflammatory root resorption (EIRR): This type of root resorption is a complication that can follow dental trauma. It begins as a surface resorption due to damage to the periodontal ligament in conjunction with the traumatic injury. The pulp is also damaged and becomes necrotic. As the surface resorption approaches the dentine, the osteoclasts will carry on their resorptive activity, as necrotic and possible infected pulp matter is released from the thus exposed dentine tubules. The pulp products will then maintain an inflammatory process in the adjacent periodontal tissues that in turn will trigger the continuance of the resorption.

Odontoclastic resorptive lesions (ORLs) may well represent the single most common dental disease seen in the cat. They account for a large proportion of the dental clinical caseload in small animal veterinary practice. It is likely that the lesions are either peripheral inflammatory root resorption (triggered by inflammation of periodontal tissues) or replacement resorption (idiopathic).

Clinically, they commonly present as a cavity at the cemento-enamel junction of the tooth. However, studies which included radiography have demonstrated that the resorption can occur anywhere on the root surfaces, i.e. not necessarily at the cemento-enamel junction. The lesions can be detected by means of a combination of visual inspection, tactile examination with a dental explorer and radiography.

Visual inspection and tactile examination with a dental explorer will only identify end-stage lesions, i.e. when the process involves the crown and has resulted in an obvious cavity. Radiography will identify lesions that are localized to the root surfaces within the alveolar bone, which would not be detected by clinical methods. Consequently, radiography is required for diagnosis of ORLs. In fact, full-mouth radiographs (using intra-oral radiographic techniques) are recommended for all cats presented for dental therapy.

Most studies have shown an increased incidence with increasing age. Differences in breed susceptibility have also been suggested in some studies, but differences in mean age among different breed groups make comparisons of significance suspect. The lesions have also been shown to occur in both feral and wild cats, and in other species, e.g. man, dog and chinchilla.

In a recent study, which investigated the incidence of ORLs in a clinically healthy population of 228 relatively young cats (mean age was 4.92 years), using a combination of clinical examination and radiography, it was found that the overall prevalence rate was 29% and that it increased with age. The mandibular third premolars (307, 407) were the most commonly affected teeth and the pattern of odontoclastic resorptive lesion (ORL) development was symmetrical in most cats. Cats with clinically missing teeth were more likely to have ORLs. Neutering, sex, age at neutering or mean whole-mouth gingivitis index did not affect the prevalence of ORL.

Currently, the suggested methods of managing odontoclastic resorptive lesions are:
1. Conservative management
2. Tooth extraction
3. Coronal amputation.

Historically, restoration of the tooth surface has been recommended for the treatment of accessible lesions that extend into the dentine and do not involve pulp tissue. However, several studies have shown that tooth resorption continues and the restorations are lost. Consequently, the use of restoration of odontoclastic lesions as a major treatment technique cannot be recommended.

Conservative management: This consists of monitoring the lesions clinically and radiographically. This approach is recommended for lesions that are not evident on clinical examination, i.e. only seen radiographically, and there is no evidence of discomfort or pain. In general practice, most lesions are only diagnosed when pathology is extensive and conservative management is rarely an option.

In most cases, extraction or coronal amputation of an affected tooth is indicated. Preoperative radiographs are mandatory to allow selection of the appropriate treatment option.

Extraction: Teeth with ORLs are notoriously difficult to extract, as the root is resorbing and being replaced by bone-like tissue. Moreover, there are areas of ankylosis, i.e. fusion of bone and tooth substance, along the root surface. In addition to preoperative radiographs to detect the lesions and determine appropriate treatment, postoperative radiographs to ensure that the whole tooth has been removed are required.

Teeth affected by ORL can be extracted using a closed technique, but an open technique is usually less traumatic to the tissues and easier to perform.

Coronal amputation: The indications for, and outcome of, coronal amputation have been well documented and the procedure is recommended for selected cases, but needs radiographic monitoring at regular intervals postoperatively to ensure that the root is resorbing and that healing is uneventful.

In brief, the technique involves raising a gingival flap both buccally and palatally/lingually to expose the margin of the alveolar bone. The crown of the affected tooth is amputated using a small round bur. A small amount of root tissue is also removed with the bur, just enough to ensure that the intentionally retained root(s) is (are) apical to the alveolar margin. The gingival flap is replaced and sutured in place.

In summary:
- ORLs are common.
- The lesions are progressive.
- Diagnosis requires radiography.
- The purpose of the treatment is the relief of discomfort or pain. In most instances, extraction of the tooth, or coronal amputation, remain the preferable treatment options.
- Successful extraction and uncomplicated healing needs clinical and radiographic monitoring.

18 No clinical signs of root resorption

INITIAL PRESENTATION

Bilateral upper lip ulcers.

PATIENT DETAILS

A 7-year-old, male, domestic short-haired cat.

CASE HISTORY

The upper canines had been extracted a few months earlier. Following the extractions of the upper canine teeth, the lower canines were impinging on the upper lip (in fact, the upper lip was trapped between the maxillary alveolar ridge and the lower canines bilaterally), causing ulcerated indentations. The lip lesions were causing discomfort as evidenced by reduced appetite and pawing at the mouth to free the trapped lip tissue. The case was referred to us for management of the lip ulcerations. The reason for extracting the upper canine teeth was not mentioned in the clinical records.

ORAL EXAMINATION – CONSCIOUS

The owner reported that the lip lesions had developed within a few weeks of extracting the upper canine teeth. They were not sure why the teeth had been extracted, but thought they could have been 'broken'.

The cat allowed conscious examination of the head and mouth, which identified the following:
1. Bilateral deep ulcerated indentation of the upper lip where the lower canines were occluding
2. Occlusion otherwise normal
3. Teeth 106 and 206 were missing
4. Mild gingivitis, localized to the upper premolars and molars bilaterally.

The cat was obviously uncomfortable, and pawed at its face and freed the trapped lip tissue several times during the examination.

ORAL EXAMINATION – UNDER GENERAL ANAESTHETIC

A thorough oral examination, including investigating periodontal parameters, was performed and all findings were noted on the dental record.

In summary, examination under general anaesthesia identified the following:
1. Bilateral deep ulcerated indentation of the upper lip where the lower canines were occluding
2. Teeth 106 and 107 were missing
3. Mild gingivitis, localized to the upper premolars and molars bilaterally.

FURTHER INVESTIGATIONS

A series of full-mouth radiographs (10 films) was taken.

RADIOGRAPHIC FINDINGS

1. The extraction sockets of 104 and 204 had healed and there was no evidence of any retained root remnants.
2. Teeth 106 and 206 were absent, with some tooth-like material remaining in the alveoli, but the teeth were almost completely resorbed and replaced by alveolar bone.

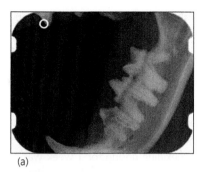

(a)

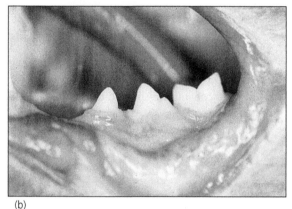

(b)

Figure 18.1 Radiograph (a) and lateral photograph (b) of the left lower premolars and molar.

(a) Note the extensive resorption of both roots of 307, with the process extending into the crown dentine. The periodontal ligament space is not apparent, and it is difficult to differentiate between tooth substance and bone.

(b) Clinically, the left premolars and molar appear healthy. The gingivae are clinically healthy and there is no evidence of disease of dental hard tissue. The resorptive process affecting the roots and crown of 307 would not have been detected without radiography.

3. External root resorption affecting 307 could be seen (Fig. 18.1a, b).

THEORY REFRESHER

Resorption of teeth is common in domestic cats. Tooth resorption has also been shown to occur in feral and wild cats.

Odontoclastic resorptive lesions (ORLs) are a type of 'idiopathic' external root resorption, where the hard tissues of the root surfaces are destroyed by the activity of multinucleated cells called odontoclasts. The destroyed root surface is replaced by cementum- or bone-like tissue. The process starts in the cementum and progresses to involve the dentine, where it spreads along the dentine tubules and eventually comes to involve the dentine of the crown as well as the root. The peri-pulpal dentine is relatively resistant to resorption and the pulp therefore only becomes involved late in the disease. The process extends through the crown dentine, eventually reaching the enamel. The enamel is either resorbed or it fractures off and a cavity becomes clinically evident. In the absence of routine radiography, the lesions are first noted clinically when they become evident in the crown, often as cavities at the cemento-enamel junction (CEJ). The first clinical manifestation of ORLs is thus a late-stage lesion. In many cases, the progressive dentine destruction with ORLs weakens and undermines the crown to such an extent that minor trauma, e.g. during chewing, causes the crown to fracture off, leaving the root in the alveolar bone. The resorbing root remnants are usually covered by intact gingiva. However, in some cases the overlying gingiva may be inflamed.

Visual inspection and tactile examination with a dental explorer will only identify end-stage lesions, i.e. when the process involves the crown and has resulted in an obvious cavity. Radiography will identify lesions that are localized to the root surfaces within the alveolar bone (as in this case), which would not be detected by clinical methods. Moreover, it is only with the aid of radiography that the extent of a resorptive process can be identified. Selection of the best treatment option thus depends on radiography. In fact, a series of full-mouth radiographs (the technique is covered in Chapter 4) is recommended for all cats presented for dental therapy. If taking a series of full-mouth radiographs is not possible, e.g. financial restrictions, then take one view of each mandibular premolar/molar region. The mandibular third premolars are the most commonly affected teeth and it has been shown that, in nine out of 10 cats with resorptive lesions, the process will be identified on these two views. If radiographs show resorption of these teeth, then a full-mouth series must be taken.

It remains a matter of debate as to whether odontoclastic resorptive lesions (ORLs) cause discomfort or pain to the affected individual. Based on the fact that pulpal inflammation occurs late in the disease process, it seems likely that lesions that are limited to the root surfaces and do not communicate with the oral environment are asymptomatic. However, once dentine destruction has progressed to such an extent that the process invades the pulp and/or a communication with the oral cavity has been established (when the enamel has been resorbed or it has fractured off to reveal the dentine to the oral cavity), then discomfort and/or pain are likely. Some cats may show clinical signs indicating oral discomfort or pain, e.g. changes in food preferences (soft rather than hard diet) and reduced food intake, but many cats do not.

TREATMENT OPTIONS

To date, there is no known treatment, which prevents development and/or progression of ORLs. It seems unlikely that such treatment can be developed without knowledge of the cause of the pathology. Currently, the suggested methods of managing odontoclastic resorptive lesions are:

1. Conservative management
2. Tooth extraction
3. Coronal (crown) amputation.

TREATMENT PERFORMED

1. Periodontal therapy to remove plaque and calculus and provide a clean environment.
2. Crown amputation of 307. A postoperative radiograph was taken as baseline for future monitoring of continued resorption.

3. Tooth shortening and endodontic therapy, and restoration of 304 and 404, to remove the traumatic occlusion and allow healing of the lip ulcers.
4. Debriding of lip indentations (epithelium removed with a scalpel and left to heal by second intention).

RECHECKS

At conscious examination 3 weeks later, the owner reported that the cat was no longer pawing at its face and had regained its appetite. The lip lesions had healed. The restorations of 304 and 404 were in place and the teeth were not discoloured. The gingiva overlying the intentionally retained roots of 307 had healed and there was no evidence of inflammation.

Examination under anaesthesia and full-mouth radiographs 6 months later confirmed successful outcome of the endodontic therapy of 304 and 404, showed continued root resorption of the root remnants of 307 (Fig. 18.2) and identified development of root resorption of 407 (Fig. 18.3a–c). Treatment consisted of crown amputation of the distal root and open extraction of the mesial root of 407.

At conscious examination 3 weeks later, the gingiva over 407 had healed with no evidence of inflammation. The cat was rebooked for examination under general anaesthesia and full-mouth radiographs in 1 year's time, to monitor the outcome of the coronal amputations of 307 and 407, and to identify and treat any new resorptive lesions that are likely to develop.

PROGNOSIS

Cats with diagnosed resorptive lesions will develop further lesions with time. The lesions can affect any

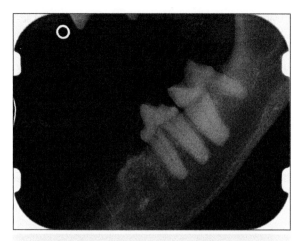

Figure 18.2 Radiograph of the left mandible 6 months after crown amputation of 307. The intentionally retained roots of 307 were covered by healthy gingiva and the radiograph confirms continued resorption of the roots.

tooth, but the pattern of development is strikingly symmetrical, i.e. if a cat has root resorption of 307, it is just a matter of time before 407 is affected.

Regular (usually annual) examinations under anaesthesia and a series of full-mouth radiographs are indicated for cats with diagnosed root resorption.

In short, this cat is guaranteed to develop root resorption of other teeth, and requires lifelong radiographic monitoring and intervention (coronal amputation or extraction) as appropriate. It is essential that the owner is aware of the need for continuous monitoring and intervention as required.

COMMENTS

External root resorption affecting the root surfaces only is not generally associated with clinical signs of discomfort or pain. The reduction in appetite experienced by

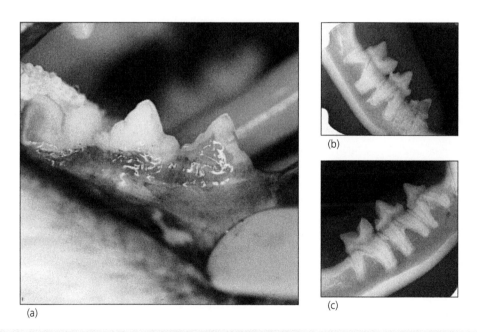

(a)

(b)

(c)

Figure 18.3 Lateral photograph (a) and radiographs (b, c) of the right mandible.

(a) The resorptive lesion affecting 407 is evident on clinical examination.

(b) The radiograph confirms extensive root resorption of the distal root and crown of 407. Note that the mesial root is not resorbing to the same extent and a periodontal ligament space can be detected. Treatment consisted of crown amputation of the distal root and open extraction of the mesial root.

(c) This radiograph was taken 6 months earlier and there is no radiographic evidence of root resorption of 407. The importance of radiographs as part of a full oral examination should not be ignored. If radiographs are not taken, pathology will not be detected.

this cat was more likely attributable to the discomfort from the lip lesions caused by the lower canine occlusion than to the root resorption.

Crown amputation has a good success rate if performed with the correct indications, namely that there is obvious loss of tooth substance and lack of a clear periodontal ligament space on the radiograph (i.e. a distinct root cannot be identified from surrounding bone). It is contraindicated where there is no radiographic evidence of root resorption, i.e. a root has a smooth contour and is clearly delineated by a periodontal ligament space. In this cat the distal root of 407 was obviously resorbing while the mesial root seemed less affected. Consequently, this tooth was treated by means of crown amputation of the distal root and open extraction of the mesial root.

Crown amputation needs to be monitored clinically and radiographically. Gingival healing over the intentionally retained roots needs to be checked 3–4 weeks after surgery. If the gingiva has not healed or there is marked inflammation, further surgery to remove tooth root substance is required. Continued root resorption needs to be evaluated radiographically, usually 6 months after initial surgery.

19 Virtually edentulous, no clinical signs of root resorption

INITIAL PRESENTATION

Inappetance and dysphagia.

PATIENT DETAILS

A 14-year-old, female, domestic short-haired cat.

CASE HISTORY

The cat had always had an extremely good appetite until roughly a month ago, when she started having trouble eating. She seemed to want to eat but had trouble swallowing and would stop eating after a few mouthfuls. In the last 2 weeks she had not been eating at all and barely drinking. She was drooling continuously. She was referred to us for evaluation and management.

The cat had never had any oral or dental problems. In fact, she had never had her teeth scaled and polished. The owner was very clear that they had restricted finances and would only want treatment if I could guarantee successful outcome at minimal cost.

ORAL EXAMINATION – CONSCIOUS

The cat was distressed and would only allow a cursory conscious examination of the face and oral cavity. She was virtually edentulous, with only the right upper canine tooth evident. All edentulous areas were covered by clinically healthy gingivae. She strongly resented attempts to open the mouth, so this was abandoned.

The owner declined pre-anaesthetic blood work-up.

ORAL EXAMINATION – UNDER GENERAL ANAESTHETIC

Examination under general anaesthesia confirmed that 104 was the only remaining tooth. There was no evi-dence of any pathology affecting 104 based on inspection and tactile exploration with a dental explorer. There was no inflammation of the gingivae and oral mucous membranes. However, a large, right-sided tonsillar mass was identified. The owner did not want any further treatment (likelihood of squamous cell carcinoma and poor prognosis) and the cat was euthanized.

FURTHER INVESTIGATIONS

I was given permission to take a series of full-mouth radiographs and submit a section of the tonsillar mass for histopathology. This was for my own interest and the client was not charged. I wanted to confirm that the mass really was a squamous cell carcinoma and I was interested in the dental findings.

RADIOGRAPHIC FINDINGS

The series of full-mouth radiographs (eight views) identified numerous teeth in different stages of replacement resorption. See Figs 19.1, 19.2, 19.3, 19.4 and 19.5 for details of radiographic findings.

HISTOPATHOLOGY

Histopathology of the tonsillar biopsy confirmed the clinical suspicion of squamous cell carcinoma.

THEORY REFRESHER

Resorption of teeth is common in domestic cats. Tooth resorption has also been shown to occur in feral and wild cats.

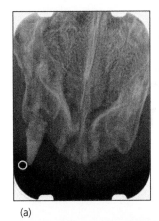

(a)

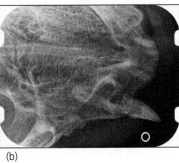

(b)

Figure 19.1 Rostrocaudal radiograph (a) and right lateral radiograph (b) of the rostral upper jaw.

(a) The upper incisors and canines are in different stages of replacement resorption. The roots of the incisors are still identifiable as 'tooth', but the absence of a clear periodontal ligament space indicates active external root resorption and replacement of lost tissue by bone. These roots are ankylosed, i.e. there is fusion between root and bone. The crown of 104 is still in place, but most of the root has been resorbed and replaced by bone. Tooth 204 has been almost completely resorbed and replaced by bone-like material. It is impossible to clearly differentiate between remaining root tissue and bone.

(b) The incisors, right upper canine and some premolars are in different stages of replacement resorption. The lateral view confirms the findings identified from the rostrocaudal view. Note that the root of 104 is more intact than one could see in the rostrocaudal view. Different projections of the same area generally give a clearer picture of the extent of the pathology than a single view. There is also evidence of resorbing root remnants in the premolar area. Their exact position is best ascertained in a lateral radiograph of the premolar and molar region (Fig. 19.2).

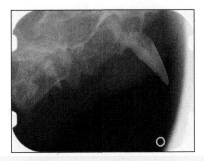

Figure 19.2 Lateral radiograph of the right upper jaw centring on the premolar and molar region. This view gives a third projection of the resorbing 104, giving a more detailed visualization of the root pathology. There is no evidence of 106, 107 and 109, but the resorbing root remnants of 108 are obvious. Clinically, all edentulous areas were covered by healthy gingiva.

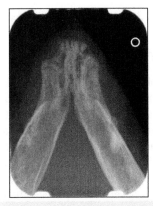

Figure 19.3 Rostrocaudal radiograph of the rostral lower jaw. Clinically, there was no evidence of teeth and the edentulous areas were covered by healthy gingiva. The replacement resorption of the lower incisors and canines is obvious. There is also evidence of resorbing root remnants in the premolar and molar regions bilaterally. Their exact position is best ascertained in a lateral radiograph of the premolar and molar region (Figs 19.4 and 19.5).

Odontoclastic resorptive lesions (ORLs) are a type of 'idiopathic' external root resorption, where the hard tissues of the root surfaces are destroyed by the activity of multinucleated cells called odontoclasts. The destroyed root surface is replaced by cementum- or bone-like tissue. The process starts in the cementum and progresses to involve the dentine, where it spreads along the dentine tubules and eventually comes to involve the dentine of the crown as well as the root. The peri-pulpal dentine is relatively resistant to resorption and the pulp

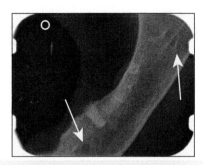

Figure 19.4 Lateral radiograph of the left mandibular premolar and molar regions. Tooth 307 has been completely resorbed and replaced by bone. The mesial root of 308 and the apical portions of both roots of 309 are still identifiable as 'tooth' undergoing active resorption. Note the obvious mental and mandibular foramina.

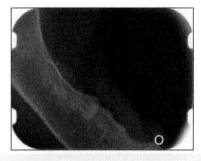

Figure 19.5 Lateral radiograph of the right mandibular premolar and molar regions. It is only the apical portion of the mesial root of 408 that is still identifiable as 'tooth'. Note the obvious mental foramen.

therefore only becomes involved late in the disease. The process extends through the crown dentine, eventually reaching the enamel. The enamel is either resorbed or it fractures off and a cavity becomes clinically evident. In the absence of routine radiography, the lesions are first noted clinically when they become evident in the crown, often as cavities at the cemento-enamel junction (CEJ). The first clinical manifestation of ORLs is thus a late-stage lesion. In many cases, the progressive dentine destruction with ORLs weakens and undermines the crown to such an extent that minor trauma, e.g. during chewing, causes the crown to fracture off, leaving the root in the alveolar bone. The resorbing root remnants are usually covered by intact gingiva, as in this case. However, in some cases the overlying gingiva may be inflamed.

It remains a matter of debate as to whether feline odontoclastic resorptive lesions (FORLs) cause discomfort or pain to the affected individual. Based on the fact that pulpal inflammation occurs late in the disease process, it seems likely that lesions that are limited to the root surfaces and do not communicate with the oral environment are asymptomatic. However, once dentine destruction has progressed to such an extent that the process invades the pulp and/or a communication with the oral cavity has been established (when the enamel has been resorbed or it has fractured off to reveal the dentine to the oral cavity), then discomfort and/or pain are likely. Some cats may show clinical signs indicating oral discomfort or pain, e.g. changes in food preferences (soft rather than hard diet) and reduced food intake, but many cats do not.

> ### CLINICAL TIPS
>
> - Resorption of teeth is common in domestic cats.
> - The first clinical manifestation of odontoclastic resorptive lesions is a late-stage lesion.

COMMENTS

This cat had run through the whole spectrum of the resorptive process, resulting in the loss of most teeth, and had never shown any signs of oral discomfort. In fact, she had never had a day off food until the last month of her life. The dysphagia and inappetance suffered in the last month is attributable to the tonsillar squamous cell carcinoma rather than the extensive root resorption.

20 Clinical lesions and signs of discomfort

INITIAL PRESENTATION

Cavities at the buccal aspects of several teeth.

PATIENT DETAILS

A 5-year-old, female, domestic short-haired cat.

CASE HISTORY

The cat had no previous history of oral or dental disease. She had been presented to the referring veterinarian due to signs of oral discomfort, i.e. reduced appetite and selecting soft foods. On conscious clinical examination, the referring veterinarian had identified cavities at the buccal aspects of several teeth and referred the cat to us for evaluation and treatment.

ORAL EXAMINATION – CONSCIOUS

The cat did not allow anything other than a cursory examination of the head and mouth. The findings were as follows:

1. Normal occlusion
2. Generalized mild gingivitis, which was more severe at buccal aspects of upper premolars
3. Obvious cavities at the buccal aspects of 307 and 404
4. Small cavity at the buccal gingival margin of 204.

ORAL EXAMINATION – UNDER GENERAL ANAESTHESIA

A thorough oral examination, including investigating periodontal parameters, was performed and all findings were noted on the dental record.

In summary, examination under general anaesthesia identified the following:

1. Generalized mild gingivitis, which was more severe at buccal aspects of upper premolars.
2. Obvious cavities at the buccal aspects of 307 (Fig. 20.1a) and 404 (Fig. 20.2a).
3. Small cavities at the buccal gingival margin of 204 (Fig. 20.3a) and 107 (Fig. 20.4). The lesion on 107 was only obvious after calculus had been removed.
4. Teeth 106, 206, 207 and 407 were missing. The gingiva at these sites was not inflamed except over 407, which was intensely inflamed.

FURTHER INVESTIGATIONS

A series of full-mouth radiographs (10 films) was taken.

RADIOGRAPHIC FINDINGS

The following teeth were affected by external root resorption: 304 (Fig. 20.2b), 307 (Fig. 20.1b), 404 (Fig. 20.2b), 104 (Fig. 20.5), 107 and 204 (Fig. 20.3b).

At the sites of the clinically missing 106 (Fig. 20.5), 206 (Figs 20.3b and 20.6), 207 (Figs 20.3b and 20.6) and 407 (Fig. 20.7), some tooth-like material remained, but most of the dental tissue had been replaced by alveolar bone.

THEORY REFRESHER

Odontoclastic resorptive lesions (ORLs) are a type of 'idiopathic' external root resorption, where the hard tissues of the root surfaces are destroyed by the activity of multinucleated cells called odontoclasts. The destroyed

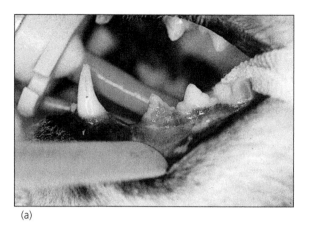
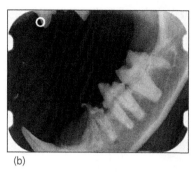

(a) (b)

Figure 20.1 Lateral photograph (a) and lateral radiograph (b) of the left lower quadrant.

(a) Note the soft tissue-filled cavity at the buccal aspect of 307.

(b) The radiograph shows that external root resorption has caused destruction and bone replacement of the mesial root. In contrast, the distal root is radiographically unaffected. The resorptive process has spread to involve the crown, resulting in the obvious clinical lesion. Once the disease is clinically apparent, i.e. a cavity is formed, root resorption is extensive. The first clinically detectable sign of resorption is already an end-stage lesion.

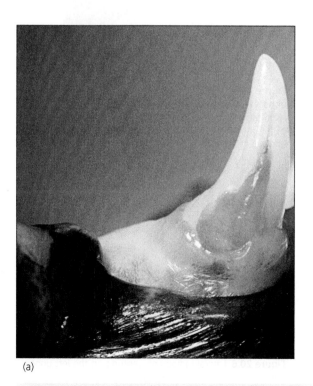
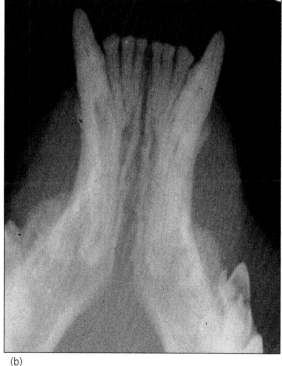

(a) (b)

Figure 20.2 Lateral photograph of the right lower canine (a) and radiograph of the rostral lower jaw (b).

(a) Note the large, soft tissue-filled cavity at the buccal aspect of 404.

(b) Both right and left canine roots are affected by replacement resorption.

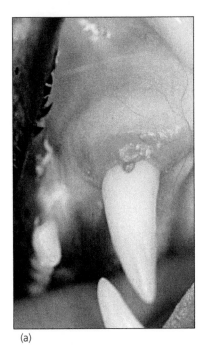

(a)

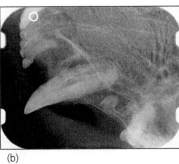

(b)

Figure 20.3 Lateral photograph of the left upper canine (a) and oblique lateral radiograph of the left rostral upper jaw (b).

(a) Note the small, soft tissue-filled cavity at the buccal aspect of 204.

(b) Replacement resorption of 204 is obvious. Note the radiolucent resorption tracks within the dentine of the root. Teeth 206 and 207 were missing on clinical examination. The radiograph shows no evidence of 206, but the resorbing roots of 207 are evident.

root surface is replaced by cementum- or bone-like tissue. The process starts in the cementum and progresses to involve the dentine, where it spreads along the dentine tubules and eventually comes to involve the dentine of the crown as well as the root. The peri-pulpal dentine is relatively resistant to resorption and the pulp therefore only becomes involved late in the disease. The

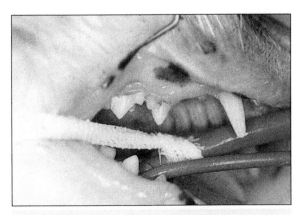

Figure 20.4 Lateral photograph of 107. Note the small buccal cavity.

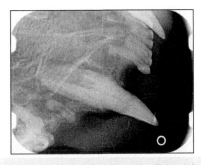

Figure 20.5 Oblique lateral radiograph of the right rostral upper jaw. Replacement resorption of 104 is obvious. Note the radiolucent resorption tracks within the dentine of the root. Tooth 106 was missing on clinical examination and the radiograph shows that it is resorbing.

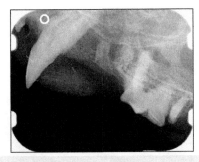

Figure 20.6 Lateral radiograph centring on the left upper premolars. Teeth 206 and 207 were missing on clinical examination. The gingiva overlying these sites was clinically healthy. There is no radiographic evidence of 206. It is likely to have been completely resorbed and replaced by bone. Both roots of 207 are resorbing.

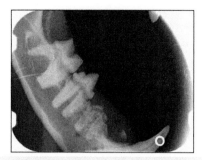

Figure 20.7 Lateral radiograph of the right mandibular premolars and molar. Tooth 407 was missing on clinical examination and the overlying gingiva was intensely inflamed, with pieces of crown material protruding.

process extends through the crown dentine, eventually reaching the enamel. The enamel is either resorbed or it fractures off and a cavity becomes clinically evident. In the absence of routine radiography, the lesions are first noted clinically when they become evident in the crown, often as cavities at the cemento-enamel junction (CEJ). The first clinical manifestation of ORLs is thus a late-stage lesion, as in this case. In many cases, the progressive dentine destruction with ORLs weakens and undermines the crown to such an extent that minor trauma, e.g. during chewing, causes the crown to fracture off, leaving the root in the alveolar bone. The resorbing root remnants are usually covered by intact gingiva. However, in some cases the overlying gingiva may be inflamed.

Visual inspection and tactile examination with a dental explorer will only identify end-stage lesions, i.e. when the process involves the crown and has resulted in an obvious cavity. Radiography will identify lesions that are localized to the root surfaces within the alveolar bone, which would not be detected by clinical methods. Moreover, it is only with the aid of radiography that the extent of a resorptive process can be identified. Selection of the best treatment option thus depends on radiography. In fact, a series of full-mouth radiographs is recommended for all cats presented for dental therapy. If taking a series of full-mouth radiographs is not possible, e.g. financial restrictions, then take one view of each mandibular premolar/molar region. The mandibular third premolars are the most commonly affected teeth and it has been shown that, in nine out of 10 cats with resorptive lesions, the process will be identified on these two views. If radiographs show resorption of these teeth, then a full-mouth series must be taken.

TREATMENT OPTIONS

To date, there is no known treatment, which prevents development and/or progression of odontoclastic resorptive lesions (ORLs). It seems unlikely that such treatment can be developed without knowledge of the cause of the pathology. Currently, the suggested methods of managing odontoclastic resorptive lesions are:

1. Conservative management, which means scaling, polishing, and monitoring clinically (development of a cavity) and radiographically. Suitable for lesions that affect the root surfaces only, i.e. with no oral communication established. Normally only applicable to larger teeth, namely canines.
2. Tooth extraction. If a periodontal ligament space can be identified, then extraction should be attempted.
3. Coronal (crown) amputation. Suitable for teeth where the roots have undergone extensive resorption (periodontal ligament space cannot be identified radiographically or clinically) at the time of diagnosis.

TREATMENT PERFORMED

1. Periodontal therapy to remove plaque and calculus, and provide a clean environment for surgery.
2. Crown amputation of 107, 204, 307 distal root, 404 and 407 (only small fragment of crown remaining). Postoperative radiographs were taken of all sites as the baseline for future monitoring of continued resorption.
3. Open extraction of the mesial root of 307. Postoperative radiographs were taken to confirm complete extraction of the root.
4. Conservative management of 104 and 304.
5. Shortening of 304 without entry into the pulp chamber, to prevent trauma to the upper lip (as the crown of 204 was removed).

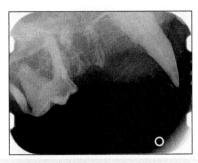

Figure 20.8 Lateral radiograph of the right upper jaw. Tooth 108 is now showing signs of root resorption extending into the crown. Note the continued replacement resorption of 107 (crown amputation performed a year earlier).

RECHECKS

At conscious examination 3 weeks later, the extraction and coronal amputation sites had healed, i.e. they were covered with clinically healthy gingivae. The owner reported that the cat seemed comfortable and was eating extremely well.

Examination under anaesthesia and full-mouth radiographs 6 months later confirmed continued resorption of the roots of the teeth that had been treated by means of crown amputation, namely 107, 204, 404, the distal root of 307 and both roots of 407. These sites were covered by clinically healthy gingiva. Also, the roots of 104 and 304 were progressively resorbing but the lesions were still localized to the root surfaces, with no obvious cavity formation at the gingival margin.

Examination under anaesthesia and full-mouth radiographs 6 months later (1 year after initial diagnosis and treatment) confirmed continued root resorption of the roots that had been intentionally retained, namely 107, 204, 404, the distal root of 307 and both roots of 407. These sites were covered by clinically healthy gingiva. At this time, there was obvious oral communication, with small cavities at the buccal and lingual gingival margin of both 104 and 304, and crown amputation was performed. Moreover, new lesions had developed on 108 (Fig. 20.8), 308 and 408. These teeth were also treated by crown amputation. All crown amputation sites healed uneventfully.

The cat is rebooked for examination under general anaesthesia and full-mouth radiographs in 1 year to monitor the outcome of coronal amputations, and to identify and treat any new resorptive lesions that are likely to develop. The owners will contact us sooner if signs of oral discomfort occur or if they see cavities developing on any of the remaining teeth.

PROGNOSIS

Resorptive lesions are progressive. Diagnosed lesions will progress and new lesions will develop. Regular examinations under anaesthesia and a series of full-mouth radiographs are indicated for cats with diagnosed root resorption.

In short, this cat is guaranteed to develop root resorption of other teeth, and requires lifelong radiographic monitoring and intervention (crown amputation or extraction) as appropriate. Moreover, the canine teeth which were treated conservatively will need crown amputation or extraction.

COMMENTS

Some cats with resorptive lesions may show no clinical signs at all, especially if the pathology is limited to the root surfaces. However, once dentine destruction has progressed to such an extent that the process invades the pulp and/or a communication with the oral cavity has been established (when the enamel has been resorbed or it has fractured off to reveal the dentine to the oral cavity), then discomfort and/or pain are likely. This cat displayed signs of discomfort in reduced appetite and selectively choosing soft food. This only occurred when the resorption was end-stage, i.e. clinical cavities were obvious.

It is essential that the owner of a cat with resorptive lesions understands that the cat is guaranteed to develop root resorption of other teeth, and will require lifelong radiographic monitoring and intervention (crown amputation or extraction).

In this case, conservative management of 104 and 304 resulted in these teeth being kept for an additional year.

21 Idiopathic canine root resorption

INITIAL PRESENTATION

Complicated crown fracture of 404.

PATIENT DETAILS

A 9-year-old, neutered male, cross-breed.

CASE HISTORY

The dog was referred to us for endodontic treatment of a complicated crown fracture of 404. The fractured tooth had been noted by the referring veterinarian at the time of vaccination. There was no history of any previous dental treatment. The owner had not been aware of the fractured tooth and did not feel that it was causing any discomfort.

ORAL EXAMINATION – CONSCIOUS

He was a nice-tempered dog that allowed conscious examination of the head and mouth. The following were identified:
1. Normal occlusion
2. Generalized moderate gingivitis
3. Teeth 101, 102, 201, 202, all lower incisors and 304 were missing
4. Complicated crown fracture of 404.

ORAL EXAMINATION – UNDER GENERAL ANAESTHESIA

A thorough oral examination, including investigating periodontal parameters, was performed and all findings were noted on the dental record.

In summary, examination under general anaesthesia identified the following:

1. Teeth 101, 102, 201, 202, 110, 210, all lower incisors, 304, 305, 310, 311, 405, 410 and 411 were missing
2. Generalized moderate gingivitis
3. Complicated crown fracture of 404
4. Cavity (filled with soft tissue) at the lingual cervical aspect just above the gingival margin of 404
5. Cavity (filled with soft tissue) at the buccal cervical aspect just above the gingival margin affecting 104, 109 (Fig. 21.1), 208, 306, 307, 308, 309, 406, 407, 408 and 409
6. Teeth 108, 109, 208 and 209 (Fig. 21.1) were discoloured pink.

FURTHER INVESTIGATIONS

A series of full-mouth radiographs (14 views) was taken.

RADIOGRAPHIC FINDINGS

The series of full-mouth radiographs showed replacement resorption of all remaining teeth. See Figs 21.2, 21.3, 21.4, 21.5, 21.6, 21.7, 21.8 and 21.9 for details of findings.

THEORY REFRESHER

Resorption of teeth is common in domestic cats. Tooth resorption has also been shown to occur in feral and wild cats. It has also been reported in man and in dogs.

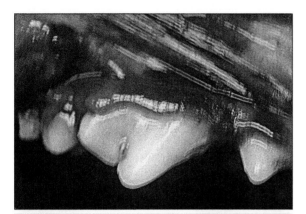

Figure 21.1 Oblique lateral photograph of 108 and 109. Both 108 and 109 are discoloured pink. This is a consequence of the destruction of the dental hard tissue extending into the crown and involving the pulp, which 'shines through' the thin enamel. Note the soft tissue-filled cavity on the buccal aspect of 109.

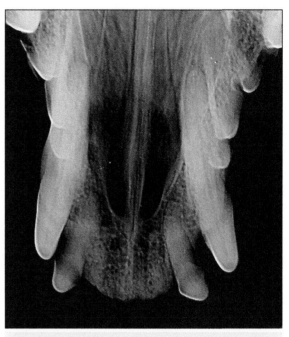

Figure 21.2 Rostrocaudal radiograph of the rostral upper jaw. Clinically, there was no evidence of 101, 102, 201 and 202, and the edentulous area was covered by healthy gingiva. The radiograph shows that these teeth have undergone resorption and been replaced by bone.

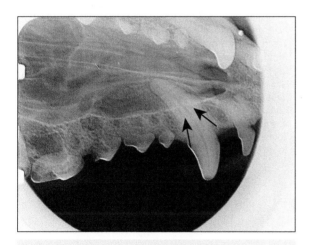

Figure 21.3 Lateral radiograph of the right upper jaw. Tooth 103 has a clear periodontal ligament space and a smooth root outline, i.e. there is no radiographic evidence of external root resorption. A clear periodontal ligament space separating the tooth from the alveolar bone can be identified for 104, but note the vertical radiolucent lines in the root, indicating ongoing resorption of dentine. The roots of 105, 106, 107 and 108 all show extensive replacement resorption. It is difficult to identify a clear periodontal ligament and the roots have the appearance of bone rather than dentine.

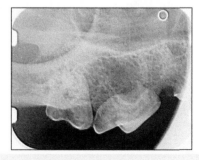

Figure 21.4 Lateral radiograph of 108 and 109. The crowns of these teeth have lost their roots and have only soft tissue attachment to the jaw. Clinically, there was a soft tissue-filled cavity at the buccal aspect of 109 just above the gingival margin and both teeth were discoloured pink as a consequence of the resorptive process spreading into the crowns of these teeth.

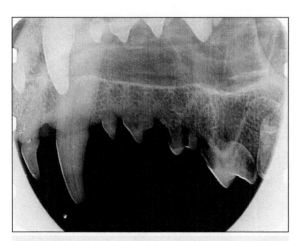

Figure 21.5 Lateral radiograph of the left upper jaw. The roots of 205, 206, 207 and 208 all show extensive replacement resorption. It is difficult to identify a clear periodontal ligament and the roots have the appearance of bone rather than dentine. Note the resorptive process spreading to involve the crowns of 207 and 208.

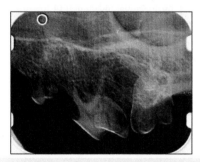

Figure 21.6 Lateral radiograph of 207, 208 and 209. The crowns of these teeth have lost their roots and have only soft tissue attachment to the jaw. Clinically, 208 and 209 had a pink discoloration due to the progressive destruction of crown dentine, allowing the pulp to 'shine through' the thin enamel.

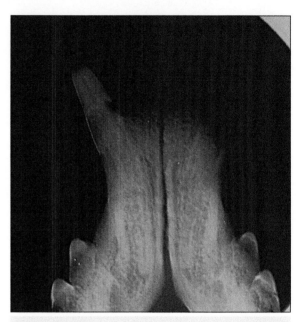

Figure 21.7 Rostrocaudal radiograph of the rostral lower jaw. Clinically, the edentulous incisor region was covered by healthy gingiva. The radiograph shows that these teeth have undergone resorption and been replaced by bone. Tooth 304 was missing clinically. The radiograph shows its root undergoing replacement resorption. The overlying gingiva was intact and non-inflamed. The root of 404 is undergoing replacement resorption and the destruction of dental hard tissue involves the crown. Clinically, this tooth had a soft tissue-filled cavity on the lingual aspect just above the gingival margin. The tooth also had a complicated crown fracture. In fact, the dog was referred to us for endodontic treatment of this tooth.

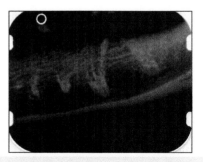

Figure 21.8 Lateral radiograph centring on 308 and 309. Both teeth are affected by extensive replacement resorption involving the crown as well as the roots. Clinically, both teeth had soft tissue-filled cavities buccally just above the gingival margin.

Odontoclastic resorptive lesions (ORLs) are a type of 'idiopathic' external root resorption, where the hard tissues of the root surfaces are destroyed by the activity of multinucleated cells called odontoclasts. The destroyed root surface is replaced by cementum- or bone-like tissue. The process starts in the cementum and progresses to involve the dentine, where it spreads along the dentine tubules and eventually comes to involve the dentine of the crown as well as the root. The peri-pulpal dentine is relatively resistant to resorption and the pulp therefore only becomes involved late in the disease. The process extends through the crown dentine, eventually

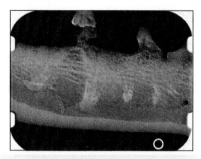

Figure 21.9 Lateral radiograph centring on 408 and 409. Both teeth are affected by extensive replacement resorption involving the crown as well as the roots. Clinically, both teeth had soft tissue-filled cavities buccally just above the gingival margin.

reaching the enamel. The enamel is either resorbed or it fractures off and a cavity becomes clinically evident. In the absence of routine radiography, the lesions are first noted clinically when they become evident in the crown, often as cavities at the cemento-enamel junction (CEJ). The first clinical manifestation of ORLs is thus a late-stage lesion. In many cases, the progressive dentine destruction with ORLs weakens and undermines the crown to such an extent that minor trauma, e.g. during chewing, causes the crown to fracture off, leaving the root in the alveolar bone. The resorbing root remnants are usually covered by intact gingiva. However, in some cases the overlying gingiva may be inflamed.

Visual inspection and tactile examination with a dental explorer will only identify end-stage lesions, i.e. when the process involves the crown and has resulted in an obvious cavity. Radiography will identify lesions that are localized to the root surfaces within the alveolar bone, which would not be detected by clinical methods. Moreover, it is only with the aid of radiography that the extent of a resorptive process can be identified. Selection of the best treatment option thus depends on radiography.

It remains a matter of debate as to whether ORLs cause discomfort or pain to the affected individual. Based on the fact that pulpal inflammation occurs late in the disease process, it seems likely that lesions that are limited to the root surfaces and do not communicate with the oral environment are asymptomatic. However, once dentine destruction has progressed to such an extent that the process invades the pulp and/or a communication with the oral cavity has been established (when the enamel has been resorbed

or it has fractured off to reveal the dentine to the oral cavity), then discomfort and/or pain are likely. Some animals may show clinical signs indicating oral discomfort or pain, e.g. changes in food preferences (soft rather than hard diet) and reduced food intake, but many do not.

CLINICAL TIPS

- The first clinical manifestation of odontoclastic resorptive lesions is a late-stage lesion.
- Visual inspection and tactile examination with a dental explorer will only identify end-stage lesions.
- Radiography is essential to identify the extent of a resorptive process.
- To date, there is no known treatment, which prevents development and/or progression of odontoclastic resorptive lesions.
- It is common for an owner to report marked improvement in general well-being of the animal once remedial dentistry has been performed.

TREATMENT OPTIONS

To date, there is no known treatment, which prevents development and/or progression of ORLs. It seems unlikely that such treatment can be developed without knowledge of the cause of the pathology. Currently, the suggested methods of managing odontoclastic resorptive lesions are:

1. Conservative management
2. Tooth extraction
3. Coronal amputation.

TREATMENT PERFORMED

The oral cavity was flushed with 10 ml of chlorhexidine preoperatively to provide a clean environment for surgery, which consisted of:

1. Crown amputation of 105, 106, 107, 108, 109, 205, 206, 207, 208, 209, 306, 307, 308, 309, 404, 406, 407, 408 and 409
2. Open extraction of 103, 104, 203 and 204.
   All flaps were replaced using 5/0 Monocryl.

- Daily chlorhexidine rinse for 1 week
- NSAIDs for 5 days
- Soft food.

RECHECKS

Conscious examination 6 weeks after treatment revealed successful healing of the extraction and coronal amputation sites. The gingivae covering the margins of the alveolar bone were non-inflamed. The owner reported a marked change in the dog's behaviour, i.e. he was much brighter, more interested in walks and more social. Also, appetite had increased. Despite having no teeth, he was actually eating kibble as well as soft food.

At examination under anaesthesia and full-mouth radiographs 6 months after initial treatment, the gingivae covering the margins of the alveolar bone were non-inflamed and the roots were continuing to resorb.

No further treatment has been required.

PROGNOSIS

The extraction sites should heal uneventfully. The gingivae at the sites where coronal amputation was performed should heal and the roots should carry on resorbing. Continued root resorption should be monitored clinically and radiographically.

COMMENTS

The only teeth unaffected by external root resorption were 103, 203 and 204. We chose to extract these as they would almost certainly develop pathology with time. Moreover, three teeth without antagonists do not provide a functional benefit. An edentulous animal has no problem with eating. Some will require soft food but many still eat kibble despite having no teeth.

It is common that an owner reports marked improvement in general well-being of the animal once remedial dentistry has been performed. At initial consultation the owner felt that the dog had no signs of oral discomfort, but at the postoperative check-up 6 weeks after surgery the first thing they said was that he was 'like a new dog – a puppy again'.

22 Malocclusion – an introduction

By definition, malocclusion is an abnormality in the position of the teeth. Malocclusion is common in the dog, but also occurs in cats. The clinical significance of malocclusion is that it may cause discomfort and sometimes pain to the affected animal. In some cases, it may be the direct cause of severe oral pathology. It is consequently important to diagnose malocclusion early in the life of the animal so that preventative measures can be taken.

Malocclusion can result from jaw length and/or width discrepancy (skeletal malocclusion), from tooth malpositioning (dental malocclusion), or a combination of both. The development of the occlusion is determined by both genetic and environmental factors. Specific genetic mechanisms regulating malocclusion are unknown. A polygenic mechanism, however, is likely and explains why not all siblings in successive generations are affected by malocclusion to the same degree, if at all. With a polygenic mechanism, the severity of clinical signs is linked to the number of defective genes.

The most reasonable approach to evaluate whether malocclusion is hereditary or acquired is as follows:
- Skeletal malocclusion is considered inherited unless a developmental cause can be reliably identified.
- Pure dental malocclusion, unless known to have breed or family predisposition, should be given the benefit of the doubt and not be considered inherited.

An outline of the more common types of malocclusion is given below.

SKELETAL MALOCCLUSION

Brachycephalic dogs have a shorter than normal upper jaw and dolicocephalic dogs have a longer than normal upper jaw; in both cases, the mandible is not responsible for any rostrocaudal discrepancy.

Mandibular prognathic bite: In the mandibular prognathic bite, often called 'undershot', the mandible is longer than the maxilla and some or all of the mandibular teeth are rostral to their normal position. If the dental interlock prevents the mandible from growing rostrally to its genetic potential, lateral or ventral bowing of the mandible may occur to accommodate the length. This results in an open bite and is characterized by increased space between the premolar cusp tips. In addition, the caudal angle of the mandible is caudal to the temporomandibular joint to accommodate the extra length of the mandible.

Mandibular brachygnathic bite: A mandibular brachygnathic bite, often called 'overshot', occurs when the mandible is shorter than normal.

Wry bite: A wry bite occurs if one side of the head grows more than the other side. In its mildest form a one-sided prognathic or brachygnathic bite develops. In more severe cases, a crooked head and bite develop with a deviated midline. An open bite may also develop in the incisor region so that the affected teeth are displaced vertically and do not occlude.

Narrow mandible: In some animals, the mandible is too narrow with respect to the upper jaw. The result is that the lower canines impinge on the maxillary gingivae or the hard palate instead of fitting into the diastema between the upper third incisor and upper canine on either side. The animal may not be able to close its mouth and injury to the gingivae or palatal mucosa commonly occurs. In untreated severe cases, an oronasal communication may develop over time. This condition is seen in both the primary (deciduous) and permanent dentition. Persistent primary canines will further exacerbate the condition, as the permanent canines erupt medially to their primary counterparts in the mandible. The incorrect dental interlock will interfere with the normal growth in width and length of the developing mandible. The condition can also be caused by persistent primary mandibular canines in a mandible of normal width.

DENTAL MALOCCLUSION

Dental malocclusion is malpositioning of teeth where there is no obvious skeletal abnormality, i.e. there is no jaw length or width discrepancy.

Anterior crossbite: This is a clinical term used to describe a reverse scissor occlusion of one, several or all of the incisors. The condition is thought to be secondary to persistent primary incisors. However, there is probably a skeletal origin as well, since affected animals often develop a mandibular prognathic bite. In other words, an anterior crossbite in an immature animal may be the first sign of a developing mandibular prognathism. Anterior crossbite is common in medium- and large-breed dogs, where persistent primary teeth are less common. The cause can be either a dental malocclusion (i.e. linguoversion of the upper incisors) or a skeletal malocclusion (i.e. mandibular prognathism or maxillary brachygnathism).

Malocclusion of the canine teeth: The two most common abnormalities in canine tooth position are:
- Rostral displacement of the maxillary canines. Persistent primary canines may be responsible for this condition. A breed predisposition has been reported in the Shetland sheepdog.
- Medial displacement of the lower canines. Persistent primary mandibular canines are thought to be the cause of this condition. However, the condition is not frequent in toy breeds, where persistent primary teeth are common. This malocclusion is frequent in dolicocephalic breeds, where it is of skeletal origin in that the mandible is too small for the long maxilla.

Malocclusion of the premolars and molars: Posterior crossbite is used to describe an abnormal relationship of the carnassial teeth, seen commonly in the dolicocephalic breeds, where the normal buccolingual relationship is reversed.

MALOCCLUSION ASSOCIATED WITH PERSISTENT PRIMARY TEETH

Persistent primary teeth, i.e. primary teeth that are still in place when the permanent counterpart starts erupting, may interfere with the normal eruption pathway of the permanent counterparts. The smaller breeds are more often affected by this condition. The mode of inheritance is not known, but it seems to be familial. The three most commonly affected areas are the lower canines, the upper canines and the incisors.

Mandibular canines: The mandibular permanent canine begins eruption medial to its primary counterpart. Once the primary tooth is lost, the permanent canine flares out laterally to occupy the diastema between the upper third incisor and upper canine. If the primary canine is not lost, the permanent canine may be forced to continue erupting medial to the persistent primary counterpart and will impinge on the hard palate, causing pain, inflammation and possibly, with time, an oronasal communication.

Maxillary canines: The maxillary permanent canine erupts rostral to its primary counterpart. If the primary tooth is retained, this may force the permanent tooth to erupt into the diastema intended for the permanent mandibular canine. The following malocclusion situations could then develop:
- The maxillary or mandibular canine may become impacted, i.e. it does not erupt fully.
- The mandibular canine may push the upper third incisor or the upper canine in a labial/buccal direction.
- The mandibular canine may be forced to erupt medial to the maxillary canine, thus impinging on the hard palate, with possible formation of an oronasal communication if left untreated.

Incisors: The permanent incisors erupt caudal to their primary counterparts. Retention of one or more of the primary teeth may interfere with scissor occlusion of the permanent teeth, with upper incisors occluding behind the mandibular incisors, i.e. an anterior crossbite, which may result in localized soft tissue trauma.

DENTAL INTERLOCK-INDUCED ABNORMALITIES

A maloccluding dental interlock may form when a growth spurt of either the maxilla or mandible coincides with the eruption of primary or permanent canines and incisors that interact to form the dental interlock. Once this interlock has been established, the maxilla and mandible are forced to grow rostrally at the same rate, irrespective of the genetic information. For example, mandibular canines that are locked rostral to the upper third incisors will cause a non-hereditary mandibular prognathic bite; mandibular canines that are locked medial and more caudal than normal will cause a narrow mandible and a mandibular brachygnathic bite.

PREVENTION AND TREATMENT OF MALOCCLUSION

Prevention is always better than treatment. Early recognition of a problem is essential to avoid discomfort and pain to the animal and prevent the development of severe pathology. Malocclusion affecting the primary dentition may require interceptive orthodontics. Malocclusion affecting the permanent dentition may need no treatment at all, if it is not causing the animal discomfort or any oral pathology. Malocclusion causing discomfort and pathology always needs treating.

MALOCCLUSION AFFECTING THE PRIMARY DENTITION

Primary teeth involved in malocclusion should be extracted as early as possible, i.e. at 6–8 weeks of age. This will allow the maxilla and mandible to develop to their full genetic potential independently before the permanent dental interlock forms. Extracting maloccluding primary teeth before eruption of their permanent counterparts is called 'interceptive orthodontics'. It will prevent dental interlock-induced malocclusion from developing. If the developing malocclusion is of skeletal origin, the value of interceptive orthodontics is negligible, since the permanent teeth will form the same incorrect interlock.

Persistent primary teeth should be extracted as soon as possible to prevent malocclusion.

The roots of primary teeth are longer and narrower than the roots of the permanent teeth. Extraction requires care and patience to avoid tooth fracture. It is essential not to fracture the root, as a remnant may continue to deviate the eruption pathway of the permanent tooth. Every attempt should be made to minimize the risk of iatrogenic damage to the developing permanent teeth. Preoperative radiographs to determine the anatomy of the primary tooth, but also the position and stage of development of the permanent counterpart, should always be taken.

MALOCCLUSION AFFECTING THE PERMANENT DENTITION

If there is no evidence of discomfort/pain or any associated oral pathology, malocclusion affecting the permanent dentition may need no treatment. Malocclusion causing discomfort and pathology, however, always need treating. The treatment options available are orthodontics, tooth shortening or extraction. In many instances, tooth shortening or extraction are preferable to orthodontics on ethical grounds. Tooth shortening often requires pulpal exposure. In this situation, endodontic therapy of the shortened tooth is mandatory.

Lingually displaced mandibular canines in young dogs can often be corrected by stimulating the dogs to play, as often as possible, with specific rubber toys of an appropriate size and shape.

ETHICAL CONSIDERATIONS

In man, medical (predisposition to periodontal diseases), functional (alteration of mastication or speech) and psychological (alteration of aesthetics) problems relating to malocclusion are the primary reason for orthodontic treatment. In human orthodontics, whether malocclusion is hereditary or acquired is not a consideration when planning treatment. This is in contrast to veterinary orthodontics, where aesthetics and ethical concerns are linked, and treatment for the sole purpose of showing dogs or cats cannot be encouraged. The aim of any treatment is primarily to make the animal comfortable; aesthetics are a secondary consideration.

It is essential to determine if the presenting malocclusion is hereditary or not. Orthodontic correction of a malocclusion is contraindicated where the malocclusion is hereditary unless the animal is also neutered. The rationale for this is to avoid spread of inherited malocclusion within a breed.

MANAGING MALOCCLUSION CASES IN GENERAL PRACTICE

Occlusal evaluation is part of the basic oral examination of a conscious animal. To make an evaluation, the practitioner needs to be able to identify normal occlusion for the species and breed, and have an understanding of the aetiology and pathogenesis of malocclusion, as detailed earlier in this chapter. It is essential to determine if the malocclusion is of skeletal, dental or combination origin. Preventive measures (such as controlled playing with an appropriate rubber toy, interceptive orthodontics or extraction of persistent primary teeth) should be carried out early in the animal's life. In most instances, treatment other than prevention is best left to a veterinarian with special skills.

SUMMARY

Malocclusion is common and may cause pain/discomfort and severe oral pathology. It is essential to diagnose malocclusion early in the life of the animal. Prevention is the best form of treatment. Skeletal malocclusions and persistent primary teeth are hereditary. Orthodontic treatment of an inheritable malocclusion should only be considered in the neutered animal. In most instances, treatment, other than prevention, is best left to a veterinarian with special skills in dentistry. The aim of any treatment is to make the animal comfortable with a functional bite; aesthetic considerations are of secondary importance.

23 Persistent primary teeth

INITIAL PRESENTATION

Persistent primary teeth and developing malocclusion.

PATIENT DETAILS

A 20-week-old, female, Yorkshire terrier.

CASE HISTORY

The owner was concerned that 'she has too many teeth'. She had a poor appetite and would not eat anything other than grilled chicken, cut into small pieces. The case was referred to us for management.

ORAL EXAMINATION – CONSCIOUS

The dog disliked having her face handled. She was tiny (weight 1.8 kg) and difficult to restrain adequately. A cursory conscious examination was performed, which revealed the following:
1. Mixed dentition with numerous persistent primary teeth
2. Generalized moderate to severe gingivitis.

ORAL EXAMINATION – UNDER GENERAL ANAESTHETIC

A thorough oral and dental examination, including investigating periodontal parameters, was performed. All findings were noted on the dental record sheet.

In summary, examination under general anaesthesia identified the following:
1. Skeletal relationship
   - The upper and lower jaw seemed to be of normal length and width for breed.

2. Persistent primary teeth
   - The primary upper incisors were solidly (no mobility) in place and the permanent counterparts were erupted caudal to them (Fig. 23.1).
   - The primary lower incisors had been shed and the erupted permanent lower incisors were occluding between the persistent primary and the permanent upper incisors (i.e. reverse scissor occlusion of permanent incisors).
   - All four primary canines were solidly in place. The diastema between the third upper incisor and upper canine was filled by the permanent upper canine erupting in front of the persistent primary canine bilaterally (Fig. 23.2). The permanent lower canines were trapped medial to the persistent primary canines, and were occluding with and traumatizing the palatal mucosa.
   - Persistent primary first premolars in all quadrants were causing crowding and rotation of the permanent successors.
3. Generalized moderate to severe gingivitis
   - The gingivitis was most severe in regions where there were persistent primary as well as permanent teeth (Fig. 23.2).

FURTHER INVESTIGATIONS

Radiographs were taken of all persistent primary canine teeth (to determine the anatomy of the primary tooth, and the position and stage of development of the permanent counterpart).

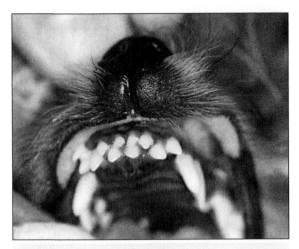

Figure 23.1 Incisor occlusion. The permanent upper incisors were fully erupted caudal to the persistent primary upper incisors. The primary lower incisors had been exfoliated and the permanent counterparts were fully erupted and occluding between the rows of upper incisors.

RADIOGRAPHIC FINDINGS

The primary teeth were fully developed with closed apices. All permanent teeth were in early development (around half of total root length formed for incisors, around one-third of the total root length formed for the canines and around two-thirds of the estimated total root length for the premolars).

THEORY REFRESHER

Persistent primary teeth, i.e. primary teeth that are still in place when the permanent counterpart starts erupting, may interfere with the normal eruption pathway of the permanent counterparts. The smaller breeds are more often affected by this condition. The mode of inheritance is not known, but it seems to be familial. The three most commonly affected areas are the lower canines, the upper canines and the incisors.

The mandibular permanent canine begins eruption medial to its primary counterpart. Once the primary tooth is lost, the permanent canine flares out laterally to occupy the diastema between the upper third incisor and upper canine. If the primary canine is not lost, the permanent canine may be forced to continue erupting medial to the persistent primary counterpart and will impinge on the hard palate, causing pain, inflammation and possibly, with time, an oronasal communication.

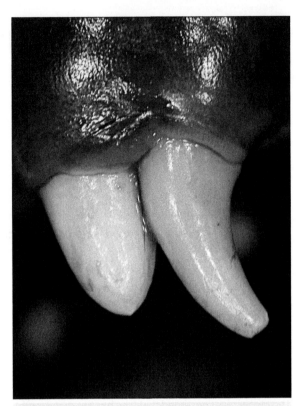

Figure 23.2 Canine occlusion. The permanent upper canines were erupting in front of the persistent primary canine bilaterally, thus closing the diastema where the permanent lower canines should occlude. Note the severe gingivitis (reddening, swelling and spontaneous haemorrhage of the gingival margin).

The maxillary permanent canine erupts rostral to its primary counterpart. If the primary tooth is retained, this may force the permanent tooth to erupt into the diastema intended for the permanent mandibular canine. The following malocclusion situations could then develop:

- The maxillary or mandibular canine may become impacted, i.e. it does not erupt fully.
- The mandibular canine may push the upper third incisor or the upper canine in a labial/buccal direction.
- The mandibular canine may be forced to erupt medial to the maxillary canine, thus impinging on the hard palate, with possible formation of an oronasal communication if left untreated.

The permanent incisors erupt caudal to their primary counterparts. Retention of one or more of the primary teeth may interfere with scissor occlusion of the permanent teeth, with upper incisors occluding behind the mandibular incisors, i.e. an anterior crossbite, which may result in localized soft tissue trauma.

CLINICAL TIPS

- Persistent primary teeth may interfere with the normal eruption pathway of the permanent counterparts.
- The mode of inheritance is not known, but it seems to be familial.
- Extraction of all persistent primary teeth is the treatment of choice.
- The owner does need to be aware that there is always a risk of iatrogenic damage to the developing permanent teeth when primary teeth are extracted.
- The owner must also be aware that further treatment may be indicated for malocclusion of the permanent teeth.
- Extracting persistent primary teeth is difficult.

TREATMENT OPTIONS

1. Wait for the primary teeth to be shed. Most of the persistent primary teeth are solidly in place and the radiographs show little evidence of root resorption of the primary teeth. In short, they are unlikely to exfoliate, and their continued presence will lead to both incisor and canine malocclusion, as well as a predisposition to periodontitis. So, this is not a good option!
2. Extract all persistent primary teeth. This is the option of choice. The owner does need to be aware that there is always a risk of iatrogenic damage to the developing permanent teeth, but careful technique under strict radiographic control (pre- and post-extraction radiographs are mandatory, also intra-extraction if there are complications) minimizes this risk. The owner must also be aware that further treatment may be indicated for malocclusion of the permanent teeth. It is, however, likely that the malocclusion of the permanent teeth will be even more severe if the persistent primary teeth are left in situ.

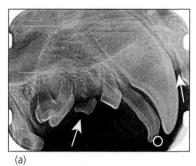

(a)

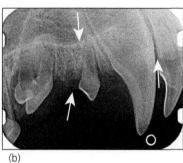

(b)

Figure 23.3 Radiographs of the right upper canine and rostral premolar region.

(a) Prior to extraction of the persistent 504 and 506. The persistent primary canine has a long, fine root and closed apex. There is little evidence of any ongoing root resorption. The roots of 506 have resorbed and only the crown is still in place. Note that the diastema between 103 and 104 is narrow. This is trapping the erupting 404 medially, where it is occluding with the palatal mucosa.

(b) Post-extraction radiograph. The persistent 504 has been successfully removed. Note the clear empty extraction socket. The crown remnant of 506 has also been removed.

TREATMENT PERFORMED

1. Periodontal therapy to remove plaque and calculus and provide a clean environment for extraction, and for the owner to start instituting home care (daily toothbrushing).
2. Extraction of persistent primary teeth 501, 502, 503, 504, 506, 601, 602, 603, 604, 606, 704, 706, 804 and 806 were extracted using an open technique, taking great care not to interfere with developing permanent tooth roots. Pre- and post-extraction radiographs were taken (Figs 23.3a, b and 23.4a, b). The flaps were replaced with 5/0 Monocryl.
3. Curettage of palatal indentations.

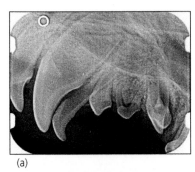

(a)

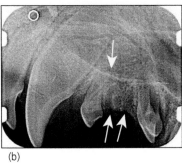

(b)

Figure 23.4 Radiographs of the left upper canine and rostral premolar region.

(a) Prior to extraction of the persistent 604 and 606. Tooth 604 has a long fragile root with little evidence of any ongoing root resorption. The persistent 606 also has a closed apex and no evidence of any ongoing root resorption. Note that 206 is rotated 90° due to the lack of space. The diastema between 203 and 204 is even narrower than on the right.

(b) Post-extraction radiograph. The persistent 604 and 606 have been successfully removed.

POSTOPERATIVE CARE

- Daily chlorhexidine rinse
- Booked for conscious examination 3 weeks later.

RECHECK

At recheck 3 weeks after extraction of all persistent primary teeth, it was obvious that the reverse scissor occlusion of the incisors was permanent. However, canine occlusion was normal, albeit a tight interlock. All extraction sites had healed uneventfully. The owner was shown how to brush the teeth and daily toothbrushing was recommended.

PROGNOSIS

It is likely that the reverse scissor occlusion of the permanent incisors is established. Similarly, the malocclusion of 304 and 404 may also be established, as there is not enough of a diastema between the upper third incisor and upper canine on either side for them to flare out and take their normal interlock position. There is, however, a chance that the prompt extraction of the persistent primary canines will allow the developing permanent teeth to achieve a normal or near normal position and interlock.

COMMENTS

Extracting persistent primary teeth is difficult (long, fragile roots, often undergoing resorption) and the risk of iatrogenic injury to the developing permanent teeth is relatively high. In fact, the owners should always be made aware of this risk. The operator needs to be familiar with radiographic techniques and interpretation, as well as skilled with extraction techniques. Referral to a specialist is often indicated.

In this case, prompt extraction of the persistent primary teeth did not prevent the establishment of an incisor malocclusion, but did prevent the developing canine malocclusion. The incisor malocclusion is not causing trauma either to soft tissue or teeth, and the dog requires no further treatment.

24 Interceptive extractions

PATIENT DETAILS

An 8-week-old, male, German shepherd.

CASE HISTORY

I saw this dog when I was working in general practice. He was presented to me for first vaccination, a healthy puppy with a severe skeletal malocclusion, of which the owner was totally unaware.

ORAL EXAMINATION – CONSCIOUS

He was a well-behaved puppy that allowed careful conscious evaluation, which revealed the following:
1. All primary teeth present
2. Skeletal malocclusion
   - The upper jaw was extremely long and narrow with respect to the lower jaw, which had a relatively normal length and width for the breed, i.e. relative mandibular brachygnathism.
   - The lower primary canines were distal to the upper primary canines and occluded with the palatal mucosa.
   - The lower primary incisors also occluded with the palatal mucosa.
3. Generalized mild gingivitis.

ORAL EXAMINATION – UNDER GENERAL ANAESTHETIC

A thorough oral and dental examination, including investigating periodontal parameters, was performed. All findings were noted on the dental record sheet.

In summary, examination under general anaesthesia identified the following:
1. Skeletal malocclusion
   - The upper jaw was extremely long and narrow with respect to the lower jaw, which had a relatively normal length and width for the breed, i.e. relative mandibular brachygnathism.
   - The lower primary canines occluded with palatal mucosa, distal to the upper primary canines, causing deep ulcerated indentations.
   - The lower primary incisors occluded with the palatal mucosa, causing small non-ulcerated indentations. There were also small non-ulcerated indentations in the palatal mucosa where the primary lower carnassials occluded.
2. Generalized mild gingivitis.

FURTHER INVESTIGATIONS

Radiographs were taken of the maloccluding primary lower canine teeth (to determine the anatomy of the primary tooth, and the position and stage of development of the permanent counterpart).

RADIOGRAPHIC FINDINGS

The primary canines were fully developed with closed apices. The permanent canines were in the normal position with respect to the primary canines (upper permanent are rostral to the primary and lower permanent are lingual to the primary). Root development of the permanent canines was in early stages, with only around one-third of the total root length formed. As expected, the permanent canines were still within the alveolar bone, i.e. not yet erupting.

THEORY REFRESHER

Primary teeth involved in malocclusion should be extracted as early as possible, i.e. at 6–8 weeks of age. This will allow the maxilla and mandible to develop to their full genetic potential independently before the permanent teeth erupt and dental interlock forms. Extracting maloccluding primary teeth before eruption of their permanent counterparts is called 'interceptive orthodontics'. It aims to prevent dental interlock-induced malocclusion from developing. However, if the developing malocclusion is skeletal in origin (as in this case), then the permanent teeth are likely to form the same incorrect interlock when they erupt. Malocclusion causing discomfort and pathology always needs treating, and interceptive orthodontics will remove discomfort or pain associated with maloccluding teeth.

The roots of primary teeth are longer and narrower than the roots of the permanent teeth. They may also be resorbing, which makes them fragile structures to handle. Extraction requires care and patience to avoid tooth fracture. It is essential not to fracture the root, as a remnant may continue to cause deviation of the eruption pathway of the permanent tooth. Preoperative radiographs to determine the anatomy of the primary tooth, but also the position and stage of development of the permanent counterpart, should always be taken.

This type of malocclusion, i.e. where the maloccluding teeth are due to a discrepancy in size of the upper and lower jaw, is inheritable and this dog should not be used for breeding.

CLINICAL TIPS

- Primary teeth involved in malocclusion should be extracted as early as possible.
- If the developing malocclusion is skeletal in origin then the permanent teeth are likely to form the same incorrect interlock when they erupt.
- It is essential not to fracture the primary root during extraction, as a remnant may continue to cause deviation of the eruption pathway of the permanent tooth.
- Malocclusion due to a discrepancy in size of the upper and lower jaw is inheritable and affected animals should not be used for breeding.
- Interceptive orthodontics for skeletal malocclusion is unlikely to be the only treatment required.

TREATMENT OPTIONS

1. No treatment. This is the poor choice! Although the primary canines will only remain for a short period of time (should be lost and permanent canines starting to erupt between 12 and 16 weeks of age), the lower primary canines are causing severe indentation and ulceration of the palatal mucosa, which is likely to be uncomfortable. Moreover, the lower canines are preventing any genetic potential for rostral growth of the mandible and may well contribute to the development of a more severe malocclusion of the permanent teeth.

2. Interceptive orthodontics. Here, this involves immediate extraction of the maloccluding lower primary canine teeth. This is the option of choice. The owner does need to be aware that this is a skeletal malocclusion and that the permanent teeth are likely to malocclude. The likelihood of further treatment (probably shortening and endodontic therapy of the permanent lower canines) is almost a certainty. It is, however, highly possible that the malocclusion of the permanent teeth will be even more severe if the maloccluding primary teeth are left in situ.

TREATMENT PERFORMED

1. Periodontal therapy to remove plaque and calculus and provide a clean environment for surgery, and for the owner to start instituting home care (daily toothbrushing).
2. Extraction of lower primary canines using an open technique, taking great care not to interfere with developing permanent canines during the extraction process. Pre- and post-extraction radiographs were taken. The flaps were closed with 5/0 Monocryl.
3. Curettage of ulcerated palatal indentations.

POSTOPERATIVE CARE

- Daily toothbrushing
- The dog was booked for conscious examination 8 weeks later (when permanent canines should be erupting).

RECHECK

At recheck 8 weeks after interceptive orthodontic treatment, it was obvious that the erupting permanent lower canines would impede on the palatal mucosa (Figs 24.1

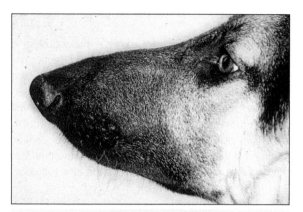

Figure 24.1 Lateral photograph of the head at 16 weeks of age. The long upper jaw is evident. You don't even have to look at the teeth to know that this dog will have a malocclusion.

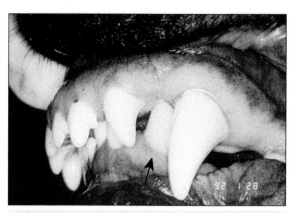

Figure 24.3 Lateral photograph of occlusion at 8 months of age. Note that there has been further rostral growth of the mandible; the lower canines are now rostral to the upper canines. The maloccluding lower canines were causing deep ulcerated indentations in the palatal mucosa and intervention (tooth shortening and endodontic therapy) was performed. The dog was neutered at the same time. To maintain pulp vitality and continued tooth development, the endodontic therapy at this time consisted of partial pulpectomy, direct pulp capping and restoration.

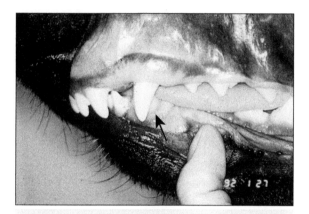

Figure 24.2 Lateral photograph of occlusion at 16 weeks of age. The lower incisors and canines are occluding with the palatal mucosa. When the dog was 8 weeks old, the primary mandibular canines were distal to the maxillary canines. At 16 weeks of age, the mandibular canines are palatal to the maxillary canines. So, extraction of the primary lower canines allowed rostral growth of the mandible.

and 24.2). There had been rostral growth of the mandible and the permanent mandibular canines were located palatal to the maxillary rather than distal to them (Fig. 24.2). So, the interceptive orthodontics had allowed rostral growth of the mandible. The owner was aware that further treatment would be required.

Further mandibular growth occurred, and by the time the dog was 8 months old the mandibular canines were rostral to the maxillary canines, but they were trapped medially causing palatal trauma (Fig. 24.3). Tooth short-

ening and endodontic therapy (partial pulpectomy, direct pulp capping and restoration – as tooth roots were not fully formed and a vital pulp is required for continued tooth root development) of 304 and 404 were performed when he was 8 months old. He was also neutered at the same time. Six months later, when the teeth were relatively mature (closed apices, good thickness of secondary dentine), conventional endodontic therapy (pulpectomy, root filling and restoration) was performed (Fig. 24.4). Postoperative radiographs 6 months after conventional endodontic therapy confirmed a successful outcome, i.e. no evidence of any periapical complications. The lower incisors and shortened canines were occluding with the palatal mucosa, causing small non-ulcerated indentations. In short, he has a functional and comfortable bite and no further treatment has been required.

PROGNOSIS

This malocclusion is of skeletal origin and the permanent teeth are likely to form the same incorrect interlock. Further treatment will be required.

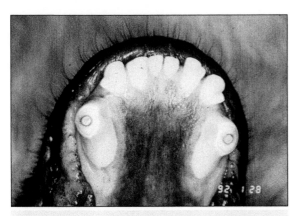

Figure 24.4 Occlusal photograph of shortened teeth at 14 months of age. When the dog was 14 months old, the lower canines were relatively mature (closed apices and good thickness of dentine), so conventional endodontic therapy (pulpectomy, root filling and restoration) was performed. Note that the restorative material used is silver amalgam. Due to the hazards associated with mercury disposal, I no longer use amalgam. Today, the restorative material of choice for this type of procedure is composite or compromer.

COMMENTS

Interceptive orthodontics for skeletal malocclusion is unlikely to be the only treatment required. The permanent teeth are likely to be involved in malocclusion and further treatment is nearly always required. It is, however, likely that the malocclusion of the permanent teeth will be even more severe if the maloccluding primary teeth are left in situ. This type of malocclusion is of genetic origin, i.e. inheritable. Consequently, it is important that the owner agrees not to breed from the affected dog.

25 Rubber toy technique and alveoloplasty

INITIAL PRESENTATION

Malocclusion – lower canine teeth erupting into palatal mucosa.

PATIENT DETAILS

A 6-month-old, male, bearded collie.

CASE HISTORY

The owner is active in the show ring and thus concerned about the malocclusion. In fact, the owner is more worried about the aesthetics than the developing pathology (palatal trauma). The dog is showing no obvious signs of discomfort. He is very active and enjoys playing with toys. The case was referred to us for evaluation and treatment.

ORAL EXAMINATION – CONSCIOUS

The dog was amenable to thorough oral examination and occlusal evaluation, which revealed the following:
1. Mild generalized gingivitis
2. Upper and lower jaw of normal length for this breed
3. The lower jaw was slightly too narrow with respect to the upper jaw
4. Lower canines not yet fully erupted
5. Lower canine occluding with gingiva at diastema between the upper third incisor and upper canine bilaterally, causing indentations and gingival hyperplasia (Fig. 25.1a, b)
6. Diastema between the upper third incisor and upper canine of adequate size for lower canine to fit bilaterally (Fig. 25.1a, b).

THEORY REFRESHER

In some animals, the mandible is too narrow with respect to the upper jaw. The result is that the lower canines impinge on the maxillary gingivae or the hard palate instead of fitting into the diastema between the upper third incisor and upper canine on either side. The animal may not be able to close its mouth and injury to the gingivae or palatal mucosa commonly occurs. In untreated severe cases (i.e. where the lower canines are upright and occluding with the palatal mucosa rather than the gingivae of the diastema), an oronasal communication may develop over time.

This malocclusion is seen in both the primary (deciduous) and permanent dentition. Persistent primary canines will further exacerbate the condition as the permanent canines erupt medially to their primary counterparts in the mandible. The incorrect dental interlock will interfere with the normal growth in width and length of the developing mandible. The condition can also be caused by persistent primary mandibular canines in a mandible of normal width.

In this case, the upper and lower jaw were of normal length; the mandible was narrow with respect to the upper jaw, but there was sufficient diastema for the lower canines to form a correct interlock if they were moved just slightly laterally.

- Incorrect dental interlock will interfere with the normal growth in width and length of the developing mandible.
- Malocclusion is seen in both the primary and permanent dentition.
- The use of a removable orthodontic appliance ('rubber toy' technique) has proved to be successful in correcting the malocclusion within 4 weeks.
- The diastema between the third incisor and canine tooth in the upper jaw should be wide enough to accommodate the mandibular canine tooth in its corrected position.
- The most appropriate objects to use are toys with a round or oval shape.
- The correct size of toy sits in between and just behind the canine teeth, and is larger than the distance between the mandibular canine teeth.
- If no movement is seen after 3 weeks, other treatment methods should be considered.
- Photographs (rostral, left and right views) should be taken to record the extent of the malocclusion prior to treatment.
- The time required for correction is longer when the teeth are fully erupted.
- This condition is probably heritable. Breeding from affected animals should be discouraged.

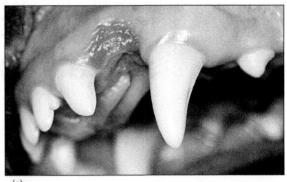
(a)

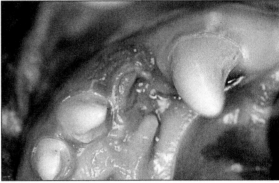
(b)

Figure 25.1 Lateral photograph (a) and occlusal photograph (b) of the malocclusion. The right lower canine is occluding with the gingival mucosa of the diastema. The malocclusion is the same on the left side.

(a) Note the inflamed hyperplastic gingiva.

(b) Note the indentation, as well as the inflamed hyperplastic gingiva.

TREATMENT

Oral examination under anaesthesia was not indicated at this stage.

For normal canine interlock to be achieved, the lower canines would need to be moved laterally.

The owner was advised to play with the dog for 15 minutes three to four times a day using a hard rubber ball of appropriate size and shape ('rubber toy technique') to encourage the lower canines to flare out laterally. All other toys were removed. The owner was also given toothbrushing instruction and advised to start daily brushing. The dog was rebooked for evaluation and possibly further treatment in 1 month.

'Rubber toy' technique

Lingually displaced mandibular canines in young dogs can often be corrected by stimulating the dogs to play, as often as possible, with specific rubber toys of an appropriate size and shape. In properly selected cases (young dogs, no major jaw discrepancies), the use of a removable orthodontic appliance ('rubber toy' technique) has proved to be successful in correcting the malocclusion, within 4 weeks in most cases. The technique also encourages development of a strong bond between owner and animal during the course of the treatment.

As with any technique, correct diagnosis is critical for success of the treatment. No major jaw discrepancies should be present. The diastema between the third incisor and canine tooth in the upper jaw should be wide enough to accommodate the mandibular canine tooth in its corrected position. In other words, the only orthodontic movement required is lateral movement of the mandibular canines, and there needs to be enough space available between the third incisor and canine in the upper jaw for them to fit into their correct positions.

The most appropriate objects to use are toys with a round or oval shape. The size is important. The correct size of toy sits in between and just behind the canine teeth, and is larger than the distance between the mandibular canine teeth. The toy thus applies primarily lateral pressure to the teeth while the dog plays. A toy that is too small will be held more caudally in the mouth and thus exert no lateral force on the canine teeth. Too large a toy might cause intrusion rather than lateral tipping. In dogs that prefer to hold a toy between the carnassial teeth rather than the canine teeth, a very large toy may be needed. It needs to be so large that it cannot be fitted between the carnassial teeth. Rostral as well as lateral tipping of the mandibular canines occurs with a toy this large.

The composition and consistency of the toy are important. It should be of hard rubber that slightly deforms on chewing. If the toy is too soft, it is unlikely to create enough pressure for lateral tipping of the mandibular canines. If it is too hard, the result is tooth damage due to abrasion. The toy should have a smooth surface to avoid excessive abrasion.

Active play for 15 minutes, three times per day, is the recommended minimum. Longer and more frequent episodes are preferable, and the owner should be recommended to play with the dog as often as possible and to take away all other toys. Assuming a 1-week learning phase, 2 additional weeks are needed before any benefit is likely to be seen. If no movement is seen after 3 weeks, other treatment methods should be considered.

In this case, the likelihood of normal canine occlusion within 4 weeks was high.

Photographs (rostral, left and right views) should always be taken to record the extent of the malocclusion prior to treatment.

Once the mandibular canines are in their correct position, the established canine dental interlock should prevent relapse. However, continued playing with the toy for several months is recommended. It appears that there is little risk of overcorrection (labioversion) of the canine teeth. The technique works in teeth that are still

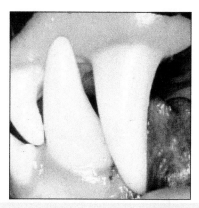

Figure 25.2 Lateral photograph of the canine occlusion (right side) after 8 weeks of treatment. Normal canine interlock has been established bilaterally. Note the normal architecture of the gingiva in the diastema, i.e. there is no evidence of inflammation or hyperplasia. Once trauma is removed, the gingiva will rapidly take on a normal appearance.

erupting as well as in fully erupted teeth. However, the time required for correction is longer when the teeth are fully erupted.

RECHECKS

The owner phoned after 3 weeks to let us know that normal canine occlusion was established. It was agreed to reschedule the recheck appointment to 8 weeks rather than the planned 4 weeks from start of treatment.

Conscious evaluation after 8 weeks revealed normal canine interlock, with no evidence of any trauma to the gingiva (Fig. 25.2). The dog was accepting daily toothbrushing and the gingivae were clinically healthy. The owner was advised to encourage the dog to carry on playing with the toy for 3 months to prevent relapse.

A telephone conversation after 3 months reported that normal interlock was maintained. The owner planned to carry on with the playing as they both enjoyed the interaction. Daily toothbrushing was also being performed and readily accepted by the dog.

PROGNOSIS

The rubber toy technique works especially well in teeth that are still erupting and where direct lateral tipping is the only movement required.

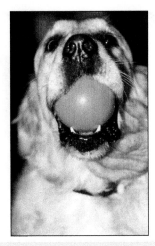

Figure 25.3 'Rubber toy' technique. The correct size of toy is critical to achieve primarily lateral pressure to the teeth while the dog plays. As shown here, the toy needs to be larger than the distance between the mandibular canine teeth, and when the dog holds it in its mouth the toy should sit in between and just behind the canine teeth. (Photograph courtesy of Dr Leen Verhaert, who described this technique.)

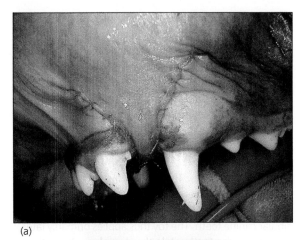

(a)

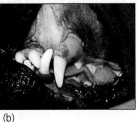

(b)

Figure 25.4 Lateral photographs of alveoloplasty procedure (a) and outcome (b). In this dog (different case), the 'rubber toy technique' had established normal canine interlock on the left side, but the right lower canine was not quite flared out (it was just touching the gingiva of the diastema). An alveoloplasty procedure was performed to correct the remaining minor malocclusion. The procedure consists of raising a full-thickness buccal mucoperiosteal flap and then recontouring the bone so that the lower canine is lateral. The flap is then advanced to close the defect and sutured in place without tension.

(a) Immediately postoperatively. Note that there is no tension in the closure.

(b) Six weeks after surgery. The lower canine is lateral in position and is not causing any damage to the gingiva.

COMMENTS

To achieve primarily lateral pressure to the teeth while the dog plays, the correct size of toy is critical. As depicted in Fig. 25.3, the toy needs to be larger than the distance between the mandibular canine teeth, and when the dog holds it in its mouth the toy should sit in between and just behind the canine teeth. A toy that is too small will be held more caudally in the mouth and thus exert no lateral force on the canine teeth. Too large a toy might cause intrusion rather than lateral tipping.

This technique is extremely useful and should be employed as soon as possible when straight lateral movement of the lower canines is required. If full correction is not achieved then alveoloplasty of the diastema (Fig. 25.4a, b) may be sufficient. In more severe cases, orthodontics or tooth shortening and endodontics may still be required.

Although this is a very minor malocclusion, it is skeletal in origin and thus likely to be inheritable. The owner was counselled not to breed from this dog.

26 Rubber toy technique and orthodontic appliances

INITIAL PRESENTATION

Malocclusion – left lower canine occluding with palate.

PATIENT DETAILS

A 6-month-old, female, bearded collie.

CASE HISTORY

The case was referred to us for evaluation and treatment of the malocclusion. The owner was active in the show ring and thus concerned about the malocclusion. While the owner was concerned about the developing pathology (palatal trauma), she was most concerned about the aesthetics and the effect on the dog's show career. She was adamant that tooth shortening would not be an option.

ORAL EXAMINATION – CONSCIOUS

This was one of the most docile and cooperative dogs that I have ever met. She readily allowed thorough oral examination and occlusal evaluation, which identified the following:

1. Mild generalized gingivitis
2. Wide spacing of teeth in the upper jaw, indicating that the upper jaw is long (Fig. 26.1)
3. Lower jaw slightly too short and narrow with respect to the upper jaw (Fig. 26.2)
4. Lower canines not yet fully erupted
5. Right lower canine flared out laterally and fitted in the diastema between 103 and 104 (Fig. 26.1)
6. Left lower canine upright in position, occluding with hard palate medial to the upper canine, causing a non-ulcerated indentation and hindering full mouth closure (Fig. 26.2)
7. Diastema between 203 and 204 of adequate size for 304 to fit (if it was moved slightly rostrally and laterally).

THEORY REFRESHER

Malocclusion can result from jaw length and/or width discrepancy (skeletal malocclusion), from tooth malpositioning (dental malocclusion), or a combination of both. This case is a skeletal malocclusion (mandibular brachygnathia) and is thus inheritable.

A mandibular brachygnathic bite, often called 'overshot', occurs when the mandible is shorter than normal. The degree of malocclusion varies as follows:

- The upper incisors are rostral to the lower incisors by 0.5 mm to 5 cm or more.
- The upper canines are caudal to but touching the mandibular canines, level with the lower canines, or rostral to the mandibular canines.
- The mandibular premolars are caudally displaced relative to the maxillary premolars, disrupting the 'pinking shear' effect. The degree of displacement is similar to that of the incisors and canines.

This case was classified as a mild relative mandibular brachygnathism, i.e. the mandible is too short (and narrow) with respect to the upper jaw. The cause of the malocclusion is the long upper jaw. The left lower canine was causing trauma to the hard palate. Malocclusion causing discomfort and pathology always needs treating.

145

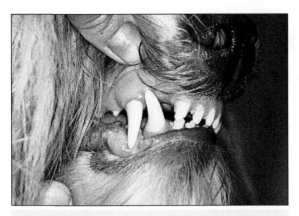

Figure 26.1 Oblique lateral photograph of the right rostral occlusion. The upper jaw is long (as evidenced by the wide spaces between the teeth and the width of the diastema) and the lower jaw is short with respect to the upper jaw. Tooth 404 is caudal in position, but has flared laterally and fits in the diastema between 103 and 104.

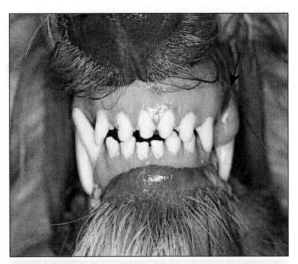

Figure 26.2 Head-on photograph of the rostral occlusion. While 404 has flared laterally and fits into the diastema, 304 is trapped medial to 104, occluding with the palate and preventing full mouth closure.

CLINICAL TIPS

- Malocclusion can result from jaw length and/or width discrepancy (skeletal malocclusion), from tooth malpositioning (dental malocclusion), or a combination of both.
- Wide spacing of teeth in the upper jaw may indicate that the upper jaw is too long.
- Orthodontic treatment is not always straightforward.
- Maintenance of oral hygiene is extremely important while an orthodontic appliance is in place.
- Orthodontic treatment may cause iatrogenic injuries.
- The effect of orthodontic treatment needs to be monitored clinically and radiographically.
- This condition is probably heritable. Breeding from affected animals should be discouraged.

TREATMENT OPTIONS

1. Extraction of the maloccluding tooth, i.e. 304. This is best avoided. The mandibular canines contribute to the bony strength of the lower jaw and should be maintained if at all possible. Also, the risk of iatrogenic jaw fracture when extracting periodontally sound lower canine teeth is a very real risk. Addition-ally, in this case extraction was in direct contradiction of the owner's clearly expressed wishes.
2. Shortening and endodontic treatment of 304. This is a good option to reduce the discomfort, but the owner was adamant that this would also destroy the dog's show career.
3. Orthodontic movement of 304. This is also a good option for this dog as the movement required is relatively small. While orthodontic movement of teeth is possible at any age, movement is easier to achieve and more rapid in the young animal. For normal canine interlock to be achieved, the lower canines would need to be moved slightly rostrally and then flared out laterally.

TREATMENT PLAN

For normal canine interlock to be achieved the left lower canine would need to be moved slightly rostrally and then flared out laterally. The plan was to achieve this in two stages: namely, to start by using the 'rubber toy technique' (see Chapter 25) and then an orthodontic appliance if necessary.

To achieve rostral as well as lateral tipping of the mandibular canines, a very large toy is needed. It needs to be so large that it cannot be fitted between the carnassial teeth.

The composition and consistency of the toy are important. It should be of hard rubber that slightly

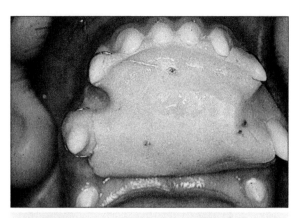

Figure 26.3 Photograph of the wire-reinforced acrylic bite plane in place in the upper jaw. Note the difference between the right and left grooves. The right groove is designed to maintain the occlusion of 404, and the left groove is designed to move 304 rostrally and laterally on chewing. This type of appliance is only effective if the dog chews.

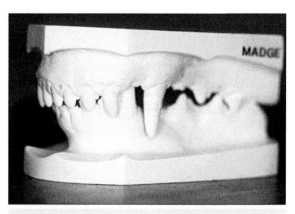

Figure 26.4 Plaster of Paris models of the occlusion. The models document the extent of the malocclusion at the start of treatment and provide an aid in designing appropriate orthodontic appliances. The models are mounted in an articulator and jaw movement can then be mimicked.

deforms on chewing. If the toy is too soft, it is unlikely to create enough pressure for lateral tipping of the mandibular canines. If it is too hard, the result is tooth damage due to abrasion. The toy should have a smooth surface to avoid excessive abrasion.

Oral examination under anaesthesia was not indicated at this stage. The owner was advised to play with the dog for 15 minutes three to four times a day using a hard rubber ball ('rubber toy technique') to encourage the lower canines to move rostrally and flare laterally. An appropriately sized hard rubber ball was selected. All other toys were removed. The owner was also given toothbrushing instruction and advised to start daily brushing. The dog was rebooked for evaluation and possibly further treatment in 1 month.

RECHECKS

The owner phoned after 1 week to let us know that the dog would not play with the ball. We then moved on to stage 2 of the planned treatment and manufactured an intra-oral maxillary acrylic bite plane under general anaesthesia (Fig. 26.3). We also took impressions, made a bite registration and produced models of the occlusion (Fig. 26.4). The dog was discharged with instructions to the owner of how to clean around the appliance (chlorhexidine rinsing and toothbrushing). She was rebooked 3 weeks later.

At the 3-week recheck, it became obvious that this type of appliance was not going to work as the dog would not close its mouth. In fact, she had not done so for 3 weeks and had refused to eat hard food. This type of appliance relies on mastication to be effective, i.e. every time the dog chews, as the lower canines contact the bite plane they will be forced rostrally and laterally. So, since the dog did not chew, the appliance had no effect.

She was again placed under general anaesthesia; the maxillary bite plane was removed, and impressions and bite registration for the manufacture of a mandibular orthodontic device were taken. Baseline radiographs were taken of 304 and 404 (orthodontic movement of teeth may induce iatrogenic pulp/periapical disease, as well as external root resorption). The mandibular expansion device (Fig. 26.5) was cemented in place 2 weeks later, again under general anaesthesia. Within 4 weeks the canines were in almost normal interlock and the expansion device was at its limit, i.e. it would not cause further tooth movement (Fig. 26.6). The dog seemed to manage well with the appliance in place. She was eating well and gaining weight. The device was left in place for a further 4 weeks to retain the canines in correct occlusion. Eight weeks after initial placement of the mandibular expansion device, the dog was again placed under general anaesthesia to remove the appliance. The outcome is depicted in Figs 26.7 and 26.8. Radiographs were again taken of 304 and 404. No abnormalities in

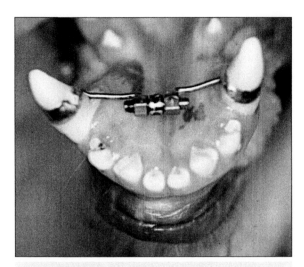

Figure 26.5 Photograph of the mandibular expansion device in place in the lower jaw. This device pushes both lower canines laterally. It is activated every 3–4 days by inserting a key. A cooperative animal is crucial.

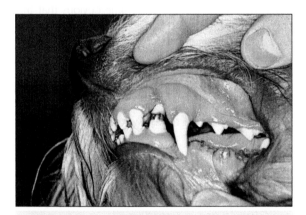

Figure 26.6 Lateral photograph of the mandibular expansion device in place. After 4 weeks the expansion device was at its limit and 304 was almost flared out laterally to fit in the diastema. Note the inflamed and hyperplastic gingiva where 304 is occluding.

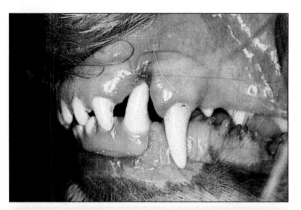

Figure 26.7 Lateral photograph of the left rostral occlusion at the time of removal of the mandibular expansion device. The left lower canine is now occluding with the gingiva in the diastema, rather than the palatal mucosa.

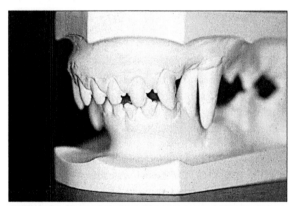

Figure 26.8 Models of occlusion at the time of removal of the mandibular expansion device. The left lower canine is now occluding with the gingiva in the diastema, rather than the palatal mucosa. It is prudent to make models of the outcome of the treatment.

tooth root development were detected and there was no evidence of any root resorption. Alveoloplasty of the left diastema (Fig. 26.9) was performed to ensure that the left canine was securely positioned laterally.

The dog was rechecked after 6 months, conscious and under general anaesthesia. Canine occlusion was normal and radiographs showed no evidence of pulp/periapical complications or root resorption.

PROGNOSIS

If the dog accepted playing with the rubber ball, then near normal or even normal canine occlusion could be achieved rapidly in such a young dog.

COMMENTS

Orthodontic treatment is not always straightforward. Revision of the initial treatment plan is not uncommon and total success is not guaranteed. The owner needs to be aware of this and also that multiple episodes of general anaesthesia are likely to be required. The owner

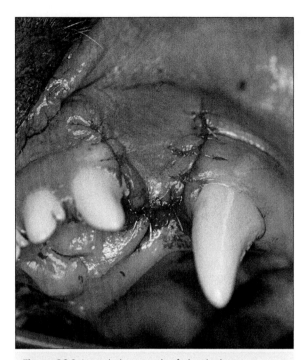

Figure 26.9 Lateral photograph of alveoloplasty. Alveoloplasty (raising a mucoperiosteal flap, recontouring the alveolar bone and replacing the flap) of the left diastema was performed to ensure that the left lower canine was securely positioned laterally.

also needs to be aware that a degree of discomfort will be present for as long as the device is in place. Maintenance of oral hygiene (daily toothbrushing and rinsing with chlorhexidine) is extremely important while an appliance is in place. Moreover, the dog is not allowed access to toys and is restricted to supervised lead walks (so she can't pick up objects to chew on) for the period that the orthodontic appliance is in place. In short, she needs to be restricted to a rather unnatural lifestyle for a dog.

Orthodontic treatment may also cause iatrogenic injuries, e.g. pulp and periapical complication, root resorption. Therefore, the effect of orthodontic treatment needs to be monitored clinically and radiographically. Appliances that supply just enough force to achieve the required movement need to be selected.

Initially, I thought that orthodontic tooth movement would be quick and easy in this case. As it turned out, this was not the case. In retrospect, tooth shortening and endodontic treatment may have been a better option from the animal's point of view, but the owner would not have agreed to that; furthermore, on initial evaluation this did not appear to be the treatment of choice. However, the dog did not appear to be in appreciable discomfort during the 8 weeks that the mandibular expansion device was in place and the outcome was successful.

This case is a mild skelelatal malocclusion and is thus likely to be inheritable. The owner was counselled not to breed from this dog.

27 Tooth shortening and endodontic therapy

INITIAL PRESENTATION

Inability to close mouth.

PATIENT DETAILS

An 11-month-old, male, bearded collie.

CASE HISTORY

The owner was concerned that the dog didn't seem to be able to close his mouth completely and drooled continuously. Also, he would not play with toys and would only eat soft food.

The dog had been involved in a slow speed accident with a car when 6 months old (the owner had accidentally backed into him). He had seemed unhurt at the time. The problem with jaw closure was noted roughly a month after the accident and had been getting progressively worse.

The dog was seen by its own veterinarian, who referred the case to us for evaluation and treatment.

ORAL EXAMINATION – CONSCIOUS

This was a nice-tempered dog that allowed thorough oral examination and occlusal evaluation (Figs 27.1 and 27.2).

The following were noted:
1. Saliva-soaked and saliva-stained fur around jaws
2. Would not allow full closure of jaws
3. Generalized gingivitis
4. Complicated crown fracture (CCF) of 101
5. Occlusion:
   - The upper jaw was longer on the left than on the right side
   - The lower jaw was of normal length and width for the breed
   - There was an obvious midline deviation of incisors

- Tooth 304 was upright in position and occluded with the palate, causing a 14-mm-deep ulcerated indentation
- Tooth 404 flared laterally and fitted into the diastema between 103 and 104.

ORAL EXAMINATION – UNDER GENERAL ANAESTHETIC

A thorough oral and dental examination, including investigating periodontal parameters, was performed. All findings were noted on the dental record sheet.

In summary, examination under general anaesthesia identified the following:
1. Generalized gingivitis
2. Complicated crown fracture (CCF) of 101
3. Occlusion:
   - The upper jaw was longer on the left than on the right side, with obvious midline deviation
   - The lower jaw was of normal length and width for the breed
   - Tooth 304 was upright in position and occluded with the palate, causing a 14-mm-deep ulcerated indentation, which was filled with debris
   - Tooth 404 flared laterally and fitted into the diastema between 103 and 104.

It was identified that it was the maloccluding 304 which prevented full mouth closure. There was no evidence of trauma associated with occlusion of any other teeth.

FURTHER INVESTIGATIONS

Radiographs of 101 (CCF), 304 and 404 were taken.

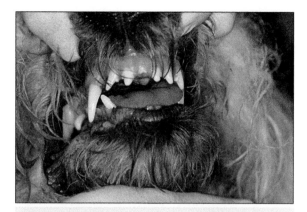

Figure 27.1 Wry bite – rostral view in the conscious animal. Occlusion is best examined in the conscious animal. The dog does not allow closure of the mouth and drools continuously. There is obvious saliva staining of the fur. Note the midline deviation of the incisors. Tooth 404 is flared out, and there is space in the diastema between 103 and 104 for this tooth to fit in normal occlusion if the jaws were able to close.

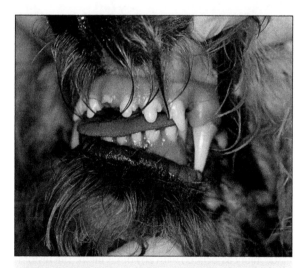

Figure 27.2 Wry bite – left lateral view of rostral occlusion in the conscious animal. Tooth 304 is trapped medially, occluding with palatal mucosa, causing a deep, ulcerated indentation.

RADIOGRAPHIC FINDINGS

1. Tooth 101 (CCF) had a wide pulp diameter and open apex.
2. Teeth 304 and 404 had complete apical closure and a substantial amount of secondary dentine formed.

THEORY REFRESHER

Malocclusion can result from jaw length and/or width discrepancy (skeletal malocclusion), from tooth malpositioning (dental malocclusion), or a combination of both. The malocclusion seen in this case is called a wry bite, and is the consequence of the discrepancy in length between the left and the right upper jaw, i.e. it is a skeletal malocclusion. A wry bite occurs if one side of the head or one side of a jaw grows more than the other side. In its mildest form, a one-sided prognathic or brachygnathic bite develops. In more severe cases, a crooked head and bite develops, with a deviated midline. An open bite may also develop in the incisor region so that the affected teeth are displaced vertically and do not occlude.

Skeletal malocclusion is considered inherited unless a developmental cause can be reliably identified. In this case, the traumatic incident at 6 months of age could explain the wry bite. The trauma may have caused cessation of growth of the right side for a period of time. The complicated fracture of 101 supports the hypothesis that it was a right-sided trauma. The left upper jaw and the lower jaw carried on growing at the normal rate. So, this skeletal malocclusion should be given the benefit of the doubt and not be considered inherited.

Malocclusion causing discomfort and pathology always needs treating.

The treatment options available are orthodontics, tooth shortening or extraction. The aim of any treatment is primarily to make the animal comfortable; aesthetics are a secondary consideration.

CLINICAL TIPS

- Malocclusion can result from jaw length and/or width discrepancy (skeletal malocclusion), from tooth malpositioning (dental malocclusion), or a combination of both.
- Malocclusion causing discomfort and pathology should always be treated.
- The aim of any treatment is to make the animal comfortable; aesthetics are a secondary consideration.
- Relatively mature teeth with a good layer of secondary dentine and apical closure can be treated by conventional endodontics (pulpectomy, root filling and restoration).
- Immature teeth should be treated by partial pulpectomy, direct pulp capping and restoration.

TREATMENT OPTIONS

1. Extraction of 304. The lower canines are large, functionally important teeth and contribute to the bony strength of the lower jaw. Maintaining 304 would be beneficial to the dog.
2. Shortening and endodontic treatment of 304. This is probably the best option for this case. It would take the canine out of occlusion and allow full closure of the mouth. The palatal defect would heal rapidly once the inciting trauma had been removed.
3. Orthodontics. No orthodontic options are applicable to this case.

TREATMENT PERFORMED

1. Periodontal therapy to remove plaque and calculus and provide a clean environment for surgery, and for the owner to start instituting home care (daily toothbrushing).
2. Shortening and conventional endodontic therapy (pulpectomy, root canal filling and restoration) of 304. Tooth 304 was shortened to level with the lower incisors.
3. Curettage of palatal indentations.
4. Extraction of 101 (CCF). Pre- and post-extraction radiographs were taken.

POSTOPERATIVE CARE

- NSAIDs for 5 days
- Daily toothbrushing
- The dog was rebooked for oral examination and radiographs of 304 (to assess periapical status) under general anaesthesia after 6 months.

RECHECK

At recheck 6 months after initial treatment, the owner reported that the dog was no longer drooling and was now eating dry food and dental hygiene treats. She was brushing his teeth almost daily. Conscious examination revealed that the dog had full mouth closure and there was no evidence of saliva staining of the fur on the muzzle. Oral examination under general anaesthesia identified mild gingivitis associated with premolars and molars, where the owner had trouble getting access

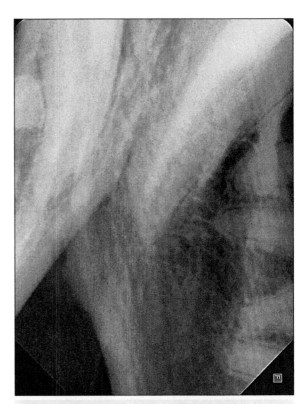

Figure 27.3 Radiograph 6 months after conventional endodontic treatment. Endodontic therapy requires radiographs (generally 6 months later) to assess the outcome. This radiograph demonstrates successful outcome in that there is no evidence of any periapical destruction, i.e. the periodontal ligament space is uniform in diameter and clearly demarcates root from alveolar bone, and there is no evidence of any radiolucent regions in the bone around the apex.

with the toothbrush. The palatal defect associated with 304 had healed and there was no evidence of any soft tissue injury associated with any other teeth. The restoration of 304 was intact and the tooth was not discoloured. Radiographs confirmed a successful outcome of the endodontic procedure performed on 304 (Fig. 27.3). No further treatment was indicated, unless the restoration is damaged or lost. The owner was given toothbrushing instruction and continued daily toothbrushing was encouraged.

PROGNOSIS

Shortening 304 removed the trauma, and healing of the palatal indentation should be rapid. The dog can close its mouth and should have pain-free occlusion as well as acceptable function.

Conventional endodontic treatment has a high success rate. As long as the restoration stays in place, 304 has an excellent prognosis. The success of the endodontic treatment needs radiographic confirmation 6 months after initial therapy.

COMMENTS

Tooth shortening and endodontic treatment is a useful method for treating certain types of malocclusion. If the tooth that requires shortening is relatively mature (good layer of secondary dentine and apical closure), then conventional endodontics (pulpectomy, root filling and restoration) is preferable to partial pulpectomy, direct pulp capping and restoration. The latter technique should be limited to immature teeth, where the goal is to keep the pulp alive for continued root development. It should be seen as a temporary procedure and conventional endodontics should be performed once the tooth is mature enough.

The skeletal malocclusion in this case was not considered inheritable as a clear cause had been identified. Breeding from her was considered acceptable.

INITIAL PRESENTATION

Malocclusion – lower canine teeth erupting into palatal mucosa, causing teeth indentations and ulceration.

PATIENT DETAILS

A 6-month-old, female, Great Dane.

CASE HISTORY

The owner was concerned about the indentations and ulcerations caused by the maloccluding lower canine teeth. The dog was showing signs of discomfort from the malocclusion (not playing with toys, selecting soft food in preference to hard, not eating very well, etc.). The dog had been examined by its own veterinarian, who referred the case to us for evaluation and treatment.

ORAL EXAMINATION – CONSCIOUS

The dog was nice tempered but anxious when the head and face were examined. Oral malodour was obvious. Cursory oral examination revealed that the upper jaw was of normal length and width for the breed, but the mandible was much too short and narrow. The lower canines occluded with the palatal mucosa, causing deep ulcerated indentations, which were filled with debris.

ORAL EXAMINATION – UNDER GENERAL ANAESTHETIC

A thorough oral and dental examination, including investigating periodontal parameters, was performed. All findings were noted on the dental record sheet. In summary, examination under general anaesthesia identified the following:

1. Skeletal malocclusion. Upper jaw of normal length and width, with short and narrow lower jaw, i.e. mandibular brachygnathism. The lower incisors were occluding with the palatal mucosa, but not causing any soft tissue lesions. The lower canines occluded with the palatal mucosa, distal to the upper canines, causing deep ulcerated indentations (12 mm), which were filled with debris. There were also non-ulcerated indentations in the palatal mucosa where the lower carnassials occluded.
2. Generalized mild gingivitis.

FURTHER INVESTIGATIONS

Radiographs of 304 and 404 were taken to determine the developmental stage.

RADIOGRAPHIC FINDINGS

Teeth 304 and 404 were immature (as expected in a 6-month-old dog) with open apices and only a thin layer of secondary dentine formed.

THEORY REFRESHER

Malocclusion can result from jaw length and/or width discrepancy (skeletal malocclusion), from tooth malpositioning (dental malocclusion), or a combination of both. This case is a skeletal malocclusion and is thus inheritable. Malocclusion causing discomfort and pathology always needs treating.

The treatment options available are orthodontics, tooth shortening or extraction. The aim of any treatment is primarily to make the animal comfortable; aesthetics are a secondary consideration.

CLINICAL TIPS

- Malocclusion can result from jaw length and/or width discrepancy (skeletal malocclusion), from tooth malpositioning (dental malocclusion), or a combination of both.
- Skeletal malocclusion is inheritable. Affected dogs should not be used for breeding.
- The aim of any treatment is primarily to make the animal comfortable; aesthetics are a secondary consideration.
- Malocclusion causing discomfort and pathology should always be treated.
- It is important to monitor partial pulpectomy, direct pulp capping and restoration procedure radiographically.

TREATMENT OPTIONS

1. Extraction of all maloccluding teeth. The lower canines are the two teeth that are causing pathology. While the lower incisors and lower carnassials do occlude with the palatal mucosa, they are causing only small indentations which are not ulcerated. The lower canines are large, functionally important teeth and contribute to the bony strength of the lower jaw. Maintaining them would be beneficial to the dog.
2. Shortening and endodontic treatment of the lower canines. This is probably the best option for this case. It would take the canines out of occlusion and allow the palatal defects to heal.
3. Orthodontics. This is not practical for this case. Theoretically, one could perform jaw lengthening surgery, but this would not be humane.

TREATMENT PERFORMED

1. Periodontal therapy to remove plaque and calculus and provide a clean environment for surgery, and for the owner to start instituting home care (daily toothbrushing).
2. Shortening and endodontic therapy (partial pulpectomy, direct pulp capping and restoration) of 304 and 404. Both teeth were shortened level with the incisors.
3. Curettage of palatal indentations.

POSTOPERATIVE CARE

- NSAIDs for 5 days
- Antibiotics for 5 days
- Daily toothbrushing
- The dog was rebooked for oral examination and radiographs of 304 and 404 (to assess periapical status) under general anaesthesia after 6 months.

RECHECK

The dog did not come back for its 6-month recheck, as she developed other, more life-threatening problems, which were treated with ovariohysterectomy. I did not see her again until 1 year after the tooth shortening and endodontic therapy. At this time, the owner was concerned about halitosis and signs of discomfort (not eating well).

Oral examination under general anaesthesia 1 year after initial treatment showed that the palatal indentations caused by the mandibular canines had healed, but there were now deep ulcerated palatal indentations from lower incisors (Fig. 28.1). The indentations were

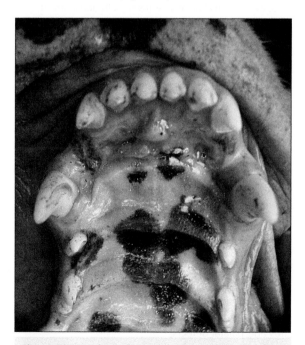

Figure 28.1 Occlusal photograph of the hard palate. The maloccluding lower incisors are causing deep, infected indentations in the palatal mucosa. Halitosis was intense. Note the pus oozing out of the indentations.

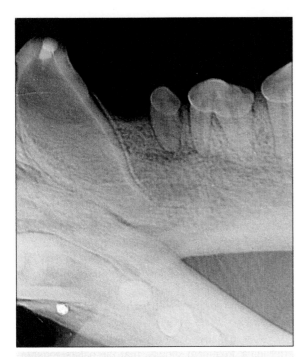

Figure 28.2 Lateral radiograph of 304. The radiograph reveals failure of the endodontic procedure (partial pulpectomy, direct pulp capping and restoration) performed a year earlier. As a consequence of pulpal disease (inflammation and necrosis) tooth development ceased, as evidenced by the wide pulp diameter and open apex.

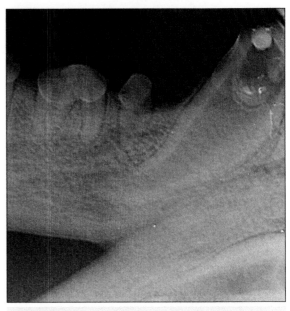

Figure 28.3 Lateral radiograph of 404. The radiograph reveals failure of the endodontic procedure (partial pulpectomy, direct pulp capping and restoration) performed a year earlier. As a consequence of pulpal disease (inflammation and necrosis) tooth development ceased, as evidenced by the wide pulp diameter and open apex. Note the hard tissue bridge separating the pulp from the direct pulp capping material. This tells us that pulpal inflammation and necrosis occurred some time after initial treatment. Note also the periapical destruction.

filled with pus and there was intense malodour. The palatal indentations from the lower carnassials were superficial and not ulcerated. The restorations of 304 and 404 were intact and the teeth were not discoloured. However, radiographs revealed failure of the endodontic treatment: both teeth had wide pulp systems and there was a periapical destruction associated with 404 (Figs 28.2 and 28.3). Treatment consisted of open extraction of the mandibular incisors and canines (Fig. 28.4), and curettage of the palatal defects. The dog was discharged with antibiotics for 1 week and advised to see their own veterinarian in 3 weeks to check healing of extraction sites and palatal defects.

A lovely thank you card from the owner 6 weeks after extraction reported that the dog was happy and functional. The extraction site and the palatal defects had healed uneventfully.

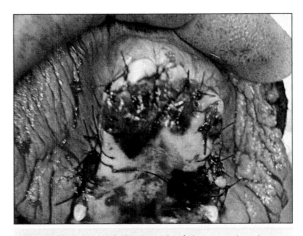

Figure 28.4 Occlusal photograph of the extraction sites. The mandibular incisors and canines were extracted using an open technique. Pre- and post-extraction radiographs were taken. The flap was replaced using 5/0 Monocryl.

PROGNOSIS

Shortening the lower canines will remove the trauma and allow healing of the palatal indentations. The dog should have pain-free occlusion as well as acceptable function.

Partial pulpectomy, direct pulp capping and restoration is a temporary procedure used in immature teeth. The purpose of the procedure is to keep the pulp vital to allow continued tooth development. Once the tooth is more mature, a total pulpectomy, root filling and restoration procedure is required. While, partial pulpectomy, direct pulp capping and restoration has a good success rate, there is always the possibility that the pulp becomes inflamed and tooth development ceases. If pulpal pathology (inflammation, necrosis) occurs, then periapical pathology will develop. If this occurs, the tooth requires either extraction or conventional endodontic therapy (pulpectomy, root filling and restoration).

COMMENTS

No further treatment is required for the malocclusion.

It is rare that the incisors cause extensive soft tissue damage with this type of malocclusion. Normally, it is only the canine teeth that cause severe pathology. In other words, shortening and endodontic therapy of the mandibular canines results in healing of the palatal ulcerations and a pain-free, functional bite.

This case highlights the importance of monitoring partial pulpectomy, direct pulp capping and restoration procedure radiographically so that interceptive treatment (further endodontic therapy or extraction) can be performed early.

Extraction of permanent teeth

INITIAL PRESENTATION

Malocclusion – long upper jaw resulting in a relative mandibular brachygnathia.

PATIENT DETAILS

A 7-month-old, female, weimaraner.

CASE HISTORY

The owner was concerned about the 'long curved nose' and the obsessive chewing on toys, furniture, etc. Their own veterinarian noted that the lower jaw was too short with respect to the upper jaw, and the dog was referred to us for evaluation and treatment of the malocclusion.

ORAL EXAMINATION – CONSCIOUS

The dog was well behaved and allowed conscious examination, which revealed the following:
1. Skeletal malocclusion
   - The upper jaw was extremely long and narrow with respect to the lower jaw, which was of relatively normal length and width for the breed, i.e. relative mandibular brachygnathism.
   - The lower canines occluded with the palatal mucosa, distal to the upper canines, causing deep indentations in palate.
   - The lower incisors occluded with the palatal mucosa, causing less severe indentations.
2. Generalized gingivitis
3. Uncomplicated crown fracture of 204.

The pulp did not seem exposed to the environment on visual examination. Exploration was not attempted, since touching an exposed pulp would have caused extreme pain and potentially aggressive behaviour.

ORAL EXAMINATION – UNDER GENERAL ANAESTHETIC

A thorough oral and dental examination, including investigating periodontal parameters, was performed. All findings were noted on the dental record sheet.

In summary, examination under general anaesthesia identified the following list:
1. Skeletal malocclusion
   - The upper jaw was extremely long and narrow with respect to the lower jaw, which was of a relatively normal length and width for the breed, i.e. relative mandibular brachygnathism.
   - The lower canines occluded with the palatal mucosa, distal to the upper canines, causing ulcerated indentations in the palate (Fig. 29.1).
   - The lower incisors occluded with the palatal mucosa, causing non-ulcerated indentations (Fig. 29.1). There were also indentations in the palatal mucosa where the lower carnassials occluded.
2. Generalized mild gingivitis (Fig. 29.1)
3. Uncomplicated crown fracture of 204.

Careful examination with a sharp explorer did not allow communication into the pulp.

FURTHER INVESTIGATIONS

Radiographs were taken of 204 (UCF) and of 104 (contralateral healthy tooth).

RADIOGRAPHIC FINDINGS

The shape and diameter of the pulp system of 104 (contralateral healthy) and 204 (UCF) were the same.

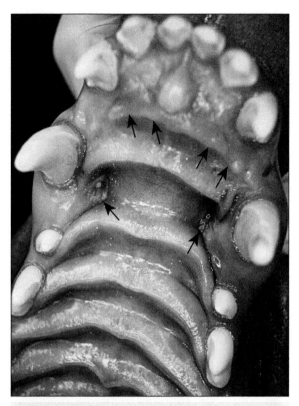

Figure 29.1 Traumatic lesions in the palatal mucosa. The upper jaw is long and narrow, while the lower jaw is of normal length and width for the breed. Consequently, the teeth are not occluding normally. Note the ulcerated indentations created by the maloccluding lower canines (they occlude with the palatal mucosa medial to the upper canines). Note also the indentations in the palatal mucosa where the lower incisors occlude. There is a generalized gingivitis as evidenced by the red and swollen gingival margins around the circumference of all teeth.

Both were immature teeth, as expected in a 7-month-old dog.

There was no evidence of periapical pathology of 204 (UCF).

THEORY REFRESHER

Malocclusion can result from jaw length and/or width discrepancy (skeletal malocclusion), from tooth malpositioning (dental malocclusion), or a combination of both. This case is a skeletal malocclusion and should therefore be considered as inheritable. Malocclusion causing discomfort and pathology always needs treating.

The treatment options available are orthodontics, tooth shortening or extraction. In many instances, tooth shortening or extraction are preferable to orthodontics on ethical grounds.

In human orthodontics, whether malocclusion is hereditary or acquired is not a consideration when planning treatment. This is in contrast to veterinary orthodontics, where aesthetics and ethical concerns are linked, and treatment for the sole purpose of showing dogs or cats cannot be encouraged. The aim of any treatment is primarily to make the animal comfortable; aesthetics are a secondary consideration.

It is essential to determine if the presenting malocclusion is hereditary or not. Orthodontic correction of a malocclusion is contraindicated where the malocclusion is hereditary, unless the animal is also neutered. The rationale for this is to avoid spread of inherited malocclusion within a breed.

Crown fractures are classified as complicated if the fracture line exposes the pulp to the oral environment and as uncomplicated if they do not involve pulpal exposure. Crown fractures are obvious visually. However, at times it can be difficult to determine if the pulp is exposed by the fracture line, and general anaesthesia for examination with a dental explorer and radiography are necessary.

An uncomplicated crown fracture usually requires minimal treatment, e.g. removal of sharp edges with a bur and sealing of the exposed dentine with a suitable liner or restorative material. However, such fractures do require monitoring (clinical examination and radiography) at regular intervals to ensure that the pulp remains vital. If pulp and periapical diseases develop, the tooth requires either extraction or endodontic therapy.

CLINICAL TIPS

- Malocclusion can result from jaw length and/or width discrepancy (skeletal malocclusion), from tooth malpositioning (dental malocclusion), or a combination of both.
- Skeletal malocclusion is inheritable. Affected dogs should not be used for breeding.
- Malocclusion causing discomfort and pathology always needs treating.
- The treatment options available are orthodontics, tooth shortening or extraction.
- It can be difficult to determine if the pulp is exposed by a crown fracture.
- Uncomplicated crown fracture usually requires minimal treatment, but ongoing monitoring is important.

TREATMENT OPTIONS

1. Shortening and endodontic treatment of the lower canines. This is a possible option to reduce the discomfort, but there would still be indentations and possibly ulceration associated with the maloccluding incisors. In other words, there would not be complete healing of the palatal defects and the dog may still be uncomfortable.
2. Shortening and endodontic treatment of the lower canines and extraction of the lower incisors. This is the best option. The traumatic occlusion would be removed and the palatal mucosa would heal. Also, the mandible would not be weakened by the removal of the lower canines and associated bone. Radiographic monitoring of the endodontic therapy (radiographs 6 months later) would be required. So, two episodes of general anaesthesia would be necessary.
3. Extraction of the lower canines and incisors. This is an acceptable choice in this case, as the lower incisors were also causing deep palatal indentations. It is a one-stage procedure, unlike option 2, which would require radiographic monitoring of the outcome of the endodontic therapy.

TREATMENT PERFORMED

1. Periodontal therapy to remove plaque and calculus and provide a clean environment.
2. Smoothing sharp fracture edges and sealing exposed dentine tubules. Since the radiographs showed no evidence of pulp/periapical disease of 204, there was no need for endodontic therapy.
3. Extraction of the lower incisors and canines. The owner wanted a quick solution to the problem and was not prepared to return for radiographic monitoring of endodontic therapy. The teeth were extracted using an open technique (Figs 29.2, 29.3 and 29.4). The flap was replaced using 5/0 Monocryl. Pre- and post-extraction radiographs were taken.
4. Curettage of palatal indentations was performed.

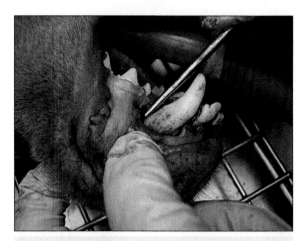

Figure 29.2 Open extraction. The mucoperiosteal buccal access flap extends from the mesial aspect of 305 to the mesial aspect of 405, with short, vertical releasing incisions at these locations. Buccal and lingual bone was removed to facilitate extraction (luxation and elevation) of lower canines and incisors. Pre- and post-extraction radiographs were taken.

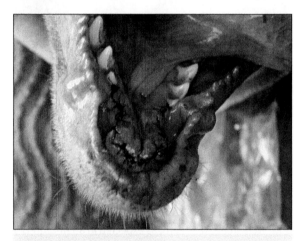

Figure 29.3 Flap closure. Once postoperative radiographs had confirmed successful extraction of the canines and incisors, the extraction sockets were closed by attaching the buccal flap to the lingual gingiva (which had been elevated off the bone to provide required tissue for anchorage) using 5/0 Monocryl. For optimal healing the flap closure must be completely free of tension.

RECHECK

Conscious examination 4 weeks later showed that the palatal ulcerations and all extraction sites had healed. Small indentations where the lower carnassials occluded were still present, but they were not deep and fully

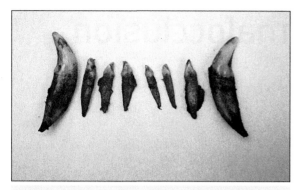

Figure 29.4 Extracted teeth. Note that all tooth roots appear intact. Radiographs to confirm successful extraction and absence of sharp bony edges are still required.

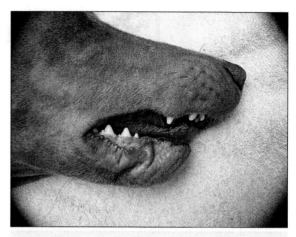

Figure 29.5 Lateral photograph after tooth extraction. The length discrepancy between the upper and lower jaw is obvious. Extraction of the lower incisors and canines will remove the traumatic occlusion and allow the palatal injuries to heal. The dog will have pain-free and relatively functional occlusion.

epithelialized. The owner was brushing the teeth daily and the gingivae were clinically healthy. The owner reported that the dog was no longer incessantly looking for objects to chew on.

The owner did not want to return for radiographic monitoring of the pulp and periapical status of 204 (UCF). It was decided that the referring veterinarian would take radiographs of 204 at the time of neutering 3 months later.

PROGNOSIS

Extraction of the maloccluding lower incisors and canines will allow healing of the palatal indentations and remove the discomfort (Fig. 29.5). The dog should have pain-free occlusion as well as acceptable function.

The malocclusion is inheritable and she should not be used for breeding.

Uncomplicated crown fractures do require monitoring (clinical examination and radiography) at regular intervals to ensure that the pulp remains vital. If pulp and periapical disease develop, the tooth requires either extraction or endodontic therapy.

COMMENTS

No further treatment is required for the malocclusion.

Pulp/periapical complications with 204 (UCF) may still occur. The owner was advised to monitor the tooth colour and seek veterinary advice if the tooth begins to discolour (pink, grey).

30 Iatrogenic malocclusion

INITIAL PRESENTATION

A dog unable to close his mouth, with atrophy of the muscles of mastication on the left side of the face.

PATIENT DETAILS

A 5-year-old, male, springer spaniel.

CASE HISTORY

The dog was referred for management of complications to jaw fracture healing. Case history was not supplied. The owner reported that the dog had been involved in a road traffic accident 6 weeks earlier. The mandible had fractured, as had multiple teeth. The mandibular fracture had been stabilized using double figure-of-eight wires around the lower canines (wires in place but loose) and some teeth had been extracted. Further extractions had been performed 3 weeks prior to referral. The dog had been unable to close his mouth since the accident (6 weeks ago) and the owner had noticed that the muscles on the left side of the face (above eye) were undergoing atrophy. The dog was eating well but selecting soft food rather than kibbles.

ORAL EXAMINATION – CONSCIOUS

This was a boisterous dog that did not cooperate sufficiently for thorough oral examination, but findings on cursory examination were as follows:
- Continuous drooling
- Normal jaw opening, but unable to fully close mouth (Figs 30.1, 30.2 and 30.3)
- Lower jaw deviating to the right (Figs 30.1, 30.2 and 30.3)
- Incisors in reverse scissor occlusion (Figs 30.1, 30.2 and 30.3)

- Tooth 404 positioned laterally to 103 (Fig. 30.2)
- Tooth 304 positioned medially to 203 (Fig. 30.3)
- Missing teeth (Fig. 30.1)
- Fractured teeth (Fig. 30.1)
- Marked muscle wastage of muscles of mastication (temporal, masseter and pterygoid) on the left side.

ORAL EXAMINATION – UNDER GENERAL ANAESTHETIC

While occlusion is best assessed in the conscious animal, in cases that are not amenable to conscious occlusal evaluation, it needs to be performed under general anaesthesia. The tongue needs to be folded caudally during the evaluation so as not to interfere with normal jaw closure. Pharyngotomy intubation rather than orotracheal intubation is useful when occlusal evaluation is required.

A thorough oral and dental examination, including investigating periodontal parameters, was performed. All findings were noted on the dental record sheet.

In summary, examination under general anaesthesia identified the following:
1. The mandibular fracture had healed. The jaw was stable and there was a palpable callus at the ventral border of the left and right mandible level with apices of canine teeth.
2. Jaw opening was normal.
3. Full closure of the mouth was not possible due to the mechanical obstruction from the malocclusion (Figs 30.1, 30.2 and 30.3):
   - Tooth 404 was positioned laterally to 103
   - Tooth 304 was positioned medially to 203.

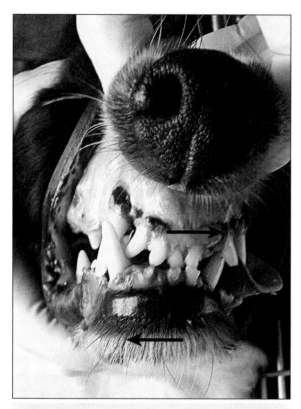

Figure 30.1 Head-on photograph of the rostral occlusion. The mandible is deviated to the right and the dog is unable to close his mouth because of the iatrogenic (mandibular fracture stabilized without considering occlusion) malocclusion; 404 is lateral to 103 and 304 is trapped medial to 203. There is also reverse scissor occlusion of incisors, which may have been present prior to jaw fracture. Note also the missing (303, 401, 403) and fractured teeth (202, 402).

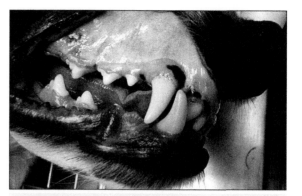

Figure 30.2 Right lateral photograph of the rostral occlusion. The deviation of the mandible to the right and the traumatic occlusion of the right lower canine (404 occluding with the lateral aspect of 103) is evident, as is the reverse scissor occlusion of the incisors.

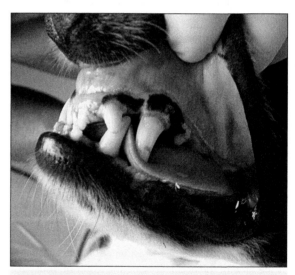

Figure 30.3 Left lateral photograph of the rostral occlusion. The deviation of the mandible to the right and the traumatic occlusion of the left lower canine (304 is occluding with the palatal aspect of 203) providing mechanical obstruction to full mouth closure is obvious, as is the reverse scissor occlusion of the incisors.

4. There was no swelling, abnormal movement or crepitus from the temporomandibular joint (TMJ) on either opening or partial closure of the jaws. When evaluating the TMJ, it is useful to place the animal in dorsal recumbency and manipulate jaw opening, closure and lateral movement while a second person holds the head and upper jaw in a fixed position. The tongue needs to be folded caudally to avoid interference with jaw closure.
5. There was marked atrophy of the muscles of mastication on the left-hand side.
6. There were complicated crown fractures (CCF) of 202 and 402 (Fig. 30.1).
7. There was an uncomplicated crown fracture (UCF) of 204.
8. There was a retained root remnant of 403.

9. The extraction sockets of 108, 208 and 309 were not fully healed (extracted 3 weeks earlier).
10. There was generalized moderate gingivitis.

FURTHER INVESTIGATIONS

Radiographs were taken of the following:
1. Mandibular fracture sites
2. Right and left temporomandibular joint (TMJ)

3. Upper incisors
4. Lower incisors
5. Extraction sites of 108, 208 and 309
6. Teeth 204 (UCF) and 104 (contralateral healthy).

RADIOGRAPHIC FINDINGS

- The fracture healed with obvious callus formation.
- TMJ radiographs revealed no abnormalities (Fig. 30.4a, b).
- Teeth 202 and 402 had complicated crown fractures, with no evidence of pulp and periapical disease as yet.
- The socket of 403 contained a root remnant.
- The extraction sockets of 108, 208 and 309 were empty.
- Tooth 204 (UCF) showed no evidence of pulp or periapical disease (as compared to healthy contralateral 104).

THEORY REFRESHER

Malocclusion in this case has resulted from an inappropriate choice of jaw fracture repair technique which did not take occlusion into account. The fracture had been stabilized with the teeth maloccluding (404 positioned laterally to 103 and 304 positioned medially to 203, i.e. the mandible deviated to the right). The fracture had been stable in this position and had healed, resulting in inability to fully close the mouth due to the mechanical obstruction from the maloccluding mandibular canine teeth.

The atrophy of the muscles of mastication on the left-hand side can be due to either neurogenic damage at the time of the accident or be the result of disuse for more than 6 weeks.

CLINICAL TIPS

- Occlusion is best assessed in the conscious animal.
- Pharyngotomy intubation rather than orotracheal intubation is useful when occlusal evaluation is required.
- Atrophy of the muscles of mastication can be due to either neurogenic damage or be the result of disuse.
- Uncomplicated crown fracture usually requires minimal treatment, but ongoing monitoring is important.

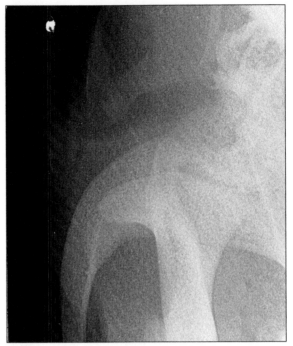

(a)

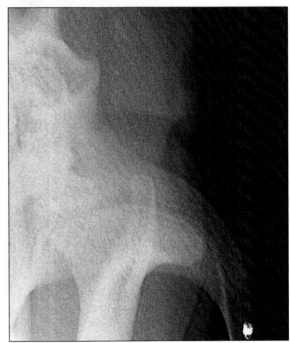

(b)

Figure 30.4 Dorsoventral (DV) radiograph of the right (a) and left (b) temporomandibular joints (TMJs). There is no evidence of pathology affecting the TMJs. Note the smooth condylar surfaces and clear joint spaces of similar width.

TREATMENT OPTIONS

1. Selective extraction of the teeth that are hindering closure of the jaws. This is the best choice in this case as it only requires extraction of 103 and 203. A buccal alveoloplasty may also be required on the left.
2. Shortening and endodontic treatment of the lower canines. This is unnecessary as jaw closure can be achieved by removing the smaller and functionally less important 103 and 203.
3. Orthodontic movement of teeth. While theoretically possible, it is not applicable in this case. It would require multiple anaesthetics and cause prolonged discomfort to the animal.
4. Refracturing the mandible and stabilizing it in correct occlusion. This is theoretically possible, but would cause discomfort to the animal during a relatively long healing period. Option 1 provides immediate relief and is thus preferable.

TREATMENT PERFORMED

1. Periodontal therapy to remove plaque and calculus and provide a clean environment for surgery, and for the owner to start instituting home care (daily toothbrushing)
2. Removal of loose orthopaedic wire (double figure-of-eight around mandibular canines)
3. Smoothing of rough edges and sealing dentine of 204 (UCF)
4. Open extraction of 202 (CCF) and 402 (CCF)
5. Open extraction of the root remnant of 403
6. Open extraction of 103 (Fig. 30.5a, b) and 203 (Fig. 30.6a, b)
7. Buccal alveoloplasty at 203.

Postoperative radiographs were taken of all extraction sites. Flaps were replaced with 5/0 Monocryl.

RECHECKS

Conscious recheck a month later revealed healing of extraction and alveoloplasty. The dog could close his mouth fully and had a functional bite. He was now

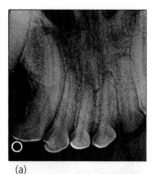

(a)

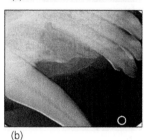

(b)

Figure 30.5 Pre-extraction (a) and post-extraction (b) radiographs of 103.

(a) The upper third incisors have long, curved roots, which make them difficult to extract using a closed technique.

(b) Successful extraction, i.e. with the whole root having been removed, should always be confirmed radiographically.

eating kibble as well as soft food. The atrophy of the muscles of mastication on the left remained unchanged. The dog was rebooked for examination under anaesthesia and radiographs of 204 (UCF) in 3 months.

At conscious examination 4 months after initial treatment, there was no evidence of muscle atrophy on the left (Fig. 30.7). The muscles of mastication had recovered fully, supporting the view that the atrophy was due to disuse rather than neurogenic damage. The owner reported that he seemed pain free and had no trouble closing his mouth (Fig. 30.8a, b). In fact, he was chewing on toys and enjoying dental hygiene chews. The owners were also brushing his teeth daily. Examination under anaesthesia revealed clinically healthy gingivae as a result of the daily toothbrushing. There was traumatic occlusion of the remaining upper incisors with the remaining lower incisors and the lingual mucosa. The malocclusion was causing lingual gingival recession and wear of 301, and inflammation of the lingual mucosa (Fig. 30.9). All remaining incisors were extracted. Radiographs of 204

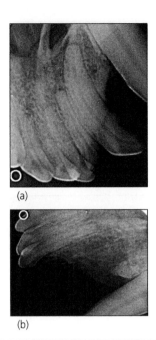

(a)

(b)

Figure 30.6 Pre-extraction (a) and post-extraction (b) radiographs of 203.

(a) Due to the long and curved root of the upper third incisors, I usually use an open extraction technique.

(b) Successful extraction, i.e. with the whole root having been removed, should always be confirmed radiographically. If an open extraction technique is used, then the radiograph should be taken before the flap is replaced and the socket sutured closed.

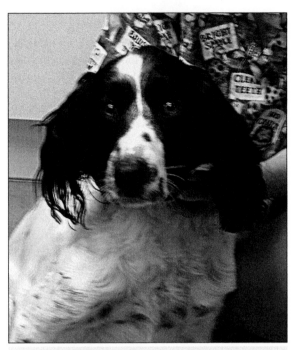

Figure 30.7 Head-on photograph of the head taken 4 months after initial treatment. The dog has pain-free and functional occlusion, with no obvious masticatory muscle atrophy. The fact that the left-sided atrophy of the muscles of mastication was reversible supports the view that it occurred as a consequence of disuse rather than neurogenic damage at the time of the jaw fracture.

(UCF) revealed no evidence of pulp and periapical disease (as compared with the contralateral healthy 104 and the previous radiograph of 204 taken 3 months earlier).

The dog was discharged with the recommendation to continue with daily toothbrushing. An uncomplicated crown fracture usually requires minimal treatment, e.g. removal of sharp edges with a bur and sealing of the exposed dentine with a suitable liner or restorative material. Pulp/periapical complications to uncomplicated crown fracture of 204 may still occur. The owners were advised to contact us immediately if 204 starts to discolour or the dog starts showing signs of discomfort, e.g. selective feeding, stops playing with toys, etc. Further radiographs of 204, e.g. after a year, would be prudent as pulp and periapical disease may occur in the absence of tooth discoloration. The dog will be recalled in 1 year, but no further treatment is anticipated.

PROGNOSIS

The extraction of 103 and extraction and buccal alveoloplasty at 203 resulted in full mouth closure. The dog should have pain-free occlusion as well as acceptable function.

The muscle wastage may be neurogenic or due to disuse. If the latter, one would expect some recovery.

COMMENTS

The method of jaw fracture repair chosen in this case had resulted in healing of the fracture but had created the malocclusion. While it is necessary to stabilize a fracture to get healing, maintaining occlusion is of paramount importance. In fact, the occlusion can be used to achieve fracture stabilization. A different device, e.g. an intra-oral acrylic splint, would have provided sufficient stability for bone healing while maintaining occlusion.

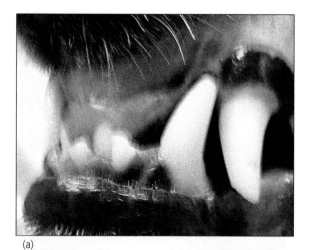

(a)

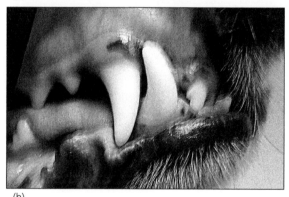

(b)

Figure 30.8 Oblique lateral photograph of left rostral occlusion (a) and of right rostral occlusion (b). The dog can close its mouth fully now the traumatic occlusion has been removed. Note the clean teeth and healthy gingivae as a consequence of daily toothbrushing.

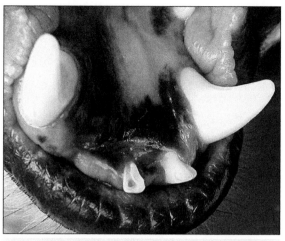

Figure 30.9 Occlusal photograph of the lower incisors. The remaining upper incisors were causing trauma to the remaining lower incisors and lingual gingivae. Note the gingival recession and wear facet on 301. Treatment consisted of extracting all remaining incisors.

The technique uses the teeth to splint the fracture. The advantages of this technique are:

- It is not invasive.
- Perfect occlusion is maintained.
- It is technically easy to do.
- It is a quick procedure, therefore only a short anaesthetic time is necessary.

The results are excellent and the technique is highly recommended.

PULP AND PERIAPICAL DISEASE

31 Pulp and periapical disease – an introduction

Trauma to a tooth (mechanical, chemical, thermal, infective) often results in pulpal inflammation (pulpitis). Depending on the type of trauma, its severity or duration, the pulpitis may be reversible, but often this is not the case and the inflammation becomes irreversible. The result of untreated irreversible pulpitis is pulp necrosis, followed by the spread of inflammation to affect the apical periodontium (apical periodontitis) and the periapical bone, resulting in bone destruction around the apex of the root (periapical disease).

A tooth affected by pulp and periapical diseases should always be treated, it cannot just be ignored. There are two available treatment options, namely to extract the tooth or to perform endodontic treatment and retain the tooth. Endodontic therapy is a specialist procedure and should not be undertaken without adequate training and supervised experience. The principles of endodontic therapy, which allows a tooth to be maintained, are outlined in Appendix 4.

PULPAL REACTIONS

The immature tooth has a wide pulp cavity. As the tooth matures, secondary dentine is laid down and the pulp cavity becomes narrower. Note that the contours of the pulp chamber mimic the shape of the crown, so the pulpal horns are always relatively close to the surface. Consequently, crown fracture very often involves exposure of the pulp in the older animal as well as the young.

As the animal gets older there is normally a reduction in the size of the pulp cavity, which is associated with continued deposition of secondary dentine. There are conditions that accelerate the rate of deposition of secondary dentine, thus prematurely reducing the size of the pulp cavity. Attrition and abrasion are two common conditions resulting in a narrow pulp cavity. Injury, orthodontic force and disease can all alter and decrease the pulp chamber and canals. In extreme cases, injury to a tooth will result in the complete obliteration of the pulp chamber and root canals. More unusually, the obliteration is partial, with the pulp chamber retaining the size and shape it had at the time of the injury, and the root canals becoming completely obliterated. On the other hand, injuries that cause inflammation and degeneration/necrosis of the pulp also account for many abnormally large pulp cavities, as dentine production ceases when the pulp is chronically inflamed or necrotic.

PERIAPICAL LESIONS

Pathology in the area surrounding the apex of a root, i.e. periapical pathology, is most commonly a sequel to chronic pulpitis or pulp necrosis. The source of the infection may be blood borne, but such cases are rare. The earliest radiographic evidence of periapical pathology is widening of the periodontal ligament space in the apical region. This widening is due to inflammation of the apical periodontal ligament. If untreated, the apical periodontitis progresses to involve the surrounding bone, resulting in destruction of the bone, which is replaced by soft tissue. This is evident as an apical rarefaction on a radiograph. The soft tissue may be granulation tissue (periapical granuloma), cyst (periapical or radicular cyst) or abscess (periapical abscess). Definitive differentiation between these three possibilities requires histopathology of the tissue. In veterinary dentistry, histopathology of periapical lesions is rarely performed. Treatment for all three entities is the same, i.e. endodontic therapy or if there are complicating factors, e.g. advanced periodontitis, then extraction. It is important to remember that not all apical rarefaction is pathological in dogs and cats. The periapical bone of normal canines often appears radiolucent in the dog. Comparison should always be made with other teeth of the same type in the same animal. A distinctly round radiolucent area, however, is usually pathological. Periapical sclerosis, instead of radiolucency, as a result of a chronically inflamed/necrotic pulp can sometimes be seen.

The periapical cyst usually occurs as a sequel to the periapical granuloma. It is a true cyst, since the lesion consists of a pathological, often fluid-filled, cavity that is lined by epithelium. Periapical cysts enlarge due to the osmotic gradient set up between the lumen of the cyst and tissue fluids in the surrounding connective tissue. These lesions can become very large at the expense of the adjacent bone tissue, which is resorbed due to pressure from the cyst.

An untreated periapical abscess can lead to complications such as osteomyelitis and cellulitis through spread of the infection. A fistulous tract opening on the skin or oral mucosa may develop.

Periapical lesions may be entirely asymptomatic or excruciatingly painful. The periapical granuloma and periapical cyst rarely cause severe discomfort, but they may undergo exacerbation and develop into a periodontal abscess, which usually is an extremely painful condition. The clinical signs indicative of periapical pathology are often insidious and not noticed by the owner. It is often only after completion of treatment that the owner reports a dramatic improvement in the animal's general demeanour. Consequently, periapical lesions confirmed by radiography should be treated even if the animal is not showing obvious signs of pain or discomfort. Similarly, discoloured teeth with a necrotic pulp need to be treated before periapical pathology develops. Once diagnosed, patients with necrotic pulps and periapical pathology should receive endodontic treatment (referral) or extraction of the affected tooth as soon as possible.

COMBINED PERIODONTIC AND ENDODONTIC LESIONS

There are possible pathways of communication between the pulp and the periodontium. These are denuded dentine tubules, lateral and/or accessory pulp canals, and at the apical foramen. Consequently, a periapical lesion may have a periodontal origin and a periodontal-type lesion may originate from the pulp. Another possibility is that a lesion is the result of a combination of endodontic and periodontal pathology. The lesions are classified according to aetiology as follows:

- A Class I lesion, or endodontic–periodontic lesion, is endodontic in origin, i.e. pathology begins in the pulp and progresses to involve the periodontium.
- A Class II lesion, or periodontic–endodontic lesion, is periodontic in origin, i.e. pathology begins in the periodontium and progresses to involve the pulp.
- A Class III lesion, or true combined lesion, is a fusion of independent periodontic and endodontic lesions.

Diagnosis depends on clinical examination and radiography. The prognosis for long-term retention of the tooth is based on the above classification. Class I lesions have a better prognosis, as endodontic treatment may lead to resolution of the periodontal extension of the inflammation. In contrast, Class II and III lesions require endodontic treatment as well as extensive periodontal therapy, and the periodontal destruction is often too extensive to be amenable to treatment.

Teeth with severe destruction of the periodontium should be extracted whatever the original cause. Other treatment options are endodontic therapy and/or periodontal therapy depending on the classification. Referral to a specialist is recommended.

OSTEOMYELITIS

Osteomyelitis of the jawbones is not a particularly common disease in dogs and cats. Infection of dental origin is not the only cause of osteomyelitis in the upper jaw or mandible, but it is probably the most frequent cause. Osteomyelitis then occurs as an extension of pulp and periapical pathology. The disease may be acute, subacute or chronic, and presents a different clinical course depending on its nature.

Osteomyelitis can be very difficult to differentiate from neoplastic bone lesions on radiography. Biopsy and histopathological examination of the bone is really the only way to reach a definitive diagnosis. Once diagnosed, osteomyelitis is treated by removing the cause (extraction or possibly endodontic therapy of teeth with pulp and periapical disease) in combination with antibiotic therapy. The choice of antibiotic should be based on the results of culture and antibiogram. The duration of antibiotic treatment required is usually longer than for other oral infections.

32 Uncomplicated crown fracture with periapical complications

INITIAL PRESENTATION

No presenting signs.

PATIENT DETAILS

A 9-year-old, neutered female, springer cross.

CASE HISTORY

This case was seen as a new client when I was in first opinion practice.

The owner was interested in oral care, and the dog had received an annual scale and polish since she was 2 years old (seven episodes of periodontal therapy under general anaesthesia). She was fed a dental diet and given daily dental hygiene chews. The owner reported that the dog was worried about having her face touched. The dog had previously allowed toothbrushing, but had not allowed it for the last year.

ORAL EXAMINATION – CONSCIOUS

The dog was aggressive when the head was approached and conscious oral examination was not possible.

ORAL EXAMINATION – UNDER GENERAL ANAESTHETIC

A thorough oral examination, including investigating periodontal parameters, was performed and all findings were entered on the dental record sheet.

In summary, examination under general anaesthesia identified the following:
1. Mild to moderate accumulation of dental deposits
2. Mild to moderate generalized gingivitis
3. Uncomplicated crown fracture (UCF) of 108 and 208 (Fig. 32.1)

4. Drainage tract at the mucogingival junction of mesial 208 (Fig. 32.1).

FURTHER INVESTIGATIONS

Radiographs were taken of 108 and 208.

RADIOGRAPHIC FINDINGS

The diameter of the pulp system of 108 was wide and the apices of the roots were open, indicating that the injury occurred during tooth development in the first year of life. There was also periapical inflammation with bone destruction and external root resorption (see Fig. 32.2 for details of the radiographic findings for 108).

The diameter of the pulp system of 208 was narrow and the apices were closed, i.e. it was a mature tooth, as expected in a 9-year-old dog. There was periapical inflammation with bone destruction. The drainage tract was shown to originate from the mesiopalatal root (see Fig. 32.3a, b for details of the radiographic findings for 208).

THEORY REFRESHER

Uncomplicated crown fractures expose dentine tubules and thus allow communication between pulp and oral environment, which can result in inflammation or death of the pulp. An uncomplicated crown fracture usually requires minimal treatment, e.g. removal of sharp edges with a bur and sealing of the exposed dentine with a suitable liner or restorative material. However, such fractures do require monitoring (clinical examination and

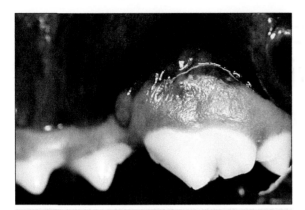

Figure 32.1 Lateral photograph of 208. The uncomplicated crown fracture involved the tip of the main cusp and can be seen in this view as a short main cusp. Note the draining tract at the mucogingival line mesial to 208.

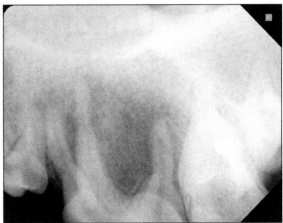

(a)

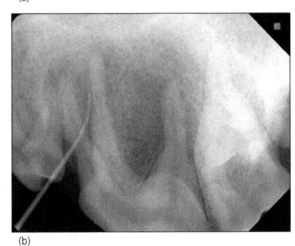

(b)

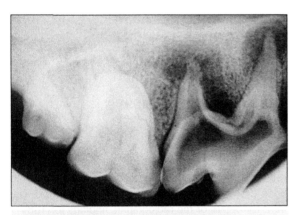

Figure 32.2 Radiograph of the right upper caudal mandible. Note the wide diameter of the pulp chamber and the distal root canal of 108, indicating pulp necrosis and cessation of dentine production. Periapical pathology is evident. There is a significant periapical destruction of the distal root of 108 and the apical segment is rough and uneven, indicating inflammatory external root resorption. A second view was taken to visualize the mesial roots, which were also found to have external root resorption and periapical bone destruction.

Figure 32.3 Radiographs centring on 208.

(a) Tooth 208 is mature with closed apices and narrow root canals, as expected in a 9-year-old dog. Lucent areas surround all three roots, indicating periapical bone destruction as a result of pulp necrosis.

(b) A gutta percha point inserted in the drainage tract shows that it originates from the mesiopalatal root.

radiography) at regular intervals to ensure that the pulp remains healthy. If pulp and periapical disease develops, the tooth requires either extraction or endodontic therapy.

The immature tooth has a wide pulp cavity. As the tooth matures, secondary dentine is laid down and the pulp cavity becomes narrower. Injuries that cause inflammation and/or necrosis of the pulp account for many abnormally large pulp cavities, as dentine production ceases when the pulp is chronically inflamed or necrotic. Necrotic immature teeth require endodontic treatment if they are to be retained. However, multiple general anaesthesia episodes are required and thus in most cases extraction of an immature tooth with a necrotic pulp, which is achieved in a single session, is usually the best course of action.

It should be noted that immature teeth might well be present in the mature animal if trauma caused pulp inflammation/necrosis during the developmental period. Treatment of immature teeth is always the same regardless of the actual age of the animal.

- Uncomplicated crown fracture usually requires minimal treatment, but ongoing monitoring is important.
- Injuries that cause inflammation and/or necrosis of the pulp account for many abnormally large pulp cavities, as dentine production ceases when the pulp is chronically inflamed or necrotic.
- Immature teeth might well be present in the mature animal if trauma caused pulp inflammation/necrosis during the developmental period.
- Pulp and periapical disease may be entirely asymptomatic or excruciatingly painful.
- The clinical signs indicative of disease are often insidious and not noticed by the owner.

TREATMENT OPTIONS

Extraction or endodontic treatment of 108 and 208.

TREATMENT PERFORMED

1. Periodontal therapy to remove plaque and calculus and provide a clean environment.
2. Open extraction of 108. Necrotic immature teeth require endodontic treatment if they are to be retained. In lieu of the extensive pathology (Fig. 32.2) present and to avoid the multiple anaesthetic episodes required for endodontic treatment of an immature tooth, extraction was the best course of action in this case.
3. Endodontic treatment (pulpectomy, root filling and restoration) of 208 (Fig. 32.4). The tooth was mature and unaffected by periodontitis, and the antagonist was present and healthy. Also, the owner was prepared to try to reinstitute daily toothbrushing. It was therefore decided to maintain the tooth.
4. Debridement of the drainage tract by means of blunt dissection from the orifice at the mucogingival junction towards the mesiopalatal root. It was left to granulate.

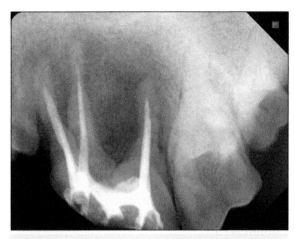

Figure 32.4 Radiograph centring on 208. This tooth has received endodontic treatment (pulpectomy and debridement of the three root canals, followed by root canal filling). This radiograph was taken to confirm adequate filling of the root canals before placing the final restorations.

- Daily chlorhexidine rinse for 1 week
- Reintroduce daily toothbrushing after 1 week
- The dog was booked for conscious recheck after 3 weeks.

RECHECK

At the recheck 3 weeks later, the owner reported a dramatic improvement in the dog's general demeanour, with increased appetite, a desire to play with toys and she was no longer protective about the face. Toothbrushing was also allowed.

The dog showed no signs of aggression on approaching the head and allowed oral examination. The extraction site of 108 had healed nicely. The restoration of 208 was intact with no evidence of discoloration of either tooth or restoration. The drainage tract had healed. There was minimal plaque accumulation on the teeth and the gingivae were clinically healthy. She was rebooked for examination under general anaesthesia and radiographs to assess the outcome of the endodontic treatment of 208 in 6 months' time.

Examination under general anaesthesia and radiographs 6 months later confirmed successful outcome of the endodontic treatment of 208 (periapical bone had regenerated). There was minimal plaque accumulation on the teeth and the gingivae were clinically healthy.

PROGNOSIS

The prognosis for this case is excellent, since the dog is allowing optimal home care, i.e. daily toothbrushing. She is also fed a dental diet and given dental hygiene chews. However, the dog will still require professional treatment at regular intervals; the specifics of the treatment need to be decided based on the efficacy of home care.

COMMENTS

Based on the developmental stage of the tooth (wide pulp system diameter, open apices), the uncomplicated crown fracture of 108 that resulted in pulp necrosis and periapical disease occurred at around 9 months of age. Although the dog received professional periodontal therapy annually (seven times), the UCF of 108 was not noted and pulp and periapical disease was allowed to develop for 8 years. The uncomplicated crown fracture of 208 was more recent, as the tooth was mature.

Pulp and periapical disease may be entirely asymptomatic or excruciatingly painful. The clinical signs indicative of disease are often insidious and not noticed by the owner. It is often only after completion of treatment (in this case, extraction of 108 and endodontic treatment of 208) that the owner reports a dramatic improvement in the animal's general demeanour, including temperament.

Complicated crown fracture with periapical disease

INITIAL PRESENTATION

Bilateral swelling on the ventral border of the mandible.

PATIENT DETAILS

A 3-year-old, neutered male, German shepherd.

CASE HISTORY

An extremely aggressive dog that only tolerates its owners! The dog needed to be muzzled at all times when in public. The first signs of aggression were noted when the dog was 16 weeks old. The aggression had become progressively worse with increasing age. The owner noticed a change in eating behaviour over the last few months. First, the dog went off its food for a few days and then started to wolf it down without chewing. They then noticed a swelling on the ventral mandible approximately a month prior to seeing us. They consulted their own veterinarian, who referred them to us for examination and treatment of the dog. The referring veterinarian had not been able to perform any examination at all.

ORAL EXAMINATION – CONSCIOUS

Conscious examination of this extremely aggressive dog was not possible.

ORAL EXAMINATION – UNDER GENERAL ANAESTHETIC

A thorough oral and dental examination, including investigating periodontal parameters, was performed. All findings were noted on the dental record sheet.

In summary, examination under general anaesthesia identified the following:

1. Occlusion normal
2. Generalized mild to moderate gingivitis
3. Complicated crown fracture (CCF) of all four canine teeth
4. Bilateral hard swelling on the ventral border of the mandible (extending from level with the first premolar to the distal aspect of the third premolar).

FURTHER INVESTIGATIONS

Radiographs were taken of all four canine teeth.

RADIOGRAPHIC FINDINGS

All four canines were mature teeth with closed apices. Periapical destruction and external root resorption were evident with all four canine teeth. The periapical lesions were more extensive in the lower jaw (Fig. 33.1), and had resulted in thinning and expansion of the ventral cortical bone.

ORAL PROBLEM LIST

Complicated crown fracture (CCF) resulting in pulpal inflammation and periapical disease affecting all four canines.

THEORY REFRESHER

The crown fracture has exposed the pulp, resulting in pulpal inflammation. The teeth are mature, i.e. the apices are closed, so the injury must have occurred when the dog was more than 1 year old. The inflammatory

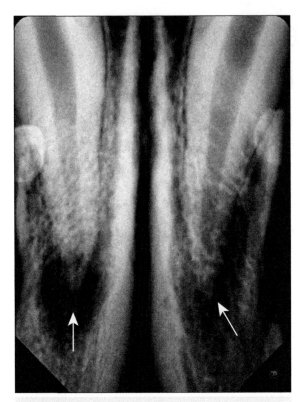

Figure 33.1 Rostrocaudal radiograph of the anterior mandible. Note the extensive periapical lesions affecting 304 and 404.

response has spread to involve the periapical region, resulting in destruction of the periapical bone. This is evident as an apical rarefaction on a radiograph. The bone defect is filled with soft tissue, which may be granulation tissue (periapical granuloma), cyst (periapical or radicular cyst) or abscess (periapical abscess). Definitive differentiation between these three possibilities requires histopathology of the tissue. The periapical cyst usually occurs as a sequel to the periapical granuloma. It is a true cyst since the lesion consists of a pathological, often fluid-filled, cavity that is lined by epithelium. Periapical cysts enlarge due to the osmotic gradient set up between the lumen of the cyst and tissue fluids in the surrounding connective tissue. These lesions can become very large at the expense of the adjacent bone tissue, which is resorbed (due to pressure from the cyst). Periapical lesions may be entirely asymptomatic or excruciatingly painful. The periapical granuloma and periapical cyst rarely cause severe discomfort, but they may undergo exacerbation and develop into a periodontal abscess, which usually is an extremely painful condition.

Periapical disease as a consequence of pulpal inflammation is treated by removing the inflamed pulp. This can be achieved in one of two ways, either endodontic therapy (the pulp is removed, the debrided root canal is filled and the access cavities restored, and the tooth is maintained) or extraction of the affected tooth (the whole tooth is removed). The presence of periapical disease is not a contraindication for endodontic treatment. Once the inflamed pulp has been removed, the periapical bone will regenerate and the defect will heal.

CLINICAL TIPS

- Bone defects are filled with soft tissue, which may be granulation tissue, cyst or abscess. Differentiating between these three possibilities requires histopathology of the tissue.
- Periapical lesions may be entirely asymptomatic or excruciatingly painful.
- The presence of periapical disease is not a contraindication for endodontic treatment.
- Endodontic therapy for teeth with pulpal necrosis is generally performed in two or more stages.

TREATMENT OPTIONS

Extraction or endodontic treatment of all four canines.

TREATMENT PERFORMED

1. Periodontal therapy to remove plaque and calculus and provide a clean environment.
2. Endodontic treatment of 104 (Fig. 33.2), 204 (Fig. 33.3), 304 and 404 (Fig. 33.4). Due to the aggressive nature of the dog, endodontic therapy and restoration of all four teeth were performed in one long session.

POSTOPERATIVE CARE

- Antiobiotics for 10 days
- NSAIDs for 5 days
- The dog was booked for recheck under anaesthesia in 6 months' time.

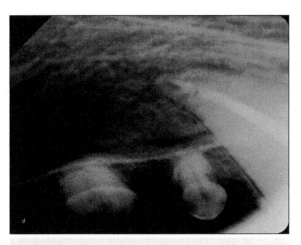

Figure 33.2 Lateral radiograph centring on the apex of 104. This radiograph was taken to confirm adequate fill of the debrided and disinfected root canal of 104 prior to placing final restorations.

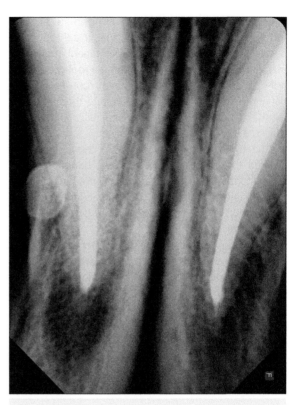

Figure 33.4 Rostrocaudal radiograph of the anterior mandible. This radiograph was taken to confirm adequate fill of the debrided and disinfected root canals of 304 and 404 prior to placing final restorations.

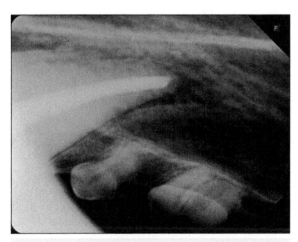

Figure 33.3 Lateral radiograph centring on the apex of 204. This radiograph was taken to confirm adequate fill of the debrided and disinfected root canal of 204 prior to placing final restorations.

RECHECK

The dog was placed under general anaesthesia for oral examination and radiography 6 months after initial treatment. There had been no improvement in temperament!

The restorations were intact and there was no evidence of tooth discoloration. The ventral border of the mandible had a normal contour. Radiographs revealed healing of the periapical defects.

PROGNOSIS

As long as the restorations stay in place, no further treatment should be required.

It was advised that radiographs of the canines should be taken if the dog required general anaesthesia for any reason.

COMMENTS

Endodontic therapy for teeth with pulpal necrosis is generally performed in two or more stages. The reason for this is that it is unlikely that adequate cleaning of the root canal can be achieved in one anaesthetic episode. The first stage consists of pulpectomy and debridement (filing and flushing), followed by filling the root canal with a temporary antiseptic material and placing a temporary restoration (to seal the root canal from the oral environment). The second stage consists of removing the temporary restoration and root-filling material, and further debridement of the root canal. If the root canal is clean it is then filled with a permanent root-filling material and the tooth is restored. If the root canal is still not clean, then an antiseptic temporary root-filling material and restoration is placed again, and the final treatment is done as a third session. Generally, two sessions spaced 3–6 weeks apart are sufficient.

Due to the aggressive nature of this dog, it was decided to perform the required endodontic therapy (pulpectomy, debridement, root canal filling and restoration) in one session. The whole procedure, including examination and radiography, took just under 5 hours to complete.

We do not routinely administer postoperative antibiotics after endodontic treatment. However, in this case, due to the extensive periapical destruction and the fact that the endodontic treatment was performed in one sitting, it seemed prudent to use antibiotics as an adjunct. It may well not have been necessary!

The choice of performing endodontic therapy and restoration rather than extraction was based on the fact that the canine teeth are functionally important teeth with no evidence of periodontitis. Also, extraction incurred the risk of iatrogenic jaw fracture exacerbated by the pre-existing bone loss.

There had not been any improvement in temperament after treatment. Although the owner did not know when the fractures had happened, the radiographs show mature teeth, so the dog must have been older than 1 year and the aggressive behaviour started at 16 weeks of age. Consequently, the two are likely to be unrelated. The owner was advised to consult an animal behaviourist to deal with the aggression.

34 Multiple tooth and jaw fracture

INITIAL PRESENTATION

Hesitation and anxiety about bite work, and multiple fractured teeth.

PATIENT DETAILS

A 6-year-old, intact male, German shepherd, working police dog.

CASE HISTORY

The dog was a working police dog that had started to hesitate during bite work a few months earlier. During bite work he firstly seemed worried about having to bite and then he would not hold on to the sleeve. He had been taken off training several times due to anxiety and hesitation.

His own veterinarian identified several fractured teeth on conscious examination and referred the case to us. There was no history of any previous oral or dental problems.

The handler reported that the dog was an obsessive cage biter and was certain that the teeth had been fractured for at least a year, i.e. this was not a new injury, but his bite work had been fine until a few months ago.

ORAL EXAMINATION – CONSCIOUS

An extremely well-behaved dog that allowed careful examination, which revealed the following:
1. Occlusion normal
2. Generalized gingivitis
3. Generalized tooth wear
4. Complicated crown fracture of 103, 104 and 203

5. Discoloured 102
6. Missing 405 and 308.

ORAL EXAMINATION – UNDER GENERAL ANAESTHETIC

A thorough oral and dental examination was performed, including investigating periodontal parameters. All findings were noted on the dental record sheet.

In summary, examination under general anaesthesia identified the following:
1. Generalized mild gingivitis
2. Generalized tooth wear (attrition and abrasion)
3. Complicated crown fracture (CCF) of 103 (Fig. 34.1), 104 (Fig. 34.1) and 203 (Fig. 34.2a)
4. Discoloured 102 (Fig. 34.1)
5. Uncomplicated crown fracture (UCF) of 105 and 107
6. Missing 405, 411, 308 and 311.

FURTHER INVESTIGATIONS

Radiographs were taken of 102 (discoloured), 103 (CCF), 104 (CCF), 203 (CCF), 204 (contralateral healthy), 105 (UCF) and 107 (UCF), as well as of the 405 and 308 regions (where the teeth were missing).

RADIOGRAPHIC FINDINGS

Most significantly, a fracture of the premaxilla level with the apex of 203 (CCF) was identified (Fig. 34.2b).

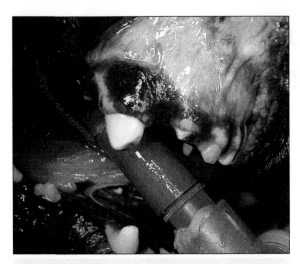

Figure 34.1 Oblique lateral photograph of the rostral right upper jaw. Note the complicated crown fracture of 103 and 104, and the discoloured 102.

There was no evidence of periapical pathology of 102 (discoloured), 103 (CCF), 105 (UCF) or 107 (UCF). There was apical periodontitis and external root resorption of 104 (CCF), and no evidence of unerupted teeth or root remnants at either the 405 or 308 regions.

ORAL PROBLEM LIST

1. Fracture of the premaxilla level with the apex of 203
2. Generalized mild gingivitis
3. Generalized tooth wear (attrition and abrasion)
4. Complicated crown fracture (CCF) of 103, 104 and 203
5. Periapical pathology associated with 104
6. Discoloured 102 (with no evidence of periapical pathology)
7. Uncomplicated crown fracture (UCF) of 105 and 107 (without evidence of pulp/periapical pathology)
8. Missing 405, 411, 308 and 311 (no evidence of unerupted teeth or root remnants).

THEORY REFRESHER

Tooth fracture may affect the crown, the crown and root, or just the root.

Crown fractures are classified as complicated if the fracture line exposes the pulp to the oral environment and as uncomplicated if they do not involve pulpal exposure. Crown fractures are obvious visually. However, at times it can be difficult to determine if the pulp is exposed by the fracture line, and general anaesthesia for examination with a dental explorer and radiography are necessary.

Complicated crown fractures always need treatment. An exposed pulp will become inflamed and may eventually undergo necrosis. The inflammation can spread from the pulp to involve the periapical area. A primary tooth with complicated crown fracture should be extracted to avoid damage to the adjacent developing permanent tooth. A permanent tooth, if unaffected by periodontal disease, can be treated by means of endodontic therapy. If the tooth has periodontitis or the fracture is too extensive, then extraction is the treatment of choice. In fact, with complicated crown fractures extraction is preferable to no treatment at all.

Uncomplicated crown fractures may also require treatment as the exposed dentine tubules allow communication between pulp and oral environment, and can thus result in inflammation or death of the pulp. An uncomplicated crown fracture usually requires minimal treatment, e.g. removal of sharp edges with a bur and sealing of the exposed dentine with a suitable liner or restorative material. However, such fractures do require monitoring (clinical examination and radiography) at regular intervals to ensure that the pulp remains vital. If pulp and periapical disease develops, the tooth requires either extraction or endodontic therapy.

Discoloured teeth usually have a necrotic pulp and possibly also periapical disease. Radiographs are mandatory. If there is pulp/periapical disease the teeth need extraction or endodontic therapy.

Teeth that are missing on clinical examination always need radiographic investigation. It is possible that there are root remnants from previous extractions (unlikely in this case, as there was no history of previous dental treatment) that may need removal or that the teeth are unerupted. Unerupted teeth may be involved in the development of follicular (dentigerous) cysts that can cause massive destruction of bone as they enlarge. An unerupted tooth should either be extracted or monitored radiographically (to detect cyst formation early) at regular intervals.

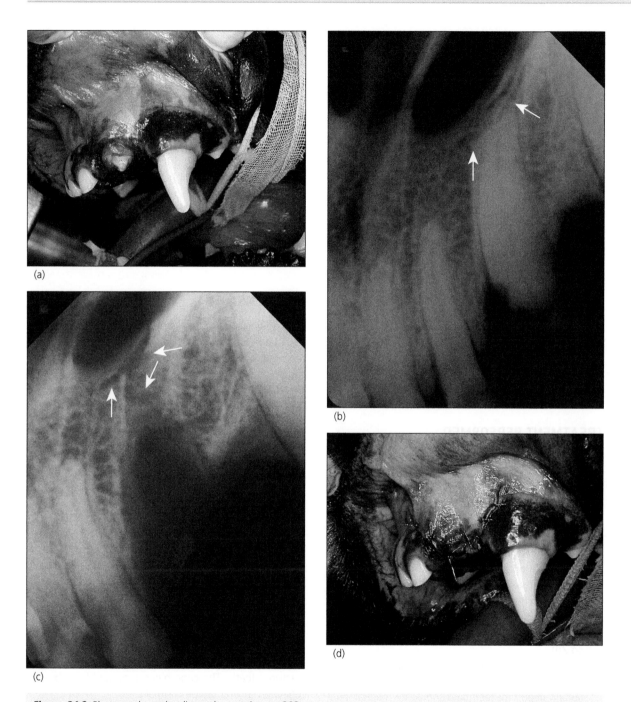

Figure 34.2 Photographs and radiographs centring on 203.

(a) Oblique lateral photograph of the rostral left upper jaw. The complicated crown fracture of 203 is obvious. Note also the wear facet on the distal aspect of 204 due to cage biting.

(b) Rostrocaudal radiograph centring on 203. Note the fracture of the premaxilla level with the apex of 203.

(c) Rostrocaudal radiograph of the extraction socket of 203. The fracture line is even more obvious after extraction of 203.

(d) Oblique lateral photograph of the extraction site. The flap used to suture the socket closed will provide stabilization during healing of the jaw fracture.

CLINICAL TIPS

- Complicated crown fractures always need treatment.
- Primary teeth with complicated crown fracture should be extracted to avoid damage to the adjacent developing permanent tooth.
- Uncomplicated crown fractures usually require minimal treatment.
- Discoloured teeth usually have a necrotic pulp and possibly also periapical disease.
- Teeth that are missing on clinical examination should always be investigated radiographically.
- Any unerupted tooth should either be extracted or monitored radiographically.
- The upper canines are functionally important teeth and should be maintained if possible.

TREATMENT OPTIONS

Extraction or endodontic treatment and restoration of 102, 103, 104 and 203.

TREATMENT PERFORMED

1. Periodontal therapy to remove plaque and calculus, and provide a clean environment for extraction, endodontic treatment and restoration.
2. Extraction of 102, 103 and 203. Since these teeth are not functionally important, extraction, a one-step procedure, was chosen rather than endodontic treatment and restoration, which requires radiographs to be taken after 3–6 months. An open technique was used to allow primary healing. Radiographs confirmed successful extraction at all sites (Fig. 34.2c). The flap sutured over the extraction socket also provided support during healing of the jaw fracture (Fig. 34.2d).
3. Endodontic treatment (pulpectomy, root canal filling and restoration) of 104. The upper canines are functionally important teeth and should be maintained if possible. This is especially important in a working police dog, as the canine teeth are used to hold on to prey. There was no evidence of periodontitis and there was more than 50% of original crown height, so this was an ideal tooth for endodontic treatment and restoration.

POSTOPERATIVE CARE

- Daily toothbrushing
- Soft food for 3 weeks
- No bite work for 3 weeks
- Analgesics for 3 weeks
- The dog was booked for conscious recheck after 3 weeks
- He was also booked for oral examination and radiographs of 104 (to assess the outcome of endodontic treatment), 105 and 107 (to check periapical status) under general anaesthesia after 6 months.

RECHECKS

Conscious examination 3 weeks postoperatively showed that the extraction sites had healed nicely. The handler reported that he was brighter in himself and had stopped cage biting.

A phone call from the handler 6 weeks postoperatively told of a completely successful return to normal bite work.

The 6-month recheck to monitor outcome of endodontic treatment of 104 and the periapical status of 105 and 107 is due in 2 months' time.

PROGNOSIS

The stable fracture of the premaxilla should heal in 3–4 weeks. Endodontic treatment and restoration is associated with a high success rate. In short, the dog should be able to return to work in 3–4 weeks' time.

COMMENTS

The anxiety and hesitancy with bite work was most likely due to the fracture of the premaxilla rather than the fractured teeth. The cage biting may well have been a reflection of oral discomfort/pain.

35 Iatrogenic tooth damage

INITIAL PRESENTATION

Swelling of the left rostral mandible and a draining fistula at the ventral border of the left rostral mandible.

PATIENT DETAILS

A 6-year-old, neutered male, Labrador retriever.

CASE HISTORY

A rostral mandibular fracture was repaired 5 years earlier, when the dog was a year old, at a specialist centre with orthopaedic expertise. The clinical notes and radiographs had been 'lost', so the details of the treatment were not available to us.

A fistula at the ventral border of the left mandible developed 3 years after the mandibular fracture repair. The dog was then referred back to the same specialist centre. Radiographs were taken, which showed a peri-apical lucency associated with 304 and a diagnosis of 'apical abscess' was made. The condition was treated with a long course of antibiotics. The problem resolved but flared up again within 3 months of ceasing antibiotic treatment. The dog was then treated intermittently with antibiotics for just over 2 years before being referred to us. Antibiotic therapy resulted in an improvement, but the fistula remained and started to drain within a few weeks of stopping an antibiotic course.

ORAL EXAMINATION – CONSCIOUS

The dog was extremely well behaved, and allowed careful conscious examination of the head and mouth, which revealed the following:
1. Occlusion normal
2. Generalized gingivitis
3. All mandibular incisors were missing
4. Some mandibular premolars were missing
5. Hard swelling of the rostral left mandible (no reaction to firm palpation)
6. Draining fistula at the ventral border of the left mandible (thick, yellow fluid).

ORAL EXAMINATION – UNDER GENERAL ANAESTHETIC

A thorough oral examination, including investigating periodontal parameters, was performed and all findings were noted on the dental record.

In summary, examination under general anaesthesia identified the following:
1. Mild generalized gingivitis
2. Hard swelling of the rostral left mandible (Fig. 35.1)
3. Draining fistula at the ventral border of the left mandible (Fig. 35.1)
4. All mandibular incisors, as well as 307, 308, 406 and 408, missing
5. Gingival inflammation at the region of the missing 406.

FURTHER INVESTIGATIONS

Radiographs were taken of the rostral mandible, 304 and 404, and at the sites of the missing 307, 308, 406 and 408.

RADIOGRAPHIC FINDINGS

The following were evident on the radiographs:
1. Bony swelling with periosteal new bone on the left rostral mandible

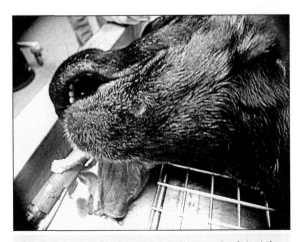

Figure 35.1 Oblique ventrolateral photograph of the left mandible. The ventral border of the left mandible is hard and swollen with a drainage tract. The drainage tract originated from the periapical inflammation of 304.

2. Teeth 304 and 404 were immature teeth with wide pulp system diameter and incomplete apical closure (Fig. 35.2a–c)
3. Lucency around the apex of 304 (Fig. 35.2a)
4. Circular lucencies at the midroot of both 304 (Fig. 35.2a, c) and 404 (Fig. 35.2a, b)
5. Root remnants of 307 (Fig. 35.2c) and 406 (Fig. 35.2b)
6. Teeth 308 and 408 absent
7. All mandibular incisors absent.

ORAL PROBLEM LIST

1. Mild generalized gingivitis
2. Pulp and periapical disease of 304 and 404 (apical lucency of 304, the draining fistula at the ventral border of the left mandible and the bony proliferation of the left rostral mandible were consequences of the pulp disease of 304)
3. All mandibular incisors missing
4. Root remnants of 307 and 406

THEORY REFRESHER

The development of 304 and 404 was incomplete, compatible with a dog younger than 1 year of age. Consequently, pulpal inflammation and necrosis (which stops further tooth development) must have occurred at around 9 months of age.

The circular lucencies in the roots of both teeth were compatible with drill holes for a pin or screw to repair the rostral mandibular fracture. Drilling through a tooth root will cause pulpal inflammation, necrosis and in time (months to years) periapical complications.

The periapical radiolucency associated with 304, as well as the bony swelling with periosteal proliferation and the draining fistula at the ventral border of the left mandible, are all complications due to pulp necrosis. In this case, it took 3 years before the consequences of the iatrogenic damage became obvious clinically. In short, the jaw fracture repair caused injury to the teeth, with subsequent development of periapical complications. It must be remembered that pulp/periapical disease is associated with discomfort and pain.

Periapical disease as a consequence of pulpal necrosis is treated by removing the cause of the inflammation, in this case the necrotic pulp. Once the cause of the inflammatory reaction has been removed, the bone defect and draining fistula will heal. Necrotic pulp can be removed in one of two ways, namely endodontic therapy and restoration (the pulp is removed, the root canal debrided and filled, the access sites restored, and the tooth is maintained) or extraction of the affected tooth (the whole tooth is removed). In this case, the drill holes through the teeth exclude endodontic treatment, as it is technically impossible to remove pulp adequately and to fill the root canal (root canal sealer will disperse into the periodontal tissue around the tooth). Consequently, extraction of the teeth becomes the only possible option to deal with the periapical pathology.

Teeth that are missing on clinical examination always need radiographic investigation. It is possible that there are root remnants from previous extractions that may need removal or that the teeth are unerupted. Unerupted teeth may be involved in the development of follicular (dentigerous) cysts that can cause massive destruction of bone as they enlarge. An unerupted tooth should either be extracted or monitored radiographically (to detect cyst formation early) at regular intervals.

This dog was missing all the mandibular incisors clinically and radiographically. These teeth were probably extracted at the time of the jaw fracture repair. The root remnants of 307 and 406 could either have been due to tooth fracture at the time of the trauma that caused the jaw fracture, but they could also have been incompletely extracted at the time of jaw fracture repair. The absence of 308 and 408 (clinically and radiographically) was considered as congenital.

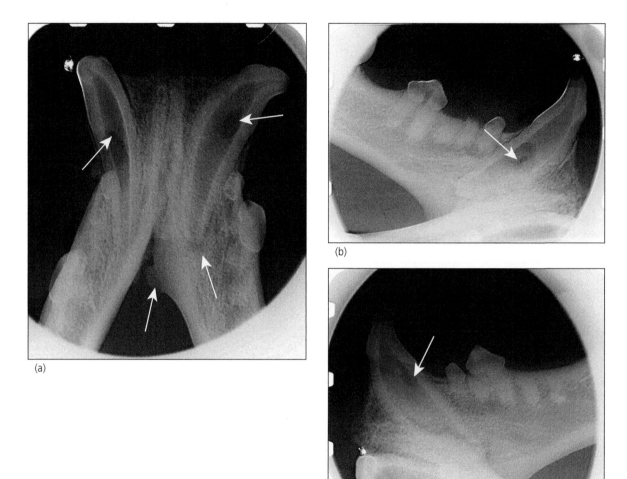

(a)

(b)

(c)

Figure 35.2 Radiographs of the rostral mandible.

(a) Rostrocaudal view. Although the dog is 6 years old, 304 and 404 are immature teeth (wide pulp system diameter and incomplete apical closure). The development of these teeth is compatible with a dog younger than a year of age. Consequently, pulpal inflammation and necrosis (which stops further tooth development) must have occurred at around 9 months of age. Note the circular lucencies at the midroot of both 304 and 404. These are compatible with drill holes for a pin or a screw to repair the rostral mandibular fracture. The pulpal inflammation and necrosis of 304 have spread to involve the periapical tissue, as evidenced radiographically by the radiolucent zone around the apex of the root. The periosteal new bone formation on the left is a consequence of the pulp and periapical disease of 304.

(b) Lateral view of the right rostral mandible. Note the circular midroot radiolucency compatible with a drill hole and the immature 404. Drilling through teeth will cause pulpitis and pulp necrosis and cessation of tooth development, as seen with 404. Clinically, there was gingival inflammation over the missing 406. The radiograph shows root remnants as the likely cause of the gingival inflammation.

(c) Lateral view of the left rostral mandible. Note the circular midroot radiolucency compatible with a drill hole and the immature 304 with a periapical destruction. Drilling through teeth will cause pulpitis and pulp necrosis and cessation of tooth development, and with time development of periapical complications, as seen with 304. Note also the root remnants of 307. The gingiva overlying the root remnants was not inflamed.

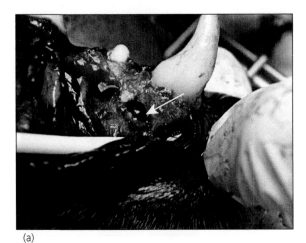

(a)

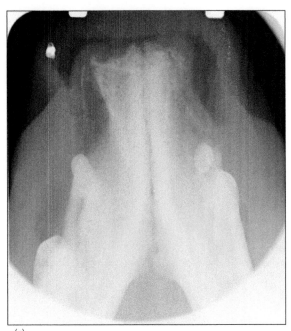

(c)

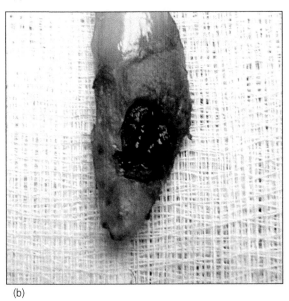

(b)

Figure 35.3 Lateral photograph during extraction of 404 (a), photograph of extracted 404 (b) and post-extraction radiograph (c).

(a) A full-thickness mucoperiosteal flap has been raised. Note the drill hole.

(b) Note the drill hole in the extracted 404.

(c) The radiograph confirms successful extraction of 304 and 404.

CLINICAL TIPS

- Drilling through a tooth root will cause pulpal inflammation, necrosis and in time (months to years) periapical complications.
- Pulp/periapical disease is associated with discomfort and pain.
- Teeth that are missing on clinical examination always need radiographic investigation.

- Unerupted teeth should either be extracted or monitored radiographically (to detect cyst formation early) at regular intervals.
- Standard orthopaedic techniques such as pinning and plating are not recommended for jaw fracture repair.
- Antibiotics alone will not cure periapical disease.

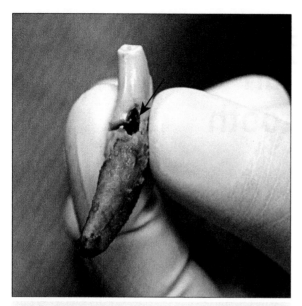

Figure 35.4 Photograph of extracted 304. Note the drill hole.

TREATMENT OPTIONS

Extraction of 304 and 404 was the only option.

TREATMENT PERFORMED

1. Periodontal therapy to remove plaque and calculus, and provide a clean environment for extraction.
2. Open extraction of 404 (Fig. 35.3a–c) and 304 (Fig. 35.4). Flaps were replaced with 5/0 Monocryl.
3. The draining fistula was debrided and left to heal by second intention.
4. The root remnants of 406 were extracted because there was inflammation of the overlying gingiva. In contrast, there was no evidence of inflammation of the gingiva overlying the root remnants of 307 and these were consequently left in situ.

POSTOPERATIVE CARE

- Daily toothbrushing
- Analgesics for 5 days
- The dog was booked for conscious recheck after 3 weeks.

RECHECK

Conscious examination 3 weeks postoperatively showed that the extraction sites had healed nicely and there was no evidence of a fistulous tract at the ventral border of the mandible.

PROGNOSIS

The prognosis for this case is excellent. The cause of the pathology has been removed.

Once the extraction sites have healed, the dog will no longer suffer discomfort or pain and will have a functional bite.

COMMENTS

Standard orthopaedic techniques, e.g. pinning and plating, are not recommended for jaw fracture repair. The likelihood of damaging teeth and oral anatomical structures (e.g. mandibular canal) is unacceptably high, and the animal will suffer discomfort and pain from the iatrogenic damage caused by these techniques. In this case, the dog lived with a focus of infection causing discomfort and possibly pain for 5 years.

Jaw fractures are best repaired using techniques such as orthopaedic wiring, external fixation and intra-oral acrylic splints. These techniques allow maintenance of occlusion and fracture fixation without damaging the teeth and oral anatomical structures.

Antibiotics alone will not cure periapical disease. Antibiotics may reduce the clinical signs, e.g. stop fistulous drainage, for a period of time, but as long as the necrotic pulp is present the disease will recur and progress. In this case, antibiotics were used intermittently for 2 years, when the appropriate treatment would have been extraction.

This case highlights the importance of understanding pulp/periapical pathophysiology in order to choose the right treatment option.

36 Complicated crown fracture of an immature tooth

INITIAL PRESENTATION

Tooth 404 fractured with exposed bleeding pulp.

PATIENT DETAILS

A 7-month-old, intact male, cross-breed.

CASE HISTORY

The dog came back from a run bleeding from the mouth. The owners took the dog to their regular veterinarian, who identified a complicated crown fracture of 404. The dog was given analgesics and referred to us. The dog was seen by us the day after the injury occurred.

ORAL EXAMINATION – CONSCIOUS

He was a boisterous but non-aggressive dog, who allowed conscious examination of the face and a quick view of the oral cavity.

Occlusion was normal and there was a mild generalized gingivitis. The tip of the crown of 404 was fractured and the pulp was exposed.

ORAL EXAMINATION – UNDER GENERAL ANAESTHETIC

A thorough oral and dental examination, including investigating periodontal parameters, was performed. All findings were noted on the dental record sheet.

In summary, examination under general anaesthesia identified the following:

1. Mild generalized gingivitis
2. Complicated crown fracture (CCF) of 404.

FURTHER INVESTIGATIONS

Radiographs were taken of 404 (CCF) and 304 (contra-lateral healthy).

RADIOGRAPHIC FINDINGS

The radiographs confirmed that both 304 and 404 were immature teeth, as expected in a 7-month-old dog.

ORAL PROBLEM LIST

1. Complicated crown fracture in an immature tooth
2. Mild generalized gingivitis.

THEORY REFRESHER

A partial pulpectomy and direct pulp capping procedure is indicated for recent tooth crown fractures with pulp exposure in immature teeth. An immature tooth has a thin dentine wall and an open apex, allowing a good blood supply to the pulp. Treatment is aimed at maintaining a viable pulp, as this is needed for continued root development.

To optimize success, a partial pulpectomy and direct pulp capping procedure needs to be performed as quickly as possible after the injury. Referral needs to be arranged on an emergency basis.

Once root development is complete, i.e. the apex has closed and sufficient dentine has been deposited, conventional endodontic therapy (pulpectomy and root filling) should be performed.

TREATMENT OPTIONS

Extraction or endodontic treatment (partial pulpectomy, direct pulp capping and restoration) of 404.

TREATMENT PERFORMED

1. Periodontal therapy to remove plaque and calculus, and provide a clean environment.
2. Partial pulpectomy, direct pulp capping and restoration of 404 (Fig. 36.1).

RECHECKS

Due to personal circumstances the owner was unable to keep the 6-month recheck appointment. Telephone conversations revealed that the dog was fine in itself, the restoration was intact and the tooth had not discoloured. A new appointment was arranged for 9 months after the original treatment.

Examination and radiographs at this time revealed a successful outcome of the partial pulpectomy and direct

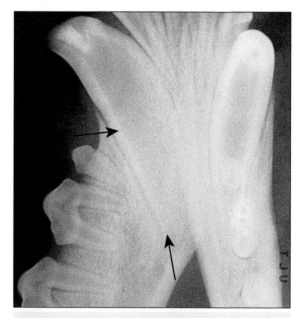

Figure 36.1 Lateral radiograph of 404. This radiograph was taken after completion of a partial pulpectomy and direct pulp capping procedure. Note the thin layer of dentine and the incomplete closure of the apex.

pulp capping procedure. The restoration was intact, with no evidence of marginal leakage (i.e. no discoloration around the edges of the restoration). The radiograph (Fig. 36.2) showed continued root development, with thick dentine walls and closed apex. Conventional endodontic therapy (total pulpectomy, debridement, root canal filling and restoration) was performed.

A recheck with radiography 6 months after the conventional endodontic therapy showed no evidence of periapical pathology (Fig. 36.3) and confirmed a successful outcome of the procedure.

PROGNOSIS

No further treatment should be required unless the restoration is damaged or lost. The owner was advised to contact us immediately should this occur.

COMMENTS

The purpose of a partial pulpectomy and direct pulp capping procedure is to keep the pulp alive to complete root development. It must be remembered that a living (vital) pulp is not necessarily a healthy pulp. In fact, it may be inflamed, and pulpal necrosis and periapical

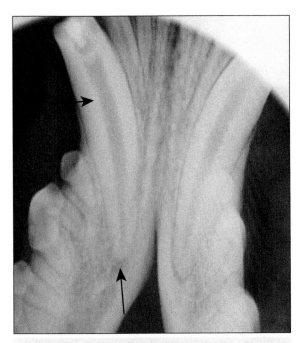

Figure 36.2 Lateral radiograph of 404. This radiograph was taken 9 months after the partial pulpectomy and direct pulp capping procedure depicted in Fig. 36.1. Note the continued tooth development, with deposition of dentine and closure of the apex. At this time, a total pulpectomy and root-filling procedure was performed.

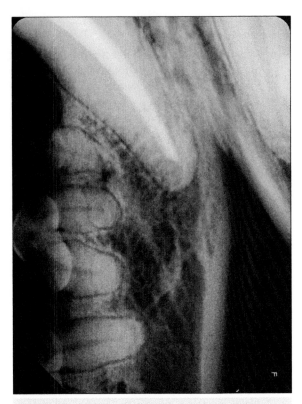

Figure 36.3 Lateral radiograph of 404. This radiograph was taken a further 6 months later, after the total pulpectomy and root-filling procedure. The radiograph indicates successful outcome of the endodontic procedure in that there is no evidence of any periapical disease. No further treatment should be necessary as long as the restoration remains intact.

pathology may develop. Consequently, a partial pulpectomy and direct pulp capping procedure needs to be monitored radiographically and, once the goal of complete root development has been achieved, the tooth should receive conventional endodontic therapy (total pulpectomy, root canal debridement and filling), which has a higher long-term success rate than a partial pulpectomy and direct pulp capping procedure.

In this case, it took three general anaesthetics and 1.5 years before it was clear that the tooth could be maintained. This is warranted for a periodontally sound, functionally important tooth such as a canine.

37 Excessive wear

INITIAL PRESENTATION

Severely worn teeth.

PATIENT DETAILS

A 6-year-old, neutered male, cross-breed.

CASE HISTORY

There was no previous history of oral/dental disease or treatment. The owner was concerned that the teeth appeared to be short and seemed to be getting shorter rapidly. The referring veterinary surgeon was concerned about possible pulpal exposure as a result of the excessive wear and referred the case to us for management.

The dog showed no evidence of discomfort or pain. He was eating well and there had been no change in eating or chewing behaviour. The owner exercised him daily on the beach by throwing tennis balls for him to retrieve. He also had a selection of toys that he chewed in the garden.

ORAL EXAMINATION – CONSCIOUS

The dog had a nice temperament, and allowed conscious examination of the face and of the oral cavity. The findings were as follows:
1. Occlusion was normal.
2. Generalized gingivitis was observed.
3. There was excessive wear of all teeth. The incisors were worn almost to the level of the gingival margin. All teeth had exposed dentine with obvious reparative dentine formation. There was no obvious pulpal exposure of any tooth.

ORAL EXAMINATION – UNDER GENERAL ANAESTHETIC

A thorough oral and dental examination, including periodontal parameters, was performed. All findings were noted on the dental record.

In summary, examination under general anaesthesia identified the following:
1. Mild generalized gingivitis was observed.
2. There was excessive wear of all teeth (Fig. 37.1a, b).
3. There was pulpal exposure of 404. Exploration with a sharp explorer allowed entry into the pulp chamber.
4. There was periodontitis of 109 and 409. Both these teeth had increased probing depths as well as gingival recession.

FURTHER INVESTIGATIONS

Radiographs were taken of 404 (pulpal exposure), 304 (contralateral without pulpal exposure), 109 (periodontitis) and 409 (periodontitis).

RADIOGRAPHIC FINDINGS

The diameter of the root canal of 404 was wider (pulpal exposure) than in 304 (contralateral, without pulpal exposure), indicating pulp necrosis and cessation of dentine production of 404. In addition, there was periapical bone destruction and external root resorption of 404. Figure 37.2 shows the important radiographic findings associated with 404.

Teeth 109 and 409 showed extensive destruction of the margin of the alveolar bone.

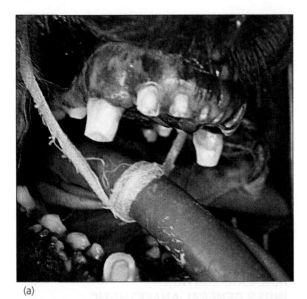

(a)

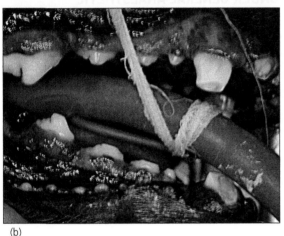

(b)

Figure 37.1 Clinical photographs.

(a) Rostrocaudal photograph centring on upper incisors and canines. The incisors were worn to gum level.

(b) Lateral photograph of the right upper and lower canines and premolars. All teeth were affected by severe wear.

ORAL PROBLEM LIST

1. Excessive tooth wear, leading to pulpal exposure, pulp necrosis and periapical complications of 404
2. Advanced periodontitis of 109 and 409.

THEORY REFRESHER

Apart from the reduction in size of the pulp cavity, which is associated with continued deposition of secondary

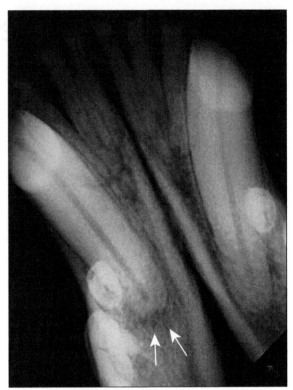

Figure 37.2 Oblique rostrocaudal radiograph centring on 404. The excessive wear had resulted in pulpal exposure of 404. Note that the root canal of 404 is wider than the root canal of 304, indicating pulp necrosis and cessation of dentine production of 404 as a consequence of the pulpal exposure. There is also periapical bone destruction and external root resorption of 404.

dentine as the animal gets older, there are also conditions that accelerate the rate of deposition of secondary dentine, thus prematurely reducing the size of the pulp cavity. Attrition and abrasion are two common conditions resulting in a narrow pulp cavity.

Attrition is the loss of tooth substance that results from wear that is produced by opposing teeth coming into contact with one another, i.e. teeth that have occlusal contact. Attrition is therefore also called occlusal wear. Incisal wear is the term used when describing attrition of the incisor region. There is progressive attrition with increasing age, resulting in the wearing away of the cusps and exposure of the dentine. The deposition of secondary dentine keeps pace with the loss of tooth substance and there is rarely pulpal exposure. In fact, the crown pulp may come close to obliteration. In other words, attrition is a physiological event that occurs, to varying degrees, in all individuals. Factors such as loss of teeth, malocclusion and habits such as stone chewing may produce excessive attrition, i.e. attrition that is so rapid that the formation of secondary dentine cannot keep pace with it, and pulp exposure results.

Abrasion is the wearing away of tooth structure which is not caused by incisal or occlusal wear. In other words, wear of tooth surfaces that are not in contact. In man, the most common cause of abrasion is incorrect use of a toothbrush, resulting in abrasion of the buccal tooth surfaces, usually just above the gingival margin. In the dog, the most common cause of abrasion is cage biting. The hard tissues on the distal aspect of the maxillary canine teeth are progressively lost, weakening the tooth until the crown fractures (generally with pulpal exposure).

In this case, the excessive wear (mainly attrition) was due to chewing on sand-coated tennis balls. A dry tennis ball is mildly abrasive, but when it becomes wet (saliva) and coated with sand from the beach, it becomes extremely abrasive and causes rapid loss of dental hard tissue as the animal chews on it.

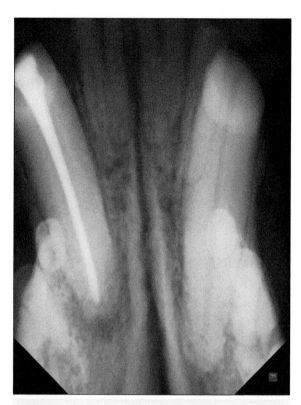

Figure 37.3 Oblique rostrocaudal radiograph centring on 404. Radiograph showing completed endodontic treatment. The pulp was removed, the root canal debrided and filled, and the access preparation restored.

CLINICAL TIPS

- Attrition and abrasion are two common conditions resulting in a narrow pulp cavity.
- Attrition is a physiological event that occurs, to varying degrees, in all individuals.
- Abrasion is the wearing away of tooth structure which is not caused by incisal or occlusal wear.
- Measures to prevent excessive attrition and abrasion should be instituted as soon as there is evidence of excessive wear.
- Stone chewing and playing with a ball on a sandy surface are common causes of excessive attrition.

2. Conventional endodontic therapy (pulpectomy, debridement and filling of root canal and restoration of access cavities) of 404 (Fig. 37.3).
3. Open extraction of 109 and 409. The flaps were replaced with 5/0 Monocryl. Successful extraction was confirmed radiographically.

TREATMENT OPTIONS

Extraction or endodontic treatment and restoration of 404, and extraction of 109 and 409.

TREATMENT PERFORMED

1. Periodontal therapy to remove plaque and calculus, and provide a clean environment.

POSTOPERATIVE CARE

- NSAIDs for 5 days
- Start daily toothbrushing
- Stop playing with tennis balls on the beach – as the dog loved chasing balls, it was advised to use a smooth rubber ball (less abrasive even if coated with a bit of sand) instead of the tennis ball, rather than stop the game completely
- The dog was booked for examination and radiography of 404 in 6 months' time.

RECHECKS

Oral examination at 6 months after initial treatment revealed clinically healthy gingivae (the owner had been brushing the teeth once daily) and no further wear of the teeth. The owner had stopped throwing balls for him. They had bought a puppy and the two of them played together energetically, so ball throwing was no longer required for exercise purposes. The restoration of 404 was intact, and the radiographs revealed no further root resorption and apical defect was filling in with new bone.

The dog was rebooked for oral examination and radiographs of 404 in 1 year's time.

PROGNOSIS

I expect to see full bony healing of the periapical lesion at 404 at the next recall in 1 year's time. No further treatment would then be required.

If full healing has not occurred, this would indicate persistent periapical inflammation and treatment options then would be further endodontic treatment (redo the conventional endodontic treatment, possibly in combination with surgical endodontics) or extraction of 404. However, the most likely outcome is full healing and no further treatment.

COMMENTS

Measures to prevent excessive attrition and abrasion should be instituted as soon as there is evidence of excessive wear. Stone chewing is a common cause of excessive attrition. Another common cause is playing with a ball on a sandy surface. The ball becomes wet and covered with sand or grit, and as the animal bites on the ball, the teeth are worn excessively. Prevention in such circumstances is restricting access to stones and playing with a ball in an environment where the ball does not become covered in abrasive material.

The advanced periodontitis with extensive bone loss of 109 and 409 was a separate condition (i.e. not a consequence of the abrasion for which the dog was initially referred), and illustrates the importance of a complete oral examination in all cases.

38 Enamel dysplasia

INITIAL PRESENTATION

Discoloured teeth and defective enamel.

PATIENT DETAILS

A 6-year-old, neutered female, Shetland sheepdog.

CASE HISTORY

The permanent teeth appeared normal when they erupted. However, within a few months sections of enamel seemed to flake off and the teeth started to discolour. The dog had received professional periodontal therapy (scaling and polishing) twice with no obvious improvement. The dog was well mannered until 4 years old, when she started avoiding having her face touched and grew progressively more wary and aggressive. It was now impossible to examine the face at all. There were no problems with a full general examination and aggressive behaviour was only manifest when approaching the head.

The owner was worried about the dog's interaction with her young children.

ORAL EXAMINATION – CONSCIOUS

The dog would not allow access to her face at all, so conscious oral examination was not performed.

ORAL EXAMINATION – UNDER GENERAL ANAESTHETIC

A thorough oral and dental examination, including investigating periodontal parameters, was performed. All findings were noted on the dental record.

In summary, examination under general anaesthesia identified the following:

1. Occlusion normal
2. Mild generalized gingivitis
3. Generalized enamel dysplasia (Fig. 38.1).

FURTHER INVESTIGATIONS

A series of full-mouth radiographs (16 films) was taken.

RADIOGRAPHIC FINDINGS

All teeth, except incisors and canines, were affected by pulp and periapical pathology (see Fig. 38.2).

ORAL PROBLEM LIST

1. Generalized enamel dysplasia
2. Pulp and periapical disease of all teeth except incisors and canines
3. Mild generalized gingivitis.

THEORY REFRESHER

Enamel dysplasia (hypoplasia) may be defined as an incomplete or defective formation of the organic enamel matrix of teeth. The result is defective (soft, porous) enamel. It can be caused by local, systemic or hereditary factors. Depending on the cause, the condition can affect one or only a few teeth (localized form), or all teeth in the dentition (generalized form). It is essential to remember that enamel dysplasia results only if the defect occurs during the formative stage of enamel development, i.e. during amelogenesis. Thus, the defect

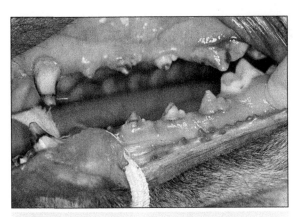

Figure 38.1 Lateral photograph of the left side of mouth. Note the generalized enamel dysplasia. The enamel is partly missing on all teeth.

occurs before the tooth erupts into the oral cavity. Crown formation lasts from the 42nd day of gestation through to the 15th day postpartum for the primary teeth, and from the second week through to the third month postpartum for the permanent teeth of dogs and cats. Depending on the time of the insult, enamel dysplasia will affect primary and/or permanent teeth. Only those areas of enamel undergoing active formation during the period of the insult will be affected. This is seen clinically as bands of dysplastic enamel encircling the crown, with areas of normal enamel elsewhere on the tooth.

Teeth with enamel dysplasia may appear normal at the time of eruption, but they soon become discoloured as the defective (porous) enamel soaks up pigments (from food, soil, etc.). In more severely affected teeth, the defective enamel may flake off with use. In very severe cases, the enamel is visibly deficient, discoloured in patches or partly missing already at the time of eruption.

As already mentioned, enamel dysplasia may be caused by local, systemic or hereditary factors. Local factors include trauma to the developing crown, e.g. a blow to the face or an infection. Usually, only one or a few teeth are affected. Systemic factors include nutritional deficiencies, febrile disorders, hypocalcaemia and excessive intake of fluoride during the period of enamel formation. Usually, most teeth are affected. Historically, enamel dysplasia in dogs occurred due to distemper infection. This is rare today, as most dogs are vaccinated against distemper. Hereditary types of enamel dysplasia

have been described in humans, but the incidence of this in cats and dogs is unknown.

Poorly protected or exposed dentine is painful. Affected teeth become less sensitive with increasing age of the animal, since secondary dentine is laid down continuously by the pulp. Another consideration is that dysplastic enamel harbours dental plaque.

In severe cases of generalized enamel hypoplasia, where the dentine is effectively exposed to the oral environment, chronic pulp disease and potentially periapical disease may occur due to pulpal irritation via the poorly protected or exposed dentine tubules.

CLINICAL TIPS

- Enamel dysplasia (hypoplasia) may be defined as an incomplete or defective formation of the organic enamel matrix of teeth. The result is defective (soft, porous) enamel.
- Enamel dysplasia can be caused by local, systemic or hereditary factors.
- Enamel dysplasia results only if the defect occurs during the formative stage of enamel development.
- Poorly protected or exposed dentine is painful.
- In severe cases of generalized enamel hypoplasia, chronic pulp disease and potentially periapical disease may occur. Radiographic assessment and monitoring are required.
- In the management of patients affected by enamel dysplasia, oral hygiene is of paramount importance.
- In young animals exhibiting signs of discomfort, topical fluoride application may be beneficial.
- Debriding the defect and replacing lost tissue with a suitable filling material is useful for smaller lesions.

TREATMENT OPTIONS

Extraction or endodontic treatment and restoration of all teeth except the incisors and canines.

TREATMENT PERFORMED

1. Periodontal therapy to remove plaque and calculus, and provide a clean environment. Calculus was carefully removed using hand instruments (scalers and

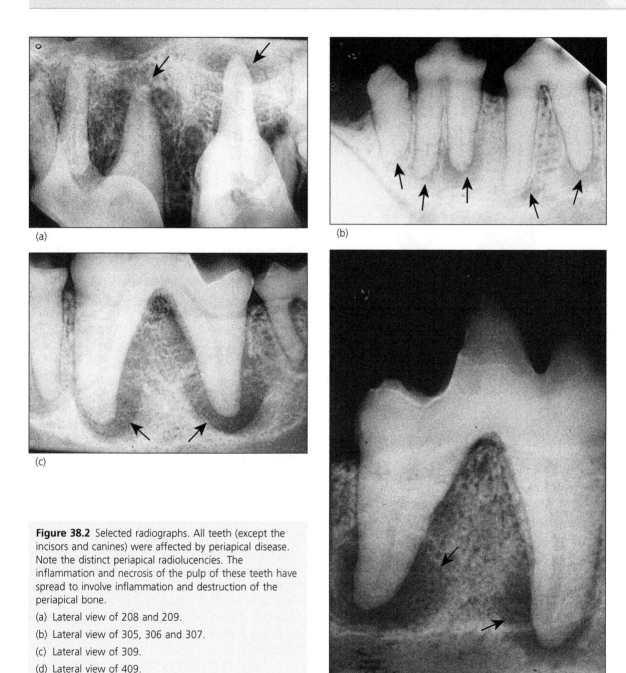

Figure 38.2 Selected radiographs. All teeth (except the incisors and canines) were affected by periapical disease. Note the distinct periapical radiolucencies. The inflammation and necrosis of the pulp of these teeth have spread to involve inflammation and destruction of the periapical bone.

(a) Lateral view of 208 and 209.

(b) Lateral view of 305, 306 and 307.

(c) Lateral view of 309.

(d) Lateral view of 409.

(a)

(b)

(c)

(d)

curettes), as the use of mechanical instruments would have resulted in the removal of the remaining soft enamel. Plaque removal and smoothing of tooth surfaces was accomplished using a soft rubber cup and a fine-grade prophy paste.

2. Open extraction of all teeth except incisors and canines. The access flaps were replaced with 5/0 Monocryl. Successful extraction was confirmed radiographically. Figure 38.3 demonstrates the clinical appearance of periapical disease.

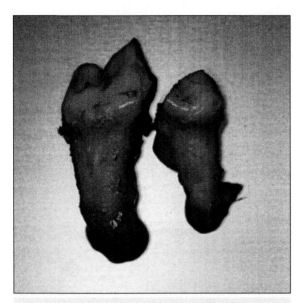

Figure 38.3 Photograph of extracted 409. Note the soft tissue attached to the apices of the roots. Histologically, this tissue is likely to be granulation tissue replacing the destroyed periapical bone.

POSTOPERATIVE CARE

- NSAIDs for 5 days
- Antibiotics for 10 days
- Soft food
- The dog was booked for examination under anaesthesia (as the dog was not allowing conscious oral examination) after 3 weeks.

RECHECKS

At recheck 3 weeks later, the owner reported a dramatic change in behaviour. The dog was no longer worried about having her face touched. Conscious examination of the oral cavity was allowed (so examination under general anaesthesia was not required) and revealed healing of all extraction sites. She did not mind gentle toothbrushing of the buccal aspects of the incisors and canines. The owner was shown how to brush and advised to do so daily. They were rebooked for check-up in 3 months.

At the 3-month recheck, the dog had clinically healthy gingivae and clean teeth (plaque disclosing solution applied). The owner reported that they both enjoyed the daily toothbrushing. A recall in 1 year was arranged.

Annual rechecks (examination under anaesthesia and radiographs) over 4 years show no evidence of any pulp/periapical disease of remaining teeth. The owner is brushing daily.

PROGNOSIS

With continued daily toothbrushing, the dog is unlikely to develop further problems.

COMMENTS

In the management of patients affected by enamel dysplasia, oral hygiene is of paramount importance. Daily plaque removal will promote periodontal health and possibly reduce pulpal irritation. Affected animals require radiographic assessment and monitoring to detect complications such as pulp and periapical disease. In fact, a series of full-mouth radiographs at regular intervals is indicated. In young animals exhibiting signs of discomfort, topical fluoride application may be beneficial. Topical fluoride application will enhance enamel remineralization and 'harden' the enamel. The main effect of fluoride incorporation into the enamel is that it makes the enamel more resistant to the acid dissolution that occurs with caries. It must be remembered that fluoride is potentially toxic, and the risk of systemic administration of fluoride products meant for topical application is greater in the dog and cat, as they will swallow these products. The use of professionally applied varnishes and gels associated with a moderate rise in plasma fluoride concentrations may well be safer than daily use of fluoride-containing toothpastes. In other words, it is useful to apply fluoride varnishes or gel at regular intervals. The best way to do this is following a dental cleaning. The product is applied while the animal is under general anaesthesia and excess is removed before the animal is allowed to recover.

In severely affected cases, the enamel is so soft that it is removed on scaling. In these patients, gross calculus accumulation is carefully removed with hand instruments (a scaler or curette) rather than powered scalers (sonic or ultrasonic). The crowns are polished with a fine-grain (to reduce abrasion) prophy paste. Restoration of lost enamel, i.e. debriding the defect and replacing lost tissue with a suitable filling material, is useful for smaller lesions as it protects against dentine sensitivity. It is not practical for extensive, generalized lesions. Restoration requires referral to a specialist.

39 Caries

INITIAL PRESENTATION

None.

PATIENT DETAILS

A 6-year-old, neutered female, Staffordshire bull terrier.

CASE HISTORY

The referring veterinarian noticed caries while performing an annual periodontal debridement.

ORAL EXAMINATION – CONSCIOUS

This was a boisterous but nice-tempered dog that allowed conscious examination, which identified the following:
1. Occlusion normal
2. Generalized gingivitis
3. Moderate accumulation of dental deposits
4. Discoloured areas on chewing surfaces of the molar teeth.

ORAL EXAMINATION – UNDER GENERAL ANAESTHETIC

A thorough oral and dental examination, including investigating periodontal parameters, was performed. All findings were entered on the dental chart.

In summary, examination under general anaesthesia identified the following:
1. Mild to moderate generalized gingivitis
2. Caries on occlusal surfaces of 109, 209, 309, 409 and 410.

FURTHER INVESTIGATIONS

Radiographs were taken of all molar teeth.

RADIOGRAPHIC FINDINGS

The occlusal caries of 109, 209 and 410 extended into the dentine, but there was no evidence of pulp and periapical involvement.

The occlusal caries of 409 extended into the pulp chamber, but there was no definitive periapical involvement.

The occlusal caries of 309 had resulted in substantial loss of dental hard tissue and extended into the pulp chamber, with definitive periapical involvement.

ORAL PROBLEM LIST

1. Caries (involving dentine but not extending into the pulp system) of 109, 209 and 410
2. Caries of 409 extending into the pulp, but with no periapical complications
3. Caries 309 extending into the pulp and with periapical disease
4. Mild to moderate generalized gingivitis.

THEORY REFRESHER

Caries usually affect the teeth that have true occlusal tables, namely the molar teeth.

While both periodontal disease and caries are caused by the accumulation of dental plaque on the tooth surfaces, the pathogenesis of the two diseases is completely different. Periodontal disease is a plaque-induced inflammation of the periodontium and caries is a plaque-induced destruction of the hard tissues of the tooth. Caries starts as an inorganic demineralization of the enamel. The demineralization occurs when plaque bacteria use fermentable carbohydrate (notably sugar) from the diet as a source of energy. The fermentation products are acidic and demineralize the enamel. Once the enamel has been destroyed, the process extends into the dentine. In the dentine, the process accelerates as an organic decay and will eventually involve the pulp, causing pulpitis and eventually pulp necrosis and/or periapical pathology. Dental caries stimulates the formation of secondary dentine on the surface of the pulpal wall, which is directly beneath it. If the carious lesion is progressing slowly, the deposition of secondary dentine may keep pace with its advance and prevent exposure of the dental pulp.

The initial inorganic demineralization can be halted as long as the process has not reached the enamel–dentine junction. However, if the process has entered the dentine it becomes irreversible and progressive. Treatment (restoration or extraction) becomes mandatory. In the dog, caries is very rarely diagnosed at the early enamel demineralization stage. It is usually diagnosed only when the process already involves the dentine, or the pulp is exposed, or there is periapical pathology. The reason why caries is rarely diagnosed at the enamel demineralization stage in dogs is twofold. Firstly, the occlusal surfaces are not generally explored with a sharp explorer during clinical examination. Secondly, dog enamel is thinner than human enamel and the process is thus likely to extend into the dentine more rapidly than in human patients.

Caries can occur on any tooth surface. However, the occlusal (grinding) surfaces of the molar teeth seem predisposed in dogs. Clinically, caries manifests as softened, often discoloured (dark brown or black) spots in the enamel. A dental explorer will 'catch' in the softened carious tooth surface. A small enamel defect covers a large cavern of decayed dentine. Note that not all lesions are grossly discoloured and all occlusal surfaces, whether discoloured or not, should be meticulously examined with a dental explorer. If the explorer sticks in the tooth surface, then caries should be suspected and radiographs are indicated. Radiographically, radiolucent defects are seen in the affected area of the crown. Radiographs will also give an indication of how close to the pulp chamber a caries lesion extends (the extent of secondary dentine formation, and the amount and thickness of dentine that separates the pulp from the carious lesion), which allows selection of the most appropriate treatment. Discoloured areas that are hard and the explorer does not 'catch' are not caries. They could be exposed dentine due to attrition or stain.

Diagnosed caries requires treatment. The options are extraction or referral to a specialist for restoration (if the process involves the pulp tissue, endodontic therapy prior to restoration is required). If the process has resulted in gross loss of tooth substance at the time of diagnosis, then extraction is the only option. Measures to prevent new lesions must be instituted in animals with diagnosed caries. In addition to home care and dietary modifications, as detailed in Appendix 1, these dogs may benefit from regular professional fluoride applications. Fluoride enhances remineralization and makes the enamel more resistant to the acid dissolution that occurs with caries.

CLINICAL TIPS

- Caries usually affect the teeth that have true occlusal tables, namely the molar teeth.
- Treatment of caries is mandatory.
- A dental explorer will 'catch' in a softened carious tooth surface.
- A small enamel defect covers a large cavern of decayed dentine.
- Radiographically, radiolucent defects are seen in the affected area of the crown.
- Discoloured areas that are hard and the explorer does not 'catch' are not caries.
- Treatment options are extraction or referral to a specialist for restoration.
- Measures to prevent new lesions must be instituted in animals with diagnosed caries.

TREATMENT OPTIONS

1. Extraction of all affected teeth.
2. Debridement and restoration of 109, 209 and 410, and extraction of 309 and 409.
3. Debridement and restoration of 109, 209 and 410; debridement and endodontic therapy (pulpectomy, root canal debridement, root filling and restoration) of 409; debridement and endodontic therapy (pulpectomy, root canal debridement of mesial root, root filling of mesial root, hemisection and extraction of distal root and restoration) of 309.

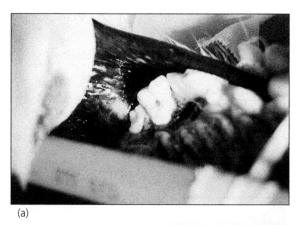

(a)

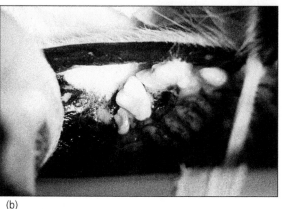

(b)

Figure 39.1 Debridement and restoration of 109.

(a) Carious tooth substance has been removed and a cavity prepared to accept a restoration.

(b) The restored occlusal tooth surface.

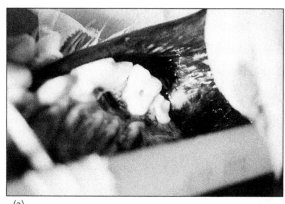

(a)

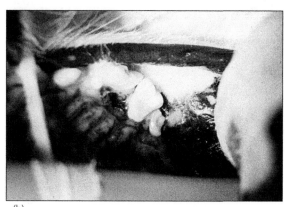

(b)

Figure 39.2 Debridement and restoration of 209.

(a) Carious tooth substance has been removed and a cavity prepared to accept a restoration.

(b) The restored occlusal tooth surface.

TREATMENT PERFORMED

1. Periodontal therapy to remove plaque and calculus, and provide a clean environment.
2. Debridement and restoration of 109 (Fig. 39.1a, b), 209 (Fig. 39.2a, b) and 410 (Fig. 39.3a, b).
3. Endodontic treatment of 409 (Fig. 39.4)
4. Endodontic treatment of the mesial root of 309, and hemisection and extraction of the distal root of 309 (Fig. 39.5a, b).
5. Application of fluoride varnish to all teeth.

POSTOPERATIVE CARE

- NSAIDs for 5 days
- Soft food
- No access to sugar-containing treats – on questioning the owner at the time of discharge, it became clear that the dog received digestive biscuits and chocolate at frequent intervals daily
- Chlorhexidine rinse once daily
- Start daily toothbrushing
- The dog was booked for recheck (examination under anaesthesia and radiographs) in 6 months' time.

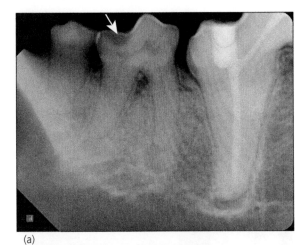

(a)

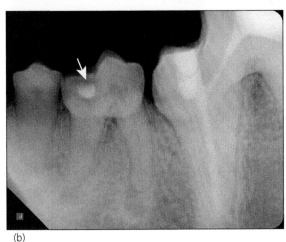

(b)

Figure 39.3 Lateral radiographs of 410.

(a) Caries manifests radiographically as a radiolucent zone in the dentine. Note that the process does not extend into the pulp system.

(b) Carious tooth substance has been removed and the cavity restored.

RECHECKS

Examination under general anaesthesia 6 months after initial treatment revealed mild generalized gingivitis (the owner was finding toothbrushing difficult to perform). All restorations were intact (Fig. 39.6a, b) and there was no discoloration of the teeth or the margins of the restorations. Radiographs confirmed successful outcome of the endodontic therapy of 409. The radiograph of 309 shows that the periapical radiolucency was smaller in size and was filling in with bone. The dog was rebooked

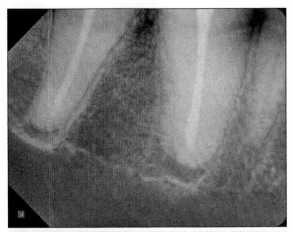

Figure 39.4 Lateral radiograph of 409. The radiograph confirms that the debrided root canals have been adequately filled with the inert root-filling material.

for recheck 6 months later to monitor periapical healing of the mesial root of 309.

PROGNOSIS

With continued dietary management and daily tooth-brushing, the dog is unlikely to develop further caries lesions. The periapical lesion of the mesial root of 309 needs further monitoring. If radiographs 6 months down the line don't show full bony healing, the tooth will probably be extracted.

COMMENTS

In simple terms, caries occurs when plaque bacteria use fermentable carbohydrate (notably sugar) from the diet as a source of energy. The fermentation by-products are acidic and demineralize the enamel. Caries can thus be prevented by removing the bacteria (toothbrushing) in combination with removing their substrate (sugar and other easily fermentable carbohydrate). Dogs should not be fed human biscuits and confectionery, as they are high in sugar.

There were three treatment options for this case. Extraction of all affected teeth would have been the least expensive option, requiring only one episode of general anaesthesia, and would have resulted in a comfortable dog with a relatively functional bite. The second alternative would have been debridement and restoration of 109, 209 and 410, and extraction of 309 and 409.

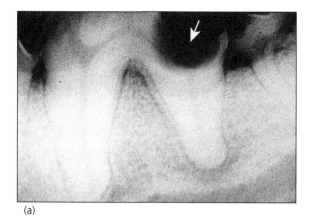

(a)

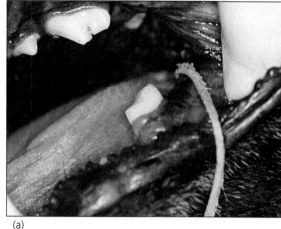

(a)

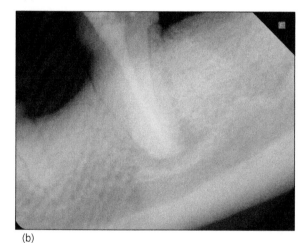

(b)

Figure 39.5 Lateral radiographs of 309.

(a) Prior to endodontic therapy. Note the extensive caries in the distal occlusal surface that clearly extends into the pulp.

(b) After endodontic therapy. The mesial root received conventional endodontic treatment (pulpectomy, root canal debridement, root filling and restoration); the tooth was then sectioned and the distal crown and root segment were extracted.

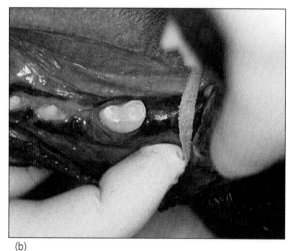

(b)

Figure 39.6 Photographs of 309 after endodontic treatment. The mesial crown root segment of 309 shows no clinical evidence of periodontitis, i.e. no increased probing depths or gingival recession. There is mild gingivitis only. The restorations are intact, with no evidence of discoloration.

(a) Lateral view.

(b) Occlusal view.

Again, this would have been a one-stage procedure and less expensive than the third option, namely: debridement and restoration of 109, 209 and 410; debridement, endodontic therapy and restoration of 409; and debridement, endodontic therapy, hemisection and restoration of 309. The owner did not want the dog to lose the teeth if other options were feasible. Consequently,

the third option was chosen. This option is more expensive and requires several anaesthetic episodes, but the dog does get to keep a functional posterior occlusion. Moreover, the opportunity to implement and monitor dietary and hygiene protocols makes it unlikely that further caries lesions on other teeth will develop in this dog.

APPENDICES

APPENDICES

MCQs

1. Which one of the following statements regarding canine and feline enamel is false?
(a) It is a thin layer as compared to man
(b) It has no nerve or blood supply
(c) It is deposited continuously throughout life
(d) Its inorganic content amounts to 96–97% of weight
(e) It is the hardest and most mineralized tissue in the body

2. Which one of the following statements regarding canine and feline dentine is false?
(a) It comprises the bulk of the mature tooth
(b) Inorganic content amounts to 70% of wet weight
(c) It has a tubular structure
(d) Dentine formation is complete when the tooth erupts
(e) It is deposited rapidly in response to trauma

3. Which of the following statements regarding canine and feline cementum is false?
(a) It is avascular bone-like tissue
(b) It is less calcified than enamel or dentine
(c) Cementum is deposited continuously throughout life
(d) It is capable of resorptive and reparative processes
(e) Cementum is produced by odontoblasts

4. Which one of the following statements is true?
(a) Ameloblasts produce enamel matrix
(b) Ameloblasts lay down mineralized enamel
(c) Odontoblasts produce dentine and cementum matrix
(d) Odontoblasts produce all the dental hard tissues
(e) Odontoclasts selectively destroy dentine

5. Which one of the following statements is true?
(a) The pulp system is lined by odontoblasts that produce dentine continuously throughout life
(b) In a multirooted tooth, each root has its own separate pulp system
(c) The root and its pulp system are fully developed by the time a tooth erupts into the oral cavity
(d) The pulp chamber is the pulp tissue contained in the roots
(e) A mature tooth has a single wide opening at the apex of the root

6. Which one of the following statements regarding the periodontium is true?
(a) The periodontium is an anatomical unit (consisting of gingiva, periodontal ligament, cementum and alveolar bone) which functions to attach the tooth to the jaw and provide a suspensory apparatus resilient to normal functional forces
(b) The periodontium is an anatomical unit (consisting of gingiva, periodontal ligament, cementum and alveolar bone) which functions to rigidly attach the tooth to the jaw
(c) The periodontium is an anatomical unit (consisting of gingiva, periodontal ligament, dentine and alveolar bone) which functions to attach the tooth to the jaw and provide a suspensory apparatus resilient to normal functional forces
(d) The periodontium is an anatomical unit (consisting of gingiva, periodontal ligament, dentine and alveolar bone) which functions to rigidly attach the tooth to the jaw
(e) The periodontium has no ability to repair

209

7. **Which one of the following statements is false?**
   (a) The gingiva forms a cuff around each tooth
   (b) The gingival sulcus is the invagination that the margin of the free gingiva forms with the tooth
   (c) Normal sulcus depth is 1–3 mm in dogs and 0.5–1 mm in cats
   (d) The periodontal ligament is connective tissue that anchors the tooth to the bone
   (e) Cementum is more calcified than enamel and/ or dentine

8. **Which one of the following statements is true?**
   (a) The dog has 26 primary teeth and 40 permanent teeth
   (b) The dog has 28 primary teeth and 42 permanent teeth
   (c) The dog has 28 primary teeth and 32 permanent teeth
   (d) The dog only has 42 permanent teeth
   (e) The dog has 26 primary teeth and 30 permanent teeth

9. **Which one of the following statements is true?**
   (a) The cat has 26 primary teeth and 40 permanent teeth
   (b) The cat has 28 primary teeth and 42 permanent teeth
   (c) The cat has 28 primary teeth and 32 permanent teeth
   (d) The cat only has 42 permanent teeth
   (e) The cat has 26 primary teeth and 30 permanent teeth

10. **Which one of the following statements is false?**
    (a) The primary teeth start forming in utero and erupt between 3 and 12 weeks of age
    (b) Resorption and exfoliation of primary teeth and replacement by permanent teeth occurs between 3 and 7 months of age in the dog
    (c) Resorption and exfoliation of primary teeth and replacement by permanent teeth occurs between 3 and 5 months of age in the cat
    (d) Enamel formation is complete before the tooth erupts
    (e) Root development occurs mainly during tooth eruption

11. **Which one of the following statements is true?**
    (a) The development of the occlusion is determined exclusively by genetic factors
    (b) The specific genetic mechanisms governing occlusion are known
    (c) The development of occlusion is determined solely by environmental factors
    (d) Jaw length, tooth bud position and tooth size are not inherited
    (e) The development of the upper jaw, mandible and teeth is independently regulated genetically

12. **Which one of the following statements is true?**
    (a) In the mesocephalic dog, the mandible is shorter and less wide than the upper jaw
    (b) In the mesocephalic dog, the mandible is shorter and wider than the upper jaw
    (c) Brachycephalic animals have a shorter than normal lower jaw
    (d) Dolicocephalic animals have a longer than normal lower jaw
    (e) The occlusion of a mesocephalic cat is the same as in the dog

13. **The periodontal probe is used for:**
    (a) Evaluating caries
    (b) Evaluating enamel/dentinal defects
    (c) Evaluating periodontal probing depths and furcation lesions
    (d) Probing for subgingival calculus
    (e) Evaluating odontoclastic resorptive lesions

14. **Which of the following statements regarding a dental explorer is false?**
    (a) It is used to evaluate caries
    (b) It is used to evaluate enamel/dentinal defects
    (c) It can be used to probe for subgingival calculus
    (d) It is a sharp-ended instrument
    (e) It is designed to be used to evaluate periodontal pocket depth

15. **Which one of the following statements is true?**
    (a) Untreated gingivitis always progresses to periodontitis
    (b) An individual with clinically healthy gingivae will not develop periodontitis

(c) Clinically healthy gingivae can be achieved by the daily use of a dental diet or dental hygiene chew

(d) Calculus accumulation is a primary cause of periodontal disease

(e) Gingivitis is irreversible

16. **Which one of the following statements is false?**

(a) Gingivitis is a plaque-induced inflammation

(b) Untreated gingivitis may progress to periodontitis

(c) Clinically healthy gingivae can be achieved by daily toothbrushing

(d) Toothbrushing is the single most effective means of removing plaque

(e) All effective dental hygiene chews have a hard texture

17. **Home care is defined as measures taken by the owner to remove/reduce the accumulation of dental deposits thus promoting periodontal health. Which of the following is not home care?**

(a) Toothbrushing

(b) Feeding a dental hygiene diet

(c) Feeding a dental hygiene chew

(d) Scaling teeth

(e) Toothbrushing and a dental hygiene diet or chew

18. **Gingivitis is best treated by which one of the following options?**

(a) Daily toothbrushing in conjunction with professional cleaning

(b) Professional cleaning and a daily dental hygiene chew or diet

(c) Professional cleaning

(d) Toothbrushing alone

(e) Dental hygiene diet or chew alone

19. **Which one of the following statements is false?**

(a) Periodontal surgery is first-line treatment for periodontal disease

(b) Periodontal surgery should only be performed when the owner has shown the ability to keep the mouth clean

(c) Conservative management of periodontitis, in combination with meticulous home care, is the first line of treatment

(d) Periodontal surgery is performed under general anaesthesia

(e) Plaque needs to be removed on a daily basis in the periodontitis patient

20. **If the dental film is positioned intra-orally (either on the occlusal plane or angled as close as possible to the tooth to be radiographed), and the X-ray beam is directed at right angles to the film plane, which of the following options will occur?**

(a) Elongation of the image

(b) Foreshortening of the image

(c) A correct reproduction of the image

(d) Magnification and elongation of the image

21. **If the dental film is positioned intra-orally (either on the occlusal plane or angled as close as possible to the tooth to be radiographed), and the X-ray beam is directed at right angles to the long axis of the tooth, which of the following options will occur?**

(a) Elongation of the image

(b) Foreshortening of the image

(c) A correct reproduction of the image

(d) Magnification and foreshortening of the image

22. **If the dental film is positioned intra-orally (either on the occlusal plane or angled as close as possible to the tooth to be radiographed), and the X-ray beam is directed at right angles to the bisecting line, which of the following options will occur?**

(a) Elongation of the image

(b) Foreshortening of the image

(c) A correct reproduction of the image

(d) Both elongation and magnification of the image

23. **Which one of the following statements relating to a persistent primary tooth is incorrect?**

(a) It is likely to affect the direction of eruption of the permanent tooth

(b) Malocclusion is a likely outcome

(c) Food and hair entrapment between the primary and permanent tooth may lead to the development of a localized periodontal defect

(d) It should be extracted early in the animal's life

(e) It should only be extracted when the animal has reached skeletal maturity

24. **Which one of the following statements is incorrect?**

(a) Untreated complicated crown fractures will inevitably result in pulpal pathology

(b) Pulpal pathology may be painful

(c) Complicated crown fractures always require treatment

(d) Complicated crown fractures do not require treatment

(e) The preferred treatment option for a periodontally sound functionally important tooth with a complicated crown fracture is endodontic therapy

25. **Which one of the following is not a complication that can occur during tooth extraction?**

(a) Tooth crown fracture

(b) Tooth root fracture

(c) Jaw fracture

(d) Haemorrhage

(e) Abscess formation

26. **Which one of the following statements relating to feline chronic gingivostomatitis is false?**

(a) Affected cats commonly have elevated serum and salivary immunoglobulins (Ig)

(b) Affected cats commonly have elevated serum immunoglobulins (IgG, IgM and IgA are all raised), and elevated salivary IgG and IgM but reduced IgA

(c) It is unclear if the Ig pattern is a cause or a result of the inflammatory disease

(d) Histological examination of affected oral mucosa shows a submucosal infiltrate consisting of plasma cells, lymphocytes, macrophages and neutrophils

(e) No underlying intrinsic immune abnormality has been identified in affected animals

27. **Which one of the following statements relating to feline chronic gingivostomatitis is false?**

(a) The extraction of all premolar and molar teeth has given the most dependable results, with 80% of cats being clinically cured or significantly improved

(b) Feline calici virus (FCV) has been isolated from up to 100% of chronic gingivostomatitis cases compared with 25% of cats in a healthy population

(c) FCV isolation from cats with chronic gingivostomatitis and then inoculated into specific pathogen-free cats produced signs of acute calici virus infection, but not chronic gingivostomatitis

(d) FCV isolation from cats with chronic gingivostomatitis and then inoculated into specific pathogen-free cats produced chronic gingivostomatitis

(e) The most common sign of feline immunodeficiency virus (FIV) infection is oral inflammation, yet most cats with chronic gingivostomatitis test negative for FIV

28. **Which one of the following statements relating to canine chronic gingivostomatitis is true?**

(a) Chronic gingivostomatitis is more common in the dog than in the cat

(b) The likely cause is an underlying vesiculo-bullous skin disease

(c) The oral inflammation is generally caused by systemic diseases, e.g. endocrine or renal disorder

(d) It is thought to be an inappropriate response to bacterial plaque present on the tooth surfaces

(e) Plaque control is unlikely to have any beneficial effect

29. **Which one of the following statements relating to tooth resorption is false?**

(a) Hard tissues are protected from resorption by their surface layer of blast cells

(b) Resorption of hard tissue requires a trigger and then a reason for the resorption to continue

(c) Internal root resorption emanates from the root canal wall

(d) External root resorption emanates from the root surface

(e) Internal root resorption is common in permanent teeth

30. **Which one of the following statements relating to external root resorption is false?**
    (a) A surface resorption is initiated by injury to the cementoblast layer
    (b) Surface resorption is self-limiting and reversible
    (c) Replacement resorption results in replacement of dental hard tissue by bone
    (d) There are two main forms of external root resorption associated with inflammation of the periodontal tissue, namely peripheral inflammatory root resorption and external inflammatory root resorption
    (e) External root resorption is uncommon in the cat

31. **Which statement relating to root resorption in the cat is false?**
    (a) Cats with clinically missing teeth were more likely to have external root resorption
    (b) Teeth 307 and 407 are the most commonly affected
    (c) The pattern of distribution of resorptive lesions is strikingly symmetrical
    (d) Neutering, sex and age at neutering did not affect the prevalence of resorptive lesions
    (e) Mean mouth gingivitis index is directly related to the prevalence of resorptive lesions

32. **Which one of the following statements relating to the treatment of root resorption in the cat is true?**
    (a) Accessible lesions which extend into dentine and do not involve the pulp are best treated by restoration
    (b) Conservative management, i.e. monitoring clinically and radiographically, is indicated when there is only a small cavity in the tooth
    (c) Coronal amputation is indicated even when there is no radiographic evidence of ongoing root resorption
    (d) Coronal amputation is only indicated when there is radiographic evidence of ongoing root resorption
    (e) Coronal amputation does not require radiographic monitoring

33. **Which one of the following statements relating to root resorption in the cat is false?**
    (a) Resorptive lesions are common
    (b) Prevention is not possible

    (c) The lesions are not progressive
    (d) Diagnosis generally requires radiography
    (e) Extraction and/or coronal amputation are the preferable treatment options

34. **Which one of the following statements relating to malocclusion is false?**
    (a) It is an abnormality in the position of the teeth
    (b) It can result from jaw length and/or width discrepancy
    (c) It can result from tooth malpositioning
    (d) The specific genetic mechanisms regulating malocclusion are unknown
    (e) A polygenic mechanism is likely, which explains why all siblings in successive generations are affected by malocclusion to the same degree

35. **Which one of the following statements relating to occlusion and malocclusion is true?**
    (a) The upper and lower jaws of brachycephalic animals are shorter than normal
    (b) The upper and lower jaws of dolicocephalic animals are longer than normal
    (c) Brachycephalic animals have a shorter than normal upper jaw and dolicocephalic animals have a longer than normal upper jaw
    (d) A mandibular prognathic bite is often called 'overshot'
    (e) A mandibular brachynathic bite is often called 'undershot'

36. **Which one of the following statements relating to malocclusion is true?**
    (a) The mandibular prognathic, the mandibular brachygnathic, the wry bite and a narrow mandible are all dental malocclusions
    (b) The mandibular prognathic, the mandibular brachygnathic, the wry bite and a narrow mandible are all skeletal malocclusions
    (c) The mandibular prognathic, the mandibular brachygnathic and a narrow mandible are all dental malocclusions
    (d) The mandibular prognathic, the mandibular brachygnathic and the wry bite are all dental malocclusions
    (e) The mandibular prognathic, the mandibular brachygnathic and a narrow mandible are all skeletal malocclusions, but the wry bite is a dental malocclusion

37. Which one of the following statements is false?
   (a) The permanent incisors erupt caudal to their primary counterparts
   (b) The maxillary permanent canine begins eruption medial to its primary counterpart
   (c) The maxillary permanent canine erupts rostral to it primary counterpart
   (d) The mandibular permanent canine begins eruption medial to its primary counterpart
   (e) Persistent primary teeth are more common in the smaller breeds

38. Which one of the following statements relating to periodontal disease is true?
   (a) The primary cause of periodontal disease is dental plaque
   (b) The cause of periodontal disease is dental calculus
   (c) Gingivitis and periodontitis are both associated with destruction of the supporting tissue
   (d) Gingivitis is irreversible
   (e) Periodontitis is generally reversible

39. Which one of the following statements relating to dental plaque is false?
   (a) It is a biofilm
   (b) Accumulation starts within minutes on a clean tooth surface
   (c) The initial accumulation is supragingival
   (d) Supragingival plaque will extend into the sulcus and populate the subgingival region if left undisturbed
   (e) Plaque accumulation starts within a few days of cleaning a tooth surface

40. Which one of the following statements relating to dental calculus is true?
   (a) Only supragingival plaque becomes mineralized
   (b) Only subgingival plaque becomes mineralized
   (c) Subgingival calculus is the primary cause of periodontitis
   (d) Dental calculus is always covered by a layer of plaque
   (e) Supragingival calculus is the primary cause of gingivitis

41. Which one of the following statements is true?
   (a) Periodontitis is always associated with increased periodontal probing depth
   (b) Gingival recession is not associated with loss of attachment
   (c) Gingival hyperplasia is always associated with loss of attachment
   (d) Horizontal bone loss is often accompanied by gingival recession so periodontal pockets may not form
   (e) Disease progression is a slow, continuous process

42. Which one of the following statements is false?
   (a) Periodontal disease is a collective term for plaque-induced inflammation of the periodontium
   (b) An individual with clinically healthy gingivae will not develop periodontitis
   (c) An individual with gingivitis will always develop periodontitis
   (d) An individual with gingivitis may or may not develop periodontitis
   (e) The aim of periodontal disease treatment is to establish and maintain clinically healthy gingivae to prevent periodontitis

43. Which one of the following statements relating to pulpitis is false?
   (a) Pulpitis is inflammation of the pulp
   (b) Pulpitis is always associated with intense pain
   (c) It may be associated with pain, but may also be asymptomatic
   (d) Untreated chronic pulpitis will result in pulp necrosis
   (e) Chronic pulpitis can cause periapical complications

44. Which one of the following is a real emergency, i.e. needs treatment as soon as possible if the tooth is to be saved?
   (a) Complicated crown fracture of a permanent tooth in a dog less than 1 year old (i.e. an immature permanent tooth)
   (b) Complicated crown fracture of a permanent tooth in an adult dog (i.e. mature permanent tooth)
   (c) Complicated crown and root fracture of a permanent tooth in an adult dog (i.e. mature permanent tooth)
   (d) Uncomplicated crown fracture of an immature tooth

(e) Uncomplicated crown fracture of a mature tooth

45. **Which one of the following alternatives is the best treatment option for a dog with a periodontally sound mature canine tooth with a complicated crown fracture?**
    (a) No treatment required
    (b) Extraction
    (c) Referral for endodontic treatment so the tooth can be maintained
    (d) Restoration without endodontic treatment
    (e) Radiographic monitoring

46. **A tooth with an uncomplicated crown fracture requires which one of the following treatment options?**
    (a) No treatment required
    (b) Smoothing of any sharp edges (possibly restoration) and radiographic monitoring
    (c) Extraction
    (d) Coronal amputation
    (e) Fixation with a splint

47. **Which one of the following statements relating to periapical pathology is false?**
    (a) Periapical pathology is a consequence of chronic pulpitis
    (b) Periapical pathology is a consequence of pulp necrosis
    (c) It manifests radiographically as a distinct radiolucent zone surrounding the apex of a tooth
    (d) The periapical lesion may be a granuloma, cyst or abscess
    (e) A cyst can be clearly differentiated from a granuloma or abscess on a radiograph

48. **Diagnosed periapical pathology should be treated by which one of the following alternatives?**
    (a) No treatment required
    (b) A long course of antibiotics
    (c) Administration of analgesics
    (d) Extraction or endodontic treatment of the affected tooth
    (e) Corticosteroids to reduce the inflammatory response

49. **Which one of the following statements relating to combined endodontic and periodontic lesions is false?**
    (a) A Class I lesion (endodontic–periodontic) is endodontic in origin, i.e. pathology begins in the periodontium and progresses to involve the pulp
    (b) A Class II lesion (periodontic–endodontic) is periodontic in origin, i.e. pathology begins in the periodontium and progresses to involve the pulp
    (c) A Class III lesion (true combined) is a fusion of independent periodontic and endodontic lesions
    (d) Class I lesions have a better prognosis than Class II or III lesions, as endodontic treatment may lead to resolution of the periodontal extension of the inflammation
    (e) Although Class II and III lesions require both endodontic treatment and periodontal therapy, they have a better prognosis than a Class I lesion

50. **Which one of the following statements relating to osteomyelitis of the jaw bone is false?**
    (a) It is not particularly common in dogs and cats
    (b) Infection of dental origin (as an extension of pulp and periapical disease) is probably the most frequent cause
    (c) Biopsy and histopathological examination of the bone is the only way to reach a definitive diagnosis
    (d) Osteomyelitis is easily differentiated from neoplastic bone lesions on radiography
    (e) Once diagnosed, osteomyelitis is treated by removing the cause (extraction or possibly endodontic treatment of teeth with pulp and periapical disease) in combination with antibiotic therapy

MCQs – Answers

1. **(c)** It is deposited continuously throughout life

2. **(d)** Dentine formation is complete when the tooth erupts

3. **(e)** Cementum is produced by odontoblasts

4. **(a)** Ameloblasts produce enamel matrix

5. **(a)** The pulp system is lined by odontoblasts that produce dentine continuously throughout life

6. **(a)** The periodontium is an anatomical unit (consisting of gingiva, periodontal ligament, cementum and alveolar bone) which functions to attach the tooth to the jaw and provide a suspensory apparatus resilient to normal functional forces

7. **(e)** Cementum is more calcified than enamel and/or dentine

8. **(b)** The dog has 28 primary teeth and 42 permanent teeth

9. **(e)** The cat has 26 primary teeth and 30 permanent teeth

10. **(e)** Root development occurs mainly during tooth eruption

11. **(e)** The development of the upper jaw, mandible and teeth is independently regulated genetically

12. **(a)** In the mesocephalic dog, the mandible is shorter and less wide than the upper jaw

13. **(c)** Evaluating periodontal probing depths and furcation lesions

14. **(e)** It is designed to be used to evaluate periodontal pocket depth

15. **(b)** An individual with clinically healthy gingivae will not develop periodontitis

16. **(e)** All effective dental hygiene chews have a hard texture

17. **(d)** Scaling teeth

18. **(a)** Daily toothbrushing in conjunction with professional cleaning

19. **(a)** Periodontal surgery is first-line treatment for periodontal disease

20. **(b)** Foreshortening of the image

21. **(a)** Elongation of the image

22. **(c)** A correct reproduction of the image

23. **(e)** It should only be extracted when the animal has reached skeletal maturity

24. **(d)** Complicated crown fractures do not require treatment

25. **(e)** Abscess formation

26. **(a)** Affected cats commonly have elevated serum and salivary immunoglobulins (Ig)

27. **(d)** FCV isolation from cats with chronic gingivostomatitis and then inoculated into specific pathogen-free cats produced chronic gingivostomatitis

28. **(d)** It is thought to be an inappropriate response to bacterial plaque present on the tooth surfaces

29. **(e)** Internal root resorption is common in permanent teeth

30. **(e)** External root resorption is uncommon in the cat

31. **(e)** Mean mouth gingivitis index is directly related to the prevalence of resorptive lesions

32. **(d)** Coronal amputation is only indicated when there is radiographic evidence of ongoing root resorption

33. **(c)** The lesions are not progressive

34. **(e)** A polygenic mechanism is likely, which explains why all siblings in successive generations are affected by malocclusion to the same degree

35. **(c)** Brachycephalic animals have a shorter than normal upper jaw and dolicocephalic animals have a longer than normal upper jaw

36. **(b)** The mandibular prognathic, the mandibular brachygnathic, the wry bite and a narrow mandible are all skeletal malocclusions

37. **(b)** The maxillary permanent canine begins eruption medial to its primary counterpart

38. **(a)** The primary cause of periodontal disease is dental plaque

39. **(e)** Plaque accumulation starts within a few days of cleaning a tooth surface

40. **(d)** Dental calculus is always covered by a layer of plaque

41. **(d)** Horizontal bone loss is often accompanied by gingival recession so periodontal pockets may not form

42. **(c)** An individual with gingivitis will always develop periodontitis

43. **(b)** Pulpitis is always associated with intense pain

44. **(a)** Complicated crown fracture of a permanent tooth in a dog less than 1 year old (i.e. an immature permanent tooth)

45. **(c)** Referral for endodontic treatment so the tooth can be maintained

46. **(b)** Smoothing of any sharp edges (possibly restoration) and radiographic monitoring

47. **(e)** A cyst can be clearly differentiated from a granuloma or abscess on a radiograph

48. **(d)** Extraction or endodontic treatment of the affected tooth

49. **(e)** Although Class II and III lesions require both endodontic treatment and periodontal therapy, they have a better prognosis than a Class I lesion

50. **(d)** Osteomyelitis is easily differentiated from neoplastic bone lesions on radiography

APPENDIX
Home care: maintenance of oral hygiene

CLIENT EDUCATION

The cause (dental plaque) and effects (discomfort, pain, loss of teeth, chronic focus of infection, systemic consequences) of periodontal disease must be thoroughly explained to the pet owner. The owner must be made aware that home care is the most essential component in both preventing and treating periodontal disease. The responsibility of maintaining oral hygiene, i.e. keeping plaque accumulation to a level compatible with periodontal health, rests with the owner of the pet. Once instituted, home care regimens need continuous monitoring and reinforcement. The veterinary nurse can play a vital role in educating clients, checking compliance and reinforcing the need for home care.

However, the owner must realize that, even with home care, most animals still need to have their teeth cleaned professionally at intervals. The intervals between professional cleaning need to be determined for each animal. With good home care, the interval between professional cleanings can be greatly extended. It is useful to draw an analogy to the situation in man, i.e. most of us brush our teeth daily but still require dental examinations and professional periodontal therapy (at a minimum scaling and polishing) at regular intervals.

TOOTHBRUSHING

Toothbrushing has been proven to be the single most effective means of removing plaque. It is the gold standard for plaque control. Every effort should be made to persuade owners to brush their pet's teeth on a daily basis. The success of toothbrushing depends on pet cooperation, owner motivation and technical ability. Toothbrushing should be introduced gradually and as early in the animal's life as possible. Adult cats are generally less amenable to the introduction of toothbrushing than adult dogs, but with patience and persistence, many will accept some degree of home care. In contrast, kittens often accept toothbrushing more readily than puppies. In both species it is much easier to introduce toothbrushing earlier rather than later in the animal's life.

Toothbrushes

There are innumerable brush-head and handle designs and sizes of human and veterinary toothbrushes available, but there is insufficient evidence to clearly recommend any particular one. The choice of brush should be based on the effectiveness of plaque control in the hands of each individual. In general, a soft to medium texture nylon filament brush of a suitable size for the intended pet seems to be the most comfortable. Many owners report that they are using a human electric motor-driven toothbrush with good results. Electric motor-driven toothbrushes are now available for dogs and cats (Fig. A1.1).

A flannel cloth folded over a finger, or a rubber 'finger brush', may be more comfortable for animals and owners, but is less effective (removes less plaque) than a nylon filament brush. The use of a finger brush or cloth during the training phase is useful, but every attempt should be made to get the animal to accept a proper toothbrush.

Toothpaste

The use of non-foaming tasty pet toothpaste is recommended, but not critical. It is the mechanical action of brushing which removes the plaque. Therefore, brushing with a toothbrush moistened with water will still do the job. Pet toothpaste tastes nice and the pet will therefore usually allow the owner to brush for longer, thus removing more plaque. The paste should be pressed down into the bristles to maintain it on the brush or the animal will just lick it off.

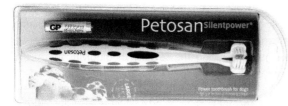

Figure A1.1 Electric motor-driven toothbrush (Petosan Silentpower) for dogs and cats. This toothbrush has been launched by Petosan AS Norway (www.petosan.com). Image courtesy of Petosan AS.

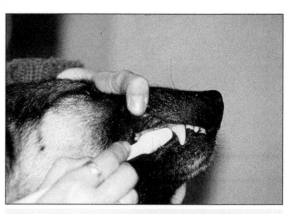

Figure A1.2 Toothbrushing technique. The teeth and gingival margin are brushed in a circular or side-to-side motion. The brush is angled at 45° to the tooth surfaces, so that the bristles enter the gingival sulcus. The circling motion should ensure that all cracks and crevices in and around the teeth are cleaned.

The use of human toothpaste is not recommended, mainly due to the high fluoride content, which may lead to acute, but more likely chronic, toxicity problems, as our pets do not rinse and spit but will swallow the toothpaste.

Frequency of toothbrushing

The current clinical recommendation is daily toothbrushing to establish and maintain clinically healthy gingivae for the whole life of the animal. Brushing less frequently is not sufficient to maintain clinically healthy gingivae.

Brushing technique

There is no one correct method of brushing, but rather the appropriate one that in each case removes plaque effectively without damaging either tooth or gingiva. Individual preference and dexterity, and the variable dentogingival morphology occurring with different stages of disease, will dictate the best method. In most instances, a combination of roll and miniscrub technique will achieve the objective.

The teeth and gingival margin are brushed in a circular or side-to-side motion. The brush is angled at 45° to the tooth surfaces, so that the bristles enter the gingival sulcus (Fig. A1.2). The circling motion should ensure that all cracks and crevices in and around the teeth are cleaned.

Some practical suggestions to give to owners are as follows:

- Start toothbrushing as early in life as possible, as prevention of disease development is the goal. The primary teeth will be exfoliated and replaced by the permanent dentition. Consequently, the benefit of introducing toothbrushing at a young age will not benefit the primary teeth, but the procedure will be accepted at the time the permanent teeth erupt.

- Make the animal comfortable and approach from the side rather than in front.
- Start with just a few teeth (premolars and molars rather than incisors, since retracting the lips is usually readily accepted, while many animals don't like having their nose lifted) and gradually increase the number of teeth cleaned each time until the whole mouth can be cleaned in a single session.
- Initially, the mouth does not need to be opened. Concentrate on brushing the buccal surfaces of the teeth, especially at the gingival margin.
- When the animal is comfortable with having the buccal surfaces of all its teeth brushed, an attempt should be made to open the mouth and carefully brush the palatal and lingual surfaces of the teeth (Fig. A1.3). If this is not accepted, there is every reason to continue with daily brushing of the buccal surfaces. However, gingivitis will occur on the palatal and lingual surfaces if these are not brushed, and periodontitis may occur at these sites, hence the need for professional check-ups at regular intervals.
- Offer a reward at the end of the procedure, e.g. a game or a walk.
- Include toothbrushing as part of the daily grooming routine. Home care is more likely to be acceptable to an older pet if it is introduced as an extension of a pre-existing routine, e.g. evening meal, walk, grooming. The owner is also more likely to remember a consistent routine.

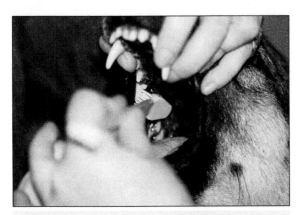

Figure A1.3 Toothbrushing technique. When the animal is comfortable with having the buccal surfaces of all its teeth brushed, an attempt should be made to open the mouth and carefully brush the palatal and lingual surfaces of the teeth.

- Owners can sit small dogs and cats on their lap whilst brushing, at the same time cuddling them to reduce their apprehension; alternatively, one person cuddles and restrains whilst a second performs the toothbrushing. Some animals may better accept the use of a 'grooming table' type situation.

DENTAL DIETS AND DENTAL HYGIENE CHEWS

The use of products (dental diets, hygiene chews and biscuits) aimed at encouraging chewing activity and designed with textural properties that maximize the self-cleansing effect of function are beneficial in reducing the accumulation of dental deposits and consequently the degree of gingivitis that develops.

None of the products in this category are as effective as daily toothbrushing. Consequently, their use cannot achieve, or maintain, clinically healthy gingivae in the absence of toothbrushing.

While every attempt should be made to ensure that daily toothbrushing is performed by the owner, dietary means of reducing the accumulation of dental deposits and thus reducing the severity of gingivitis is a useful adjunctive measure and is highly recommended. In selecting an appropriate dental diet or dental hygiene chews for patients, I would recommend using either a product that has been shown to be effective in peer-reviewed publications, or a product that has been awarded a VOHC® Seal of Acceptance.*

CHEMICAL PLAQUE CONTROL

In addition to mechanical plaque control, chemical plaque control does have a role in treating periodontitis. They are not indicated to prevent or treat gingivitis.

SUMMARY

There is no magic bullet that we can feed our pets to prevent periodontal disease. Daily toothbrushing remains the single most effective method of restoring inflamed gingivae to health and of then maintaining clinically healthy gingivae. Compliance may be an issue for some people. Compliance failure has not been critically investigated in veterinary dentistry; however, it is not difficult to imagine that many factors may prevent owners from brushing their pets' teeth. Such factors include lack of skill, questionable perceived benefit, unpleasantness of the procedure and lifestyle (lack of time). Our experience is that a combination of client education, continuous reinforcement and individually determined recalls to check efficacy yields surprisingly good compliance.

---

*The Veterinary Oral Health Council (VOHC®) Seal of Acceptance system identifies products that meet pre-set standards for prevention of accumulation of dental plaque and calculus (tartar). It is a product effectiveness recognition system, with no regulatory function, and is limited to considering products designed to control plaque and calculus.

2 APPENDIX
Equipment and instrumentation

GENERAL CONSIDERATIONS

Many dental procedures result in the creation of a bacterial aerosol, so ideally a separate room should be designated for oral and dental procedures. The room must have adequate light and ventilation. A bright light source is required. Investing in a dental light is mandatory. A good dental light is expensive, but definitely worth the money.

Ergonomic considerations are of paramount importance in the layout of the dental operatory. All equipment and instruments should be within easy reach of the operator. Posture is important! Ideally, the operator should be seated.

It is essential to protect operator and staff. The veterinarian and the assistant should wear facemasks and appropriate eye wear (spectacles or face shield) to protect themselves from the bacterial aerosol and other debris. There is a risk of infection of skin wounds if the operator works in a dirty environment without gloves. The oral cavity is never a sterile site, so the use of surgical gloves is recommended.

Important patient considerations are as follows:
- General anaesthesia with endotracheal intubation is essential. This prevents inhalation of aerosolized bacteria (and other debris) and asphyxiation on irrigation and cooling fluid.
- A pharyngeal pack is also recommended during oral and dental treatment. Remember to remove the pharyngeal pack prior to extubation! The animal should be positioned on a surface that will allow drainage to prevent it becoming wet and hypothermic. This can be achieved by the use of a 'tub-tank' or placing the animal's head on a towel or disposable 'nappy'. Most animals benefit from a heating pad.

Some important equipment and instrumentation considerations are as follows:
- Clean, sterilized instruments should be available for each patient. Ideally, several pre-packed kits with the required instruments for different procedures, e.g. examination, periodontal therapy, extraction, should be available.
- Power equipment requires regular maintenance (daily, weekly) in the practice and regular servicing by the supplier. Draw up checklists for these chores. Check maintenance and servicing requirements with the supplier.

EQUIPMENT AND INSTRUMENTATION FOR ORAL AND DENTAL EXAMINATION

There is a wide selection of dental equipment and instrumentation available on the market. My recommendation is to identify your needs and then invest in a bit more than you think you will require. The better you get at performing dentistry and oral surgery, the more demanding of your equipment you will become. There is also an element of personal preference, so test different options before making a decision. Finally, be prepared to upgrade!

The details of how to perform oral examination and recording are covered in Section 2, Chapter 3. The following will outline equipment and instrumentation requirements. Personal preferences have been inserted as a guide, where appropriate.

Periodontal probe

The periodontal probe is a rounded narrow or flat, blunt-ended, graduated instrument. Due to its blunt end, it can be inserted into the gingival sulcus without causing trauma (Fig. A2.1). The periodontal probe is used to:
- Measure periodontal probing depth
- Determine the degree of gingival inflammation
- Evaluate furcation lesions
- Evaluate the extent of tooth mobility.

A rounded narrow, rather than flat, probe (e.g. No. 14 Williams B) is my preferred choice, as it is easier to

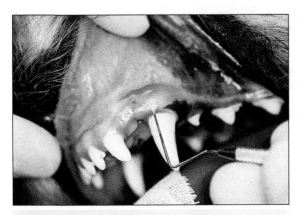

Figure A2.1 The periodontal probe is a blunt-ended, graduated instrument, which can be inserted into the gingival sulcus without causing trauma.

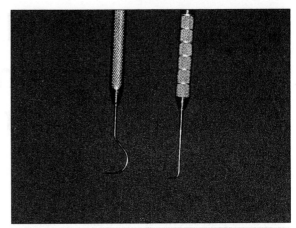

Figure A2.2 The dental explorer is either straight or curved (shepherd's hook). I don't like the double-ended explorers/probes due to the risk of inadvertent damage to the animal with the end you are not using in the oral cavity.

enter the gingival sulcus without causing damage with the rounded probe, especially in cats, where the flat probe is impossible to use.

Dental explorer

The dental explorer or probe, a sharp-ended instrument, is used to:
- Determine the presence of caries
- Explore other enamel and dentine defects, e.g. fracture, odontoclastic resorptive lesions.

The explorer is also useful for tactile examination of the subgingival tooth surfaces. Subgingival calculus and odontoclastic resorptive lesions may be identified in this way.

Dental explorers are either straight or curved (Fig. A2.2). They are also either single-ended or double-ended, usually combined with a periodontal probe, i.e. one end is an explorer and the other end is a periodontal probe. My preference is the Explorer probe No. 6, which is a single-ended straight explorer.

Dental mirror

A dental mirror is a vital, but traditionally rarely used, tool. It allows the operator to visualize palatal/lingual surfaces while maintaining posture, reflect light onto areas of interest, and retract and protect soft tissue. Orientation may cause confusion and the use of a dental mirror requires practice. The time taken to learn how to use a dental mirror is a worthy investment. To prevent condensation occurring on the mirror, it can be wiped across the buccal mucous membranes before use. Dental

mirrors are available in several sizes. A small (paediatric size) mirror for cats and small dogs and a larger one for medium to large dogs should be available.

Dental record sheets

Recording and dental record sheets are covered in Section 2. A complete dental record is required for diagnostic and therapeutic purposes, as well as for medico-legal reasons.

EQUIPMENT AND INSTRUMENTATION FOR PERIODONTAL THERAPY

Scaling

Scaling describes the procedure whereby dental deposits (plaque, but mainly calculus) are removed from the supra- and subgingival surfaces of the teeth. Scaling may be performed using either hand instruments or mechanical instruments, or a combination of both.

Hand scaling instruments: Scalers and curettes (Fig. A2.3) are used to remove dental deposits from the tooth surfaces.

Scalers are used for the supragingival removal of calculus. A scaler has a sharp working tip and should thus only be used supragingivally. If a scaler is used subgingivally, the result is laceration of the gingival margin. The scaler should always be pulled away from the gingiva

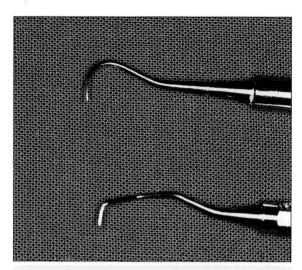

Figure A2.3 Scaler (top) and curette (bottom). The scaler can only be used to remove supragingival dental deposits. The curette is used to remove subgingival deposits and restore the root surface to smoothness. It can also be used to remove supragingival dental deposits.

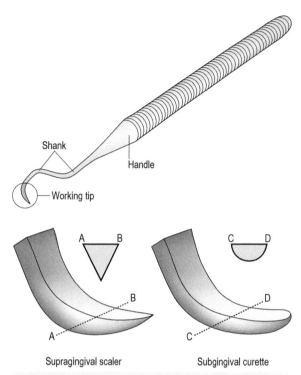

Figure A2.4 Scaler and curette design. Each has a handle, a shank and a working tip. The working tip of a scaler is more robust than that of a curette. Curettes are less bulky, with rounded back and tip, for use in gingival pockets. Both hand scalers and curettes require frequent sharpening to maintain their cutting edges. From Gorrel C (2004): Veterinary Dentistry for the General Practitioner, with permission of Elsevier.

towards the tip of the crown. Scalers require frequent sharpening to maintain their cutting edges.

Curettes are used for the subgingival removal of dental deposits and for root planing. They can also be used supragingivally. The working tip of a curette is more slender than that of a scaler. Also, the back and tip are rounded to minimize gingival trauma. Curettes also require frequent sharpening.

The differences between a scaler and a curette are summarized in Fig. A2.4.

A selection of curettes is required. My preferred curettes are the Gracey 7/8 and the Columbia 13/14. I don't recommend a separate scaler as curettes can be used both above and below the gingiva, while scalers are limited to supragingival use.

Mechanical scaling instruments: Mechanical or powered scalers enable fast and easy removal of calculus. They have a great potential for iatrogenic damage if used incorrectly. There are three types of mechanical scalers, namely sonic, ultrasonic and rotary. Gross supragingival calculus deposits are best removed with hand instruments (scaler, curette) prior to using mechanical scaling equipment.

Sonic scalers are driven by compressed air, so they require a compressed air-driven dental unit for operation. The tip oscillates at a sonic frequency and is effi-

cient at removing dental calculus. Sonic scalers are generally less effective than ultrasonic scalers, but generate less heat and are thus safer to use. Depending upon the design of the tip of the scaler, these instruments may be used for supra- and subgingival scaling. A thin, pointed tip, sometimes called a perio, sickle or universal insert, is the recommended insert.

Ultrasonic scalers are commonly used in veterinary practice. The tip oscillates at ultrasonic frequencies. They are driven by a micromotor, so do not require a compressed air-driven unit for operation. The tip vibration is generated either by a magnetostrictive mechanism, or a piezoelectric mechanism in the handpiece. The ultrasonic oscillation of the tip causes cavitation of the coolant, which aids in the disruption of the calculus on the tooth surface. Ultrasonic scalers are generally designed for supragingival use, but tips designed for subgingival scaling are available. A thin, pointed insert is recommended for supragingival use. Inserts specifically designed for subgingival use are recommended for sub-gingival scaling.

I have no real preference between sonic or ultrasonic scalers and use both.

Rotary scalers are best avoided, but are included here for completeness. In this system, roto pro burs are inserted in the high-speed handpiece of a compressed air-driven unit. They are so-called 'non-cutting' burs, which when applied to calculus cause it to disintegrate while the coolant flushes the debris away. In man, the use of these burs to scale teeth is associated with significant postoperative pain. They are thus no longer used for scaling. In addition to postoperative pain, roto pro burs can cause extensive damage to tooth enamel and hence their use in veterinary dentistry is not recommended.

Calculus forceps

Calculus forceps have been designed to aid removal of heavy calculus from the surface of teeth. It is essential to use these forceps with extreme care and in the described manner, as inappropriate use will result in fractured teeth. These forceps must not be used to extract teeth.

Polishing

Polishing removes plaque and restores the scaled tooth surfaces to smoothness, which is less plaque retentive. Scaled teeth must be polished. It is often suggested that teeth may be 'polished' by hand using a toothbrush and prophy paste. This method is inefficient and therefore not recommended. Efficient polishing can be performed using either prophy paste in a prophy cup or in a brush in a slow-speed contra-angle handpiece, or by means of particle blasting (air polishing).

Prophy paste in a cup/brush in a slow-speed contra-angle handpiece: The speed of rotation of the cup/brush can be regulated. To minimize the amount of heat generated, the prophy cup or brush should not rotate faster than 1000 revolutions per minute.

Air polishing (particle blasting): This technique, based on the sandblasting principle, is used to polish the supragingival parts of the teeth. The particles used (e.g. bicarbonate of soda) will polish the tooth surface without causing damage to the enamel. It is essential to protect the soft tissues (gingivae and oral mucosa) during air polishing. A simple way of protecting the soft tissues is to cover them with a piece of gauze.

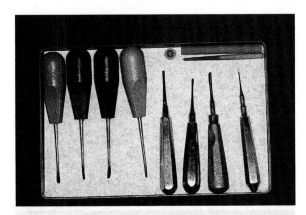

Figure A2.5 Luxators and elevators. My favourite luxators and elevators are depicted. On the left are four Svensk luxators (coloured handles) and on the right four different sizes of Coupland elevators.

Prophy paste: Prophy paste is available in bulk containers and in individual patient tubs. The latter are inexpensive and should be used to prevent contamination and the iatrogenic transmission of pathogens.

EQUIPMENT AND INSTRUMENTATION FOR TOOTH EXTRACTION

Hand instruments

Luxators and elevators: A selection of dental luxators and elevators of varying sizes is required. My preferred selection is shown in Fig. A2.5.

Luxators and elevators are used to cut/break down the periodontal ligament, which holds the tooth in the alveolus. The different sizes are required so that an appropriate range for each size of root can be selected. Always start with a small instrument and move up to a larger one as more space is created between the tooth and the alveolar bone. Luxators have a very thin working end and are used to cut the ligament, but should not be used for leverage or they may break. Elevators have a relatively thick shank. They are used to break down the periodontal ligament with a combination of apical pressure and leverage. An extraction can be started with a luxator and completed with an elevator. A very small (2 mm) luxator or a root tip elevator will assist removal of fractured root tips and should be available for all extractions – just in case!

Periosteal elevator: A periosteal elevator (Fig. A2.6) is required for open (surgical) extractions to expose the

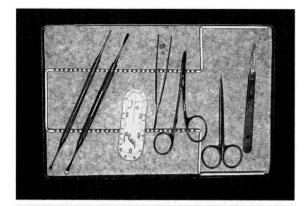

Figure A2.6 Equipment for tooth extraction. My preferred periosteal elevators and suturing kit (small instruments are required) are depicted. The two periosteal elevators depicted on the left are the Fine P24GSP (for cats) and the Howard P9H (for dogs). Also useful for dogs are the Molt P9 and the Periosteal No. 9. The size 15 blade shown in the handle is my preferred choice.

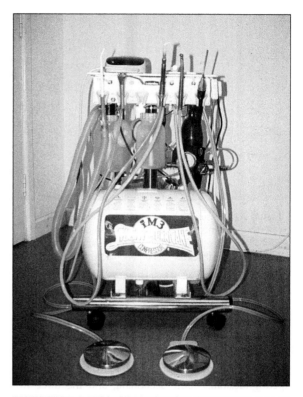

Figure A2.7 Compressed air-driven unit. This unit (IM3/Kruuse) has suction, a three-way syringe, a slow-speed outlet (with prophy handpiece attached), a high-speed outlet (with a high-speed handpiece with fibre-optic light attached) and a light for trans-illuminating teeth.

alveolar bone by raising a muco-periosteal flap. However, even if a closed (non-surgical) extraction technique has been used, the gingiva may be sutured over the extraction socket. In this situation, a periosteal elevator is invaluable to free the gingiva, allowing suturing over of the extraction socket without tension.

Extraction forceps: Although forceps can be used to aid ligament breakdown by rotational force on the tooth, it is very easy to snap the crown off by using excessive force. There is some truth in the saying that the only extraction forceps required are your fingers. If the tooth cannot be lifted out with your fingers, then the periodontal ligament has not been adequately broken down. In short, dental forceps are not essential, but if they are to be used then a selection of sizes, to fit the root anatomy of the tooth being extracted, is required.

Power equipment

Power equipment is required to perform dentistry and oral surgery. Regular maintenance is essential to avoid problems with equipment failure.

Micromotor unit: A micromotor unit can be used for polishing teeth as well as sectioning teeth. For sectioning teeth, the micromotor should be set at maximum speed (30 000 rpm). Micromotor units do not generally include water cooling of the bur and an external source (e.g.

assistant applying coolant continuously to the tissues) is required to prevent thermal damage.

Compressed air-driven unit: The basic compressed air-driven unit consists of a high-speed handpiece with water cooling, a slow-speed handpiece (with or without water cooling) and a combination air/water syringe (Fig. A2.7). A high-speed handpiece, although not essential for sectioning multirooted teeth prior to extraction, facilitates the process and allows accurate application of coolant water. Investing in a high-speed handpiece with fibre-optic light is strongly recommended. The slow-speed handpiece accommodates the contra-angle handpiece used for polishing the teeth. The three-way syringe can deliver either a stream of water or a spray of water and air, or air only. It is used to irrigate/lavage the mouth (water or water/air spray) and to dry the teeth (air only). Some units come with two high-speed outlets (Fig. A2.7)

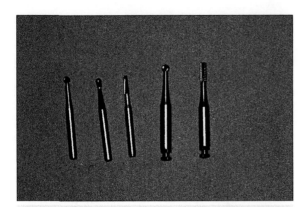

Figure A2.8 A selection of tungsten carbide burs. From the left are round, pear-shaped and tapered fissure high-speed handpiece burs. Round and cross-cutting straight fissure burs for the slow-speed handpiece are shown on the right.

and one of these can be used with a sonic scaler. Suction is also available with some units (Fig. A2.7).

Investing in a compressed air-driven unit from the outset is recommended. The high-speed handpiece greatly facilitates tooth sectioning, and the three-way syringe (for lavage and drying) will aid in the removal of debris and improve visibility during examination and any procedure. Suction is a real bonus. Investigate the maintenance and service options offered before making your choice.

Burs: Dental burs are made of a variety of materials, including stainless steel, tungsten carbide steel and 'diamond'. There is a wide selection of burs available to fit both the slow- and the high-speed handpieces (Fig. A2.8). A selection of round, pear-shaped, tapered fissure and straight fissure burs will be required for sectioning of teeth and removal of alveolar bone. 'Diamond' burs abrade rather than cut and may be safer for the inexperienced user.

MISCELLANEOUS

Sharpening

Scalers, curettes, luxators and elevators all require regular sharpening. Dental instrument sharpening kits (stones and oil), with instructions, are available through veterinary wholesalers.

Scalers and curettes should be sharpened before each use, i.e. after cleaning and sterilization. Sterilization will blunt the instruments and sharpening of dirty instruments will contaminate the sharpening stone. Sharpening is performed to retain the 70–80° angle between the face and the lateral surface of the working tip.

Luxators and elevators need to be sharpened regularly, usually after each use, with a cylindrical Arkansas stone. If either have damage to the working end they should be professionally reground.

Scalpel blade

The use of a scalpel blade to free the gingival attachment to the tooth is recommended for both closed and open extraction techniques. A size 15 or 11 blade, used in the handle, is ideal (Fig. A2.6).

Suture kit and suture material

A suture kit with small (ophthalmic) instruments should be available (Fig. A2.6). An absorbable suture material should always be used in the oral cavity. Monocryl® (Polyglecaprone, manufactured by Ethicon) is currently my suture material of choice.

Suction

Suction is invaluable. Excess water and debris can easily be removed, improving visibility for the operator and increasing safety for the patient (reducing the risk of aspiration). In addition, blood loss can be estimated more accurately. Invest in either a compressed air-driven unit that incorporates suction (Fig. A2.7) or a separate suction unit.

3 APPENDIX
Antibiotics and antiseptics

Antibiotics and antiseptics have a role to play in the management of oral diseases, but their use should be limited and selective. Dosing regimens and strategies that lead to optimal efficacy of antimicrobial agents must be implemented.

ANTIBIOTICS

Antibiotics can be used for prevention and for therapy.

Preventive use of antibiotics

The main objective of preventive (prophylactic) antibiotics is to prevent treatment-induced bacteraemia. Periodontal therapy, tooth extraction and surgical treatment of oral trauma cause a considerable bacteraemia, which typically clears in around 20 minutes. The preventive or prophylactic use of antibiotics should only be necessary in patients that cannot cope with the treatment-induced bacteraemia.

Animals that should receive preventive antibiotic administration are:
- Geriatric or debilitated animals
- Patients with pre-existing heart and/or systemic diseases
- Immunocompromised patients.

In addition to preventing treatment-induced bacteraemia, preventive antibiotic administration helps control wound infection. Consequently, animals that may benefit from receiving preventive antibiotic administration are those affected by:
- Gross infection
- Chronic stomatitis.

The choice of both type of prophylactic antibiotic and precise protocol remain controversial. A wide variety of microorganisms is found in the flora of the mouth and saliva. Antibiotic prophylaxis requires a drug with antimicrobial activity against Gram-positive and Gram-negative aerobes and anaerobes. The timing of administration of antibiotics is critical. It is generally accepted that antibiotics should be administered within 2 hours of the surgery and not continued for more than 4 hours after the procedure. In addition, antibiotics must be given at a high enough dose to reach a tissue level four times higher than the MIC of the causative organisms. A number of studies have shown that ampicillin, amoxicillin–clavulanic acid, certain cephalosporins and clindamycin meet the above requirements in dogs, cats and humans.

In our referral practice in the UK, we use either one of the following protocols.

In the presence of severe infection, we use 20 mg/kg i.v. of ampicillin prior to surgery (at the time of catheter placement for anaesthesia). This dose is repeated after 6 hours if the catheter is still in place. Metronidazole is given intravenously in addition to ampicillin to ensure a wider anaerobic spectrum.

Twice the therapeutic dose of amoxicillin or amoxicillin–clavulanic acid is given by intramuscular injection at the time of premedication for anaesthesia. This gives 20–30 minutes for the drug to disperse before the animal is anaesthetized and the surgical procedure is started. In fractious animals, who are unlikely to tolerate an intramuscular injection while conscious, we may choose to administer the antibiotic immediately after induction of anaesthesia. Examination and patient preparation will ensure that at least 20 minutes have elapsed before the surgical procedure is started.

Therapeutic use of antibiotics

The therapeutic use of antibiotics is indicated in patients with local and systemic signs of established infection, i.e. marked swelling, pus formation, fever, lymphadenopathy and an elevated white blood cell count. Clinical judgement is important in making the diagnosis of infection and deciding on antibiotic therapy. Antibiotic administration just 'to be on the safe side' is not prudent use of antimicrobials!

Principles for prudent use of therapeutic antibiotics:

1. *The causative agent should be identified and the antibiotic sensitivity determined.* In the oral cavity, the organisms involved have been well defined and are known to include a mixed flora of aerobic and anaerobic, Gram-positive and Gram-negative bacteria. Empirical antibiotic treatment based on previous susceptibility studies is therefore acceptable. Amoxicillin–clavulanic acid and clindamycin, and to a lesser extent cephalosporins, provide broad antibacterial activity against oral infections in dogs and cats. Culture is indicated for infection not responding to the initial treatment, recurrent infection, postoperative wound infection and osteomyelitis.

2. *The antibiotic with the narrowest antibacterial spectrum should be used.* This will minimize the risk of development of resistant bacteria.

3. *Combinations of antibiotics are discouraged.* The exception to this rule is the combination of amoxicillin or cephalosporins with metronidazole in severe mixed infections in which anaerobes are believed to play a major role.

4. *A bactericidal antibiotic is preferable to a bacteriostatic agent.* A bactericidal antibiotic (amoxicillin, cephalosporins and metronidazole) is preferred over a bacteriostatic antibiotic (clindamycin), mainly because there is less reliance on host inflammatory and immune reactions. Other considerations include the toxicity of the antibiotic and the patient's history of previous allergic reactions to a particular antibiotic.

5. *The antibiotic of choice must be administered at the proper dose and correct time interval.* Refer to a current Compendium of Data Sheets for Veterinary Products for correct dosing and time interval. A 7-day course of antibiotics is generally recommended. Osteomyelitis generally requires a longer period of treatment, often 21–28 days. Suboptimal dosing and/or pulse therapy is not generally recommended.

6. *The patient must be monitored for response to treatment and the potential development of adverse reactions.* Re-evaluation of the diagnosis is required if there is no response to treatment. Culture and antibiogram may well be indicated. Minor adverse reactions (e.g. mild gastrointestinal side-effects and

inappetence, due to changes in the gut flora as a result of systemic antibiotics, with amoxicillin and clindamycin) occasionally occur.

ANTIBIOTICS AND PERIODONTAL DISEASE

In veterinary practice, antibiotics are often used indiscriminately (incomplete diagnostic work-up, incorrect dose and time intervals, inadequate monitoring of response to treatment) for patients with periodontal disease.

The indication for preventive (prophylactic) use of antibiotics in animals with gingivitis and/or periodontitis is well defined (indicated for individuals that cannot cope with treatment-induced bacteraemia). In contrast, the indication for therapeutic use of antibiotics in the management of periodontal disease is not well defined. A thorough understanding of the aetiology and pathogenesis of periodontal disease is required for discriminate (limited and selective) therapeutic use of antibiotics. Periodontal disease is a clinical descriptive term for inflammation of the periodontium caused by the accumulation of dental plaque (a bacterial biofilm) on the tooth surfaces. It is essential to differentiate between gingivitis (inflammation limited to the gingiva) and periodontitis (inflammation involves periodontal ligament and alveolar bone) prior to instituting any treatment.

Gingivitis

In gingivitis, daily mechanical removal of dental plaque (toothbrushing) will restore inflamed gingivae to health and continued regular plaque removal will maintain gingival health. Antibiotics are thus not indicated for the treatment of gingivitis. Adjunctive use of antiseptics may be indicated in some patients.

Periodontitis

The role of antibiotics for treatment of periodontitis is not clear and requires further investigation. The two main questions that need to be answered before any general recommendation can be made are: can antimicrobial agents enhance the effect of mechanical plaque removal, and can they be a substitute for such treatment?

Can antimicrobial agents enhance the effect of mechanical plaque removal?: There are many similarities between human and canine periodontal disease.

Consequently, data from human studies do have relevance to canine periodontal disease.

In human dentistry, it is recognized that antimicrobial treatment is of secondary importance in the treatment of periodontitis, compared to conservative periodontal therapy. Conservative periodontal therapy involves professional cleaning (supragingival scaling and polishing, subgingival scaling and root planing) in combination with meticulous daily plaque removal by the patient. Where follow-up mechanical plaque control is successfully instituted (after professional cleaning), no benefit can be shown by including antimicrobial therapy with professional mechanical debridement as compared to mechanical debridement alone. No similar study has been performed in dogs or cats.

Various antibiotic regimens have been tested for the treatment of human patients not responding to conservative periodontal therapy. Although favourable short-term effects have been reported, a great variability in treatment response among patients has been noted. Re-emergence of putative pathogens has been observed and has been considered the reason for recurrence of disease. In dogs where no post-scaling home care is provided, a demonstrable long-term retardation effect following short-term antimicrobial therapy has been reported in one study. The ultimate evidence for the efficacy of systemic antibiotics must be obtained from longer-term treatment studies in animals with periodontitis. At present, no such data is available.

To summarize, reducing the bacterial load postoperatively can be achieved by mechanical plaque control. The use of systemic antibiotics in combination with conservative periodontal therapy will at best achieve a retardation of the disease process.

Can periodontitis be treated with antimicrobial agents alone?: There are some specific features of periodontal disease which suggest that treatment by antimicrobial agents alone, i.e. in the absence of professional periodontal therapy and home care, will not be sufficient. First, there is generally a lack of bacterial invasion of the tissues in periodontal disease. Bacteria in the subgingival plaque interact with host tissues even without direct tissue penetration. Thus, for any microbial agent to have an effect there is the requirement that the agent is available at a sufficiently high concentration in the subgingival environment outside the periodontal tissues. Secondly, periodontal pockets contain a large number of different bacteria. This may cause problems for antimicrobial agents to work properly

because they may be inhibited, inactivated or degraded by non-target microorganisms. Thirdly, subgingival plaque is a biofilm and it is known that biofilms effectively protect bacteria from antimicrobial agents. Finally, the majority of microorganisms associated with periodontal disease can frequently be detected at low numbers in the absence of disease. In the therapy of opportunistic infections, elimination is not a realistic goal. Successfully suppressed putative pathogens are likely to grow back if favourable ecological conditions (e.g. deep periodontal pockets) persist. Therefore, continuous control of ecological factors will be necessary after initial treatment.

It is important to understand that in vitro tests cannot be directly correlated to clinical efficacy, as they do not reflect the true conditions found in periodontal pockets. In particular, they do not account for the biofilm effect. Demonstration of in vitro susceptibility is therefore no proof that an agent will work in the treatment of periodontal disease.

At our present level of understanding, systemic antimicrobial therapy cannot be recommended as prevention and/or first-line treatment of periodontal disease for any species, and definitely not in the absence of mechanical periodontal therapy. Professional periodontal therapy followed by meticulous mechanical plaque control by the patient (owner) remains the way to treat periodontitis. In some very specific situations, e.g. severe local infection, or a systemically ill or immunocompromised individual, *antibiotics may be a* useful adjunctive modality. However, the adjunctive use of antiseptics rather than antibiotics is likely to achieve the same result and is associated with fewer hazards, e.g. resistance development. In short, antibiotics have not been shown to prevent periodontitis, neither have they been shown to have any significant role in the treatment of periodontitis.

Antibiotic delivery: In the few specific situations where antibiotics may be a useful adjunctive modality, the method of delivery needs to be determined. Antibiotic agents may be delivered by direct placement into the periodontal pocket (local route) or via the systemic route. Each method of delivery has specific advantages and disadvantages.

Local therapy may allow the application of an agent at a concentration that cannot be achieved by the systemic route. Local application may thus be particularly successful if the treatment of target microorganisms is confined to the clinically visible lesions.

On the other hand, systemically administered agents may reach widely distributed microorganisms. Studies in man have shown that periodontal bacteria may be distributed throughout the whole mouth in some patients, including non-dental sites such as the dorsum of the tongue and/or the tonsillary crypts. Disadvantages of systemic antibiotic therapy relate to the fact that the drug is dispersed over the whole body and only a small portion of the dose actually reaches the subgingival flora. In addition, adverse drug reactions, e.g. resistance, are more likely to occur if drugs are distributed via the systemic route.

ANTISEPTICS

Antiseptics have two major roles in veterinary dentistry and oral surgery, namely to:
1. Reduce the number of bacteria in the oral cavity prior to and during a procedure
2. Supplement mechanical plaque control.

It is good practice to rinse the oral cavity with a suitable antiseptic prior to and during dentistry and oral surgery. This reduces the number of potential pathogens, providing a cleaner environment to work in and thus reducing the bacteraemia induced by dental procedures. It also reduces the number of bacteria in the aerosol generated by dental equipment, e.g. ultrasonic scalers. This is beneficial to the operator and assistant.

Chlorhexidine gluconate, an aqueous, non-alcohol-containing solution, is generally regarded to be the oral antiseptic of choice in animals. The correct concentration should be used. A 0.2% solution is generally recommended as being safe, but a 0.05% solution may be indicated if the oral mucosa is exposed to the solution throughout the procedure. Care should be taken to avoid the eyes.

Numerous chemical agents have been evaluated for the supplementation of mechanical plaque control. Clinically effective antiplaque agents are characterized by a combination of intrinsic antibacterial activity and good oral retention properties. Agents that have been evaluated include chlorhexidine, essential oils, triclosan, sanguinarine, fluorides, oxygenating agents, quaternary ammonium compounds, substituted amino-alcohols and enzymes. Of these, the greatest effect on the reduction of plaque and gingivitis can be expected from chlorhexidine. Chlorhexidine is the gold standard and the agent against which all antiplaque agents are tested. Anti-

plaque agents delivered from toothpastes, gels or mouth rinses can augment mechanical oral hygiene to control the formation of supragingival plaque and the development of early periodontal disease. It must be emphasized that none of these agents will prevent gingivitis on their own, i.e. in the absence of mechanical plaque removal. Moreover, all these agents are associated with adverse side-effects. These effects vary according to the chemical agent, and include poor taste, a burning and/or numbing of oral mucous membranes, staining of teeth and soft tissues, and allergic reactions. The use of chemical antiplaque agents should be seen as adjunctive to the mechanical removal of plaque.

Some examples of situations where adjunctive use of topical chlorhexidine is useful are:
- Immediately postoperatively when discomfort from treatment (deep subgingival debridement, multiple extractions) may prevent mechanical plaque removal with a toothbrush
- Intermittent use when an inflammatory process flares up, e.g. cats with chronic gingivostomatitis
- Adjunct to toothbrushing when toothbrushing is performed suboptimally, e.g. the animal won't allow proper brushing or the owner is not technically capable of efficient brushing.

Chlorhexidine gluconate is available as aqueous solution and as a semi-fluid gel. It can be applied with a syringe, a piece of gauze or a toothbrush.

My preferred method of administering chlorhexidine is to use the aqueous solution as an oral rinse once or twice daily (depending on the severity of inflammation). The solution is dispensed into the oral cavity using a syringe. The owners are shown how to elevate the lip to expose the teeth and gums, and how to apply a gentle stream of chlorhexidine as a rinse. This is done on both sides of the mouth. For cats and small dogs we recommend 3 ml per side (total of 6 ml); for medium-sized dogs 5–8 ml per side and for large dogs 10 ml per side.

SUMMARY

The prevention and treatment of periodontal disease relies on mechanical plaque control. If an owner is either unwilling or incapable of mechanically removing dental plaque, they need to be aware that periodontitis and tooth loss are likely to occur. Their pet will require professional intervention at regular time intervals and teeth affected by periodontitis need to be extracted.

4 APPENDIX
Endodontics

Endodontics is the treatment of the pulp of the tooth (endo- = inside; -dontic = tooth). Endodontic therapy is a specialist procedure, and should not be undertaken without adequate training and supervised experience. The following outlines the more common endodontic treatments that are required in small animal dentistry.

There are three pulpal treatments, each of which has specific indications. They are:

1. Pulp capping
2. Partial pulpectomy with direct pulp capping
3. Root canal therapy.

Conventional root canal therapy is the most commonly indicated type of endodontic treatment. It involves total removal of pulp tissue, i.e. total pulpectomy, cleaning and filling of the root canal, followed by tooth restoration.

Root canal therapy is indicated when there is or may be irreversible pulp pathology (e.g. generalized pulpitis or pulp necrosis, often in combination with periapical involvement) in the mature permanent tooth. Immature permanent teeth are a special consideration and are dealt with separately.

The objectives of conventional root canal therapy are:

- To clean and disinfect the pulp chamber and root canals
- To fill the root canal(s) with a non-irritant, antibacterial material, thus sealing the apex
- To close the access and exposure sites with a suitable restorative material.

Many different methods are employed in the preparation and filling of root canals. In simple terms, root canal therapy involves removing the pulp, replacing it with an inert material and restoring the tooth. The inflamed or dead pulp is removed using special files. Once the pulp has been removed, the root canal is cleaned, both mechanically with files but also chemically with a disin-

fectant. The clean and disinfected root canal is then filled with inert material and the crown is restored with a suitable restorative material. The tooth is not restored to its original shape and size, as the biting forces in the dog are much greater than those in man and the restoration would be likely to fail if this was attempted.

The whole procedure is performed under general anaesthesia with strict radiographic control. It is time-consuming, as each step needs to be performed with meticulous detail to ensure a successful outcome.

The outcome of conventional root canal therapy should be monitored radiographically 6–12 months postoperatively. This will also require general anaesthesia. Evidence of disease around the tip of the root at this time indicates the need for further endodontic therapy or extraction of the tooth. Further endodontic treatment usually consists of redoing the root canal therapy, often in conjunction with surgical endodontics (usually removing the tip of the root and sealing the root canal from this direction as well).

SPECIAL CONSIDERATIONS WITH IMMATURE TEETH

A partial pulpectomy and direct pulp capping procedure is indicated for recent tooth crown fractures with pulp exposure in immature teeth. An immature tooth has a thin dentine wall and an open apex, allowing a good blood supply to the pulp. Treatment is aimed at maintaining a viable pulp, as this is needed for continued root development.

Necrotic immature teeth require endodontic treatment if they are to be retained. The procedure is an adaptation of conventional root canal therapy, as already described for the mature permanent tooth. The necrotic pulp tissue is gently removed, and the pulp chamber and root canal thoroughly cleaned. It is important to remove all the necrotic tissue, which usually extends slightly beyond the radiographically verifiable open apex. Sterile calcium hydroxide powder or paste is packed into the root canal, extending just beyond the apex. A degree of apexogenesis (normal root length and apex development) or apexification (treatment-stimulated root closure) can be stimulated if this procedure is performed. The exposure site is sealed with a restorative material. The tooth is monitored closely and the calcium hydroxide dressing is changed approximately every 6 months, as a fresh dressing is more effective in stimulating apexogenesis and apexification. When no further root development can be seen radiographically and if the apex is closed, a conventional root canal treatment should be performed. A conventional root canal treatment can only be carried out if the apex is closed. If the apex is still open and closure cannot be stimulated by repeated calcium hydroxide dressings, it may be possible to obtain an apical seal using a surgical approach and placing a root filling in a retrograde manner.

It must be noted that multiple general anaesthesia episodes are required and thus in most cases extraction of an immature tooth with a necrotic pulp is the best course of action. The salvage procedure as described above is really only indicated for the strategic permanent teeth that have undergone some degree of maturation.

It should be noted that immature teeth might well be present in the mature animal if trauma caused pulp necrosis during the developmental period. Treatment of such teeth is the same as for any immature permanent teeth, regardless of the actual age of the animal.

Further reading

Books

Crossley D, Penman S (Eds) (1995): Manual of Small Animal Dentistry, 2nd Edition. British Small Animal Veterinary Association, Gloucestershire, UK.

Gorrel C (2004): Veterinary Dentistry for the General Practitioner. WB Saunders, Philadephia.

Harvey CE, Emily P (1993): Small Animal Dentistry. Mosby, Missouri.

Holmstrom S (Ed.) (1998): The Veterinary Clinics of North America Small Animal Practice: Canine Dentistry. WB Saunders, Philadelphia.

Tutt C (2007): Small Animal Dentistry – A manual of techniques. Blackwell Publishing, Oxford.

Tutt C, Deeprose J and Crossley D (Eds) (2007): Manual of Canine and Feline Dentistry, 3rd Edition. British Small Animal Veterinary Association, Gloucestershire, UK.

Verstraete FJM (Ed.) (1999): Self-assessment Colour Review of Veterinary Dentistry. Manson Publishing, London.

Wiggs RB, Lobprise HB (1997): Veterinary Dentistry Principles and Practice. Lippincott-Raven, Philadelphia.

Articles

Andersson L, Lindskog S, Blomlöf L, et al. (1985): Effect of masticatory stimulation on dentoalveolar ankylosis after experimental tooth replantation. Endod Dent Traumatol 1, 13–16.

Andreasen JO (1985): External root resorption: its implications in dental traumatology, paedodontics, periodontics, orthodontics and endodontics. International Endodontic Journal 18, 109–118.

Andreasen JO (1988): Review of root resorption systems and models. Etiology of root resorption and the homeostatic mechanisms of the periodontal ligament. In: Davidovitch Z, Ed. Proceedings of the International Conference on the Biological Mechanisms of Tooth Eruption and Root Resorption. Ebesco Media, Birmingham, pp. 9–21.

Andreasen JO, Kristerson L (1981): The effect or limited drying or removal of the periodontal ligament. Periodontal healing after replantation of mature incisors in monkeys. Acta Odontol Scand 39, 1–13.

Arnbjerg J (1996): Idiopathic dental root replacement resorption in old dogs. Journal of Veterinary Dentistry 13 (3), 97–99.

Berger M, Schawalder P, Stich H, Lussi A (1996): Feline dental resorptive lesions in captive and wild leopards and lions. Journal of Veterinary Dentistry 13 (1), 13–21.

Boyce EN, Logan EI (1994): Oral health assessment in dogs: study design and results. Journal of Veterinary Dentistry 11 (2), 64–74.

Clarke DE, Cameron A (1997): Feline dental resorptive lesions in domestic and feral cats and the possible link with diet. In: Proceedings of the 5th World Veterinary Dental Congress, Birmingham, UK, pp. 33–34.

Coles S (1990): The prevalence of buccal cervical root resorptions in Australian cats. Journal of Veterinary Dentistry 7 (4), 14–16.

Crossley D, Dubielzig R, Benson K (1997): Caries and odontoclastic resorptive lesions in a chinchilla (Chinchilla lanigera). Veterinary Record 141, 337–339.

DeBowes LJ, et al. (1996): Association of periodontal disease and histologic lesions in multiple organs from 45 dogs. Journal of Veterinary Dentistry 13, 57.

DuPont G (1995): Crown amputation with intentional root retention for advanced feline resorptive lesions – a clinical study. Journal of Veterinary Dentistry 12 (1), 9–13.

Egelberg J (1965): Local effects of diet on plaque formation and gingivitis development in dogs. I. Effect of hard and soft diets. Odontologisk Revy 16, 31–41.

Egelberg J (1965): Local effects of diet on plaque formation and gingivitis development in dogs. II. Effect of frequency of meals and tube feeding. Odontologisk Revy 16, 50–60.

Gaskell RM, Gruffydd-Jones TJ (1977): Intractable feline stomatitis. Veterinary Annual 17, 195.

Gold SI, Hasselgren G (1992): Peripheral inflammatory root resorption. A review of the literature with case reports. Journal of Clinical Periodontology 19, 523–534.

Gorrel C (1994): The effects of fluoride and its possible uses in veterinary dentistry. In: Proceedings of the World Veterinary Dental Congress, Philadelphia.

Gorrel C, Bierer T (1999): Long term effects of a dental hygiene chew on the periodontal health of dogs. Journal of Veterinary Dentistry 16 (3), 109–113.

Gorrel C, Larsson Å (2002): Feline odontoclastic resorptive lesions: unveiling the early lesion. Journal of Small Animal Practice 43, 482–488.

Gorrel C, Rawlings JM (1996): The role of a 'dental hygiene chew' in maintaining periodontal health in dogs. Journal of Veterinary Dentistry 13 (1), 31–34.

Gorrel C, Rawlings JM (1996): The role of tooth-brushing and diet in the maintenance of periodontal health in dogs. Journal of Veterinary Dentistry 13 (3), 139–143.

Gorrel C, Inskeep G, Inskeep T (1998): Benefits of a 'dental hygiene chew' on the periodontal health of cats. Journal of Veterinary Dentistry 15 (3), 135–138.

Gorrel C, Warrick J, Bierer T (1999): Effect of a new dental hygiene chew on periodontal health in dogs. Journal of Veterinary Dentistry 16 (2), 77–81.

Gruffydd-Jones TJ (1991): Gingivitis and stomatitis. In: August JR, Ed. Consultations in Feline Internal Medicine. WB Saunders, Philadelphia, pp. 387–402.

Hammarström L, Blomlöf L, Lindskog S (1989): Dynamics of dentoalveolar ankylosis and associated root resorption. Endod Dent Traumatol 5, 163–175.

Hamp SE, et al. (1984): A macroscopic and radiologic investigation of dental diseases in dogs. Veterinary Radiology 25, 86.

Harvey CE, Thornsberry C, Miller BR, et al. (1995): Antimicrobial susceptibility of subgingival bacterial flora in dogs with gingivitis. Journal of Veterinary Dentistry 12, 151–155.

Harvey CE, Thornsberry C, Miller BR, et al. (1995): Antimicrobial susceptibility of subgingival bacterial flora in cats with gingivitis. Journal of Veterinary Dentistry 12, 157–160.

Harvey CE, Shofer FS, Laster L (1996): Correlation of diet, other chewing activities and periodontal disease in North American client-owned dogs. Journal of Veterinary Dentistry 13 (3), 101–105.

Hennet P (1997): Chronic gingivo-stomatitis in cats: long term follow-up of 30 cases treated by dental extractions. Journal of Veterinary Dentistry 14 (1), 15.

Hennet PR, Harvey CE (1991): Anaerobes in periodontal disease in the dog: a review. Journal of Veterinary Dentistry 2, 8.

Hennet PR, Harvey CE (1992): Craniofacial development and growth in the dog. Journal of Veterinary Dentistry 9 (2), 11.

Hennet PR, Harvey CE (1992): Diagnostic approach to malocclusions in dogs. Journal of Veterinary Dentistry 9 (3), 23.

Hopewell-Smith A (1930): The process of osteolysis and odontolysis, or so-called 'absorption' of calcified tissues: a new and original investigation. The evidences in the cat. Dental Cosmos 72, 1036–1048.

Ingham KE, Gorrel C (2001): Effect of long-term intermittent periodontal care on canine periodontal disease. Journal of Small Animal Practice 42 (2), 67–70.

Ingham KE, Gorrel C, Blackburn JM, et al. (2001): Prevalence of odontoclastic resorptive lesions in a clinically healthy cat population. Journal of Small Animal Practice 42, 439–443.

Ingham KE, Gorrel C, Bierer TL (2002): Effect of a dental chew on dental substrates and gingivitis in cats. Journal of Veterinary Dentistry 19 (4), 201–204.

Jensen L, Logan EI, Finney O, et al. (1995): Reduction in accumulation of plaque, stain and calculus in dogs by dietary means. Journal of Veterinary Dentistry 12 (4), 161–163.

Johnessee JS, Hurvitz AI (1983): Feline plasma cell gingivitis–pharyngitis. Journal of the American Animal Hospital Association 19, 179.

King GN, Hughes FJ (1999): Effects of occlusal loading on ankylosis, bone and cementum formation during morpho-genetic protein-2-stimulated periodontal regeneration in vivo. Journal of Periodontology 70, 1125–1135.

Knowles JO, et al. (1989): Prevalence of feline calicivirus, feline leukaemia virus and antibodies to FIV in cats with chronic stomatitis. Veterinary Record 124, 336.

Knowles JO, et al. (1991): Studies on the role of feline calicivirus in chronic stomatitis in cats. Veterinary Microbiology 27, 205.

Levin J (1996): Tooth resorption in a Siberian tiger. In: Proceedings of the 10th Annual Veterinary Dental Forum, Houston, Texas, pp. 212–214.

Lindhe J, Hamp S-E, Löe H (1975): Plaque induced periodontal disease in beagle dogs. A 4-year clinical, roentgenographical and histometrical study. Journal of Periodontal Research 10, 243–255.

Lindskog S, Hammarström L (1980): Evidence in favour of an anti-invasion factor in cementum or periodontal membrane. Scandinavian Journal of Dental Research 88, 161–163.

Lindskog S, Blomlöf L, Hammarström L (1983): Repair of periodontal tissues in vitro and in vivo. Journal of Clinical Periodontology 10, 188–205.

Lindskog S, Blomlöf L, Hammarström L (1987): Cellular colonization of denuded root surfaces in vivo: cell morphology in dentin resorption and cementum repair. Journal of Clinical Periodontology 14, 390–395.

Loesche WJ (1979): Clinical and microbiological aspects of chemotherapeutic agents used according to the specific plaque hypothesis. Journal of Dental Research 58, 2404–2414.

Logan EI, Finney O, Hefferren J (2002): Effects of a dental food on plaque accumulation and gingival health in dogs. Journal of Veterinary Dentistry, 19 (1), 15–18.

Lommer MJ, Verstraete FJM (2000): Prevalence of odontoclastic resorption lesions and periapical radiographic lucencies in cats: 265 cases (1995–1998). Journal of the American Veterinary Medical Association 217, 1866–1869.

Love DN, et al. (1989): Bacteroides species from the oral cavity and oral associated diseases of cats. Veterinary Microbiology 19, 275.

Love DN, et al. (1990): The obligative and facultatively anaerobic bacterial flora of the normal feline gingival margin. Veterinary Microbiology 22, 267.

Lund EM, Bohacek LK, Dahlke JL, King VL, Kramek BA, Logan EI (1998): Prevalence and risk factors for odontoclastic resorptive lesions in cats. Journal of the American Veterinary Medical Association 212, 392–395.

Mallonee DH, et al. (1988): Bacteriology of periodontal disease in the cat. Archives of Oral Biology 33, 677.

Miller BR, Harvey CE (1994): Compliance with oral hygiene recommendations following periodontal treatment in client-owned dogs. Journal of Veterinary Dentistry 11 (1), 18–19.

Ne RF, Witherspoon DE, Gutmann JL (1999): Tooth resorption. Quintessence International 30, 9–25.

Nyman S, et al. (1986): Role of 'diseased' root cementum in healing following treatment of periodontal disease. An experimental study in the dog. Journal of Periodontal Research 21, 496.

Okuda A, Harvey CE (1992): Etiopathogenesis of feline dental resorptive lesions. In: Harvey CE, Ed. Veterinary Clinics of North America, Small Animal Practice: Feline Dentistry. WB Saunders, Philadelphia, pp. 1385–1404.

Reichart PA, Durr U-M, Triadan H, et al. (1984): Periodontal disease in the domestic cat. Journal of Periodontal Research 19, 67–75.

Reindel JF, et al. (1987): Recurrent plasmacytic stomatitis–pharyngitis in a cat with esophagitis, fibrosing gastritis and gastric nematodiasis. Journal of the American Veterinary Medical Association 190, 65.

Reiter A, Mendoza KA (2002): Feline odontoclastic resorptive lesions: an unsolved enigma in veterinary dentistry. Veterinary Clinics of North America Small Animal Practice 32, 791–837.

Richardson RL (1965): Effect of administering antibiotics, removing the major salivary glands and toothbrushing on dental calculi formation in the cat. Archives of Oral Biology 10, 245–253.

Rosin E, Dow SW, Daly WR, et al. (1993): Surgical wound infection and use of antibiotics. In: Slatter DH, Ed. Textbook of Small Animal Surgery, 2nd Edition. WB Saunders, Philadelphia, pp. 84–95.

Sangnes G (1976): A pilot study on the effect of toothbrushing on the gingiva of a beagle dog. Scandinavian Journal of Dental Research 84, 106–108.

Sarkiala E, Asikainen SEA, Kanervo A, et al. (1993): The efficacy of tinidazole in naturally occurring periodontitis in dogs: bacteriological and chemical results. Veterinary Microbiology 36, 273–288.

Sato R, et al. (1996): Oral administration of bovine lactoferrin for treatment of intractable stomatitis in feline immunodeficiency virus (FIV)-positive and FIV-negative cats. American Journal of Veterinary Research 10, 1443.

Shigeyana Y, Grove TK, Strayhorn C, et al. (1996): Expression of adhesion molecules during tooth resorption in feline teeth: A model system for aggressive osteoclastic activity. Journal of Dental Research 75, 1650–1657.

Sims TJ, et al. (1988): Serum antibody responses to antigens of oral gram-negative bacteria in the cat. Archives of Oral Biology 33, 677.

Sims TJ, et al. (1990): Serum antibody response to antigens of oral gram-negative bacteria in cats with plasma cell gingivitis–stomatitis. Journal of Dental Research 69, 877.

Southerden P, Gorrel C (2007): Treatment of a case of refractory feline chronic gingivostomatitis with feline recombinant interferon mega. Journal of Small Animal Practice 48, 104–106.

Stockard CR (1941): The genetic and endocrinic basis for differences in form and behaviour. The American Anatomical Memoirs No. 19. The Wistar Institute of Anatomy and Biology, Philadelphia.

Tenorio AT, et al. (1991): Chronic oral infection of cats and their relationship to persistent oral carriage of feline calici, immunodeficiency, or leukaemia viruses. Veterinary Immunology and Immunopathology 23, 1.

Thompson RR, et al. (1984): Association of calicivirus infection with chronic gingivitis and pharyngitis in cats. Journal of Small Animal Practice 25, 207.

Tromp JA, van Rijn LJ, Jansen J (1986): Experimental gingivitis and frequency of tooth-brushing in the beagle dog model. Clinical findings. Journal of Clinical Periodontology 13, 190–194.

Van Wessum R, Harvey CE, Hennet P (1992): Feline dental resorptive lesions. Prevalence patterns. In: Harvey CE, Ed. Veterinary Clinics of North America Small Animal Practice: Feline Dentistry. WB Saunders, Philadelphia, pp. 1405–1416.

Verhaert L (1999): A removable orthodontic device for the treatment of lingually displaced mandibular canine teeth in young dogs. Journal of Veterinary Dentistry 16 (2), 69–75.

Verstraete FJM, Aarde Van RJ, Nieuwoudt BA, Mauer E, Kass PH (1996): The dental pathology of feral cats on Marion Island, Part II: periodontitis, external odontoclastic resorptive lesions and mandibular thickening. J Comp Pathol 115, 283–297.

Verstraete FJM, Kass PH, Terpak CH (1998): Diagnostic value of full mouth radiography in cats. American Journal of Veterinary Research 59, 692–695.

Waters L, et al. (1993): Chronic gingivitis in a colony of cats infected with feline immunodeficiency virus and feline calicivirus. Veterinary Record 132, 340.

White SD, et al. (1992): Plasma cell stomatitis–pharyngitis in cats: 40 cases (1973–1991). Journal of the American Veterinary Medical Association 200, 1377.

Williams CA, Aller MS (1992): Gingivitis/stomatitis in cats. In: Harvey CE, Ed. The Veterinary Clinics of North America Small Animal Practice: Feline Dentistry. WB Saunders, Philadelphia, p. 1361.

Yamamoto JK, et al. (1989): Epidemiologic and clinical aspects of feline immunodeficiency virus infection in cats from the continental United States and Canada and possible mode of transmission. Journal of the American Veterinary Medical Association 194, 213.

Zetner K, et al. (1989): Comparative immunological and virological studies of chronic oral diseases in cats. Weiner Tierarztliche Monatsschrift 76, 303.

Index

Notes

Page numbers in **bold** refer to figures and tables.

Readers are advised to refer to specific breeds for real-life studies related to each condition presented within this book.

Theory refresher information can be located for each condition within each chapter.

Printed and bound by CPI Group (UK) Ltd, Croydon, CR0 4YY

03/10/2024

01040349-0012